Immunology and Serology

THIRD EDITION

PHILIP L. CARPENTER

University of Rhode Island

1975

Philadelphia • London • Toronto

W. B. SAUNDERS COMPANY

W. B. Saunders Company: West Washington Square
Philadelphia, PA 19105

12 Dyott Street
London, WC1A 1DB

833 Oxford Street
Toronto, Ontario M8Z 5T9, Canada

Cover: Scanning electron micrograph of a human monocyte, a type of macrophage, cultured *in vitro* for 24 hours. Magnification: 8400×. (Micrograph and blood specimen courtesy of Ralph Albrecht, University of Wisconsin.)

Library of Congress Cataloging in Publication Data

Carpenter, Philip L

Immunology and serology.

Includes index.

1. Immunology. 2. Serology. [DNLM: 1. Immunology. 2. Serology.   QW504 C296i]

QR181.C3 1975   615'.37   74–31833

ISBN   0–7216–2422–7

Listed here is the latest translated edition of this book together with the language of the translation and the publisher.

Spanish (*1st edition*) — La Prensa Medica, Mexicana, Mexico

Immunology and Serology   ISBN 0-7216-2422-7

Last digit is the print number: 9   8   7   6   5   4   3   2   1

PREFACE

Research in immunology is accelerating at such a rapid pace and the field is so unstable that anyone who ventures to write a textbook must be either brave or foolhardy. Since I make no claim to bravery, I must perforce admit a degree of foolhardiness and the realization that some of the "facts" and concepts presented will be proven false before the date of publication. In self-justification, I feel that it is important for the student to have some idea of what seemed to be true, so that he can better appreciate and understand the direction in which the science is evolving.

The past decade has been a period of great progress. It was principally within this interval that the structure of immunoglobulins was learned. So, too, was the fact that those lymphoid cells known as T cells and B cells participate in humoral and cell-mediated immunologic processes. The physical and chemical properties, interrelations, and activities of complement components are much better understood now than ten years ago. The nature of the interaction between antigenic determinant sites and antibody or lymphoid cell reactive sites has been partially elucidated, together with the mechanism by which significant effects are produced in vitro or in vivo.

Whereas immunologic and serologic reactions were formerly attributed to mysterious properties of unknown body constituents, they are increasingly found to conform to familiar physiologic patterns. It is of interest that a surprising number of present concepts and beliefs were postulated by or developed from ideas expressed many years ago by Ehrlich, Marrack, Pauling, Burnet, and others.

The third edition of *Immunology and Serology*, like its predecessors, is intended for use in an introductory course by senior and first-year graduate students. It is assumed that they have a background in organic chemistry, college physics, zoology or biology, physiology, and an introduction to microbiology. Although the approach continues to be traditional, emphasis has been placed upon the biologic aspects of immunity and the immune response to "not-self" agents. Topics from various chapters in the earlier editions have been rearranged: in vitro antigen-antibody reactions are grouped together in two chapters, and in vivo immunologic reactions are also combined in two chapters. In keeping with recent advances, considerable discussion is devoted to cell-mediated immunologic reactions.

The serious student will wish to supplement the text with more up-to-date material. Excellent review articles are found in *Advances in Immunology*, published annually (or more often), and in *Transplantation Reviews*. A valuable guide to periodical literature is the biweekly *Current Titles in Immunology, Transplantation, and Allergy*, which surveys some 800 journals. The following are particularly useful: *Journal of Immunology, Journal of Experimental Medicine, Immunology, European Journal of Immunology, Cellular Immunology*, and *International Archives of Allergy and Applied Immunology*.

The feedback from many generations of students to whom much of the text has been given in lecture and laboratory has been very helpful. I am also indebted to the many authors, publishers, and equipment manufacturers who donated and permitted use of illustrative material, as acknowledged individually. Particular mention should be made of the scanning electron micrograph of a macrophage that appears on the cover—the work of Ralph Albrecht of the University of Wisconsin. As always, the staff of the W. B. Saunders Company have been of tremendous assistance throughout, especially Mr. Richard H. Lampert, Biology Editor; it is a pleasure to be associated with a group who take pride in good workmanship.

Special thanks are due my wife, Helen E. Carpenter, for her encouragement and forbearance and for her invaluable help in production of the final manuscript.

Errors of fact will inevitably be found, together with omissions due to oversight or to the rapid expansion of the field. I apologize for these and will appreciate being informed of them.

PHILIP L. CARPENTER

Kingston, R. I.
July 16, 1975

CONTENTS

Chapter Eleven

APPENDIX: EXPERIMENTS IN SEROLOGY 305

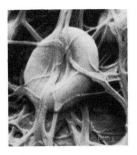

CHAPTER ONE

BIOLOGIC BASIS OF IMMUNITY

Immunity (Latin, *immunis*, safe) against infectious disease is an incidental manifestation of a physiologic process important in regulating the structure and function of body cells and tissues. The growth of cells and tissues is controlled by various homeostatic mechanisms, such as contact inhibition, hormone action, and the balance of various repressor-depressor systems. Under normal conditions, growth is regulated so that each tissue or organ consists of those cells necessary to maintain a size and shape suitable for its function, and further replication of cells occurs as required to maintain the tissue in its proper active state.

The process of cell replication includes synthesis of structural and enzymatic proteins, in accordance with the information supplied by mRNA, under the ultimate control of DNA, which is formed by the familiar process of nucleotide assembly. Errors in the latter process result in mutations. When mutation occurs in a germ-line cell, it is inherited from one generation to the next, but when it occurs in a somatic (nongermline) cell, only the progeny of that cell display the mutant character. Somatic mutations occur with a low frequency (e.g., 10^{-8} to 10^{-10}), and some of the mutant cells die because they are physiologically deficient. Others display greater growth potential than normal cells and may even cease to be subject to the usual controls and multiply without restraint. Wildly multiplying cells may produce tumors or cancerous masses, which occlude the passages or channels in various organs, or they may upset normal physiologic processes in some other way.

The chemical composition of the cells of a normal animal is characteristic of the animal, and all cells are mutually compatible; that is, when two cells make contact with one another, neither incites an untoward response by the other. Circulating blood cells and mobile tissue macrophages, for example, do not irritate or "attack" the blood vessel or tissue cells that they encounter, and vice versa. Each cell "recognizes" and accepts the others as characteristic of "self." After mutation, however, the composition of newly formed cells may differ significantly from that of normal cells, and they are no longer recognized as "self" components. Some of the other cells that they encounter —specifically, the lymphoid cells—are equipped to respond more or less vigorously to "nonself" components, the final result being destruction of the latter.

According to one school of thought, this lymphocytic "surveillance" mechanism, whose primary function is to assist in the control of tissue structure, provides the immunologic system responsible for recovery from and prevention of infectious disease.

A foreign or "nonself" substance that incites a specific immune response when introduced into the tissues of an animal is called an antigen (Greek, *anti*, against + *gennan*, to produce). The lymphoid cell response may consist of the liberation of low molecular weight chemicals that directly or indirectly destroy the antigen; it may consist of the production of a protein (immunoglobulin), known as an *antibody*, that can react specifically with the antigen that incited its production, destroying or inactivating it; or the response may be *immunologic tolerance*, in which the animal's lymphoid tissues develop specific immunologic *nonreactivity* to the antigen.

An antigen can usually react specifically with the sensitized cells or antibodies that it has induced, either in vivo or in vitro. The reactive portion of an antigen comprises only three to five amino acid residues or the equivalent in monosaccharide residues. It is known as a *determinant* site or *epitope*. The corresponding portion of an antibody is a *receptor* site.

HISTORICAL PERSPECTIVE

The first modern development in immunology (1798) was Jenner's use of cowpox vaccine to immunize humans against smallpox. Smallpox immunization had been practiced thousands of years earlier, when Chinese physicians took pustular material from a mild case of the disease and scratched it into the skin of a person who had never had smallpox. The recipient usually became slightly ill, recovered, and was immune thereafter. Occasionally, however, he had a virulent case, sometimes fatal, or became infected with bacterial contaminants in the inoculated material. Jenner discovered that smallpox and cowpox are essentially identical diseases, showing different symptoms in different hosts. Pus from infected cattle, when introduced into the skin of humans, creates a mild disease, which engenders protection against smallpox.

Metchnikoff, in 1882, discovered a cellular process by which animals combat infection. In microscopic studies of digestion by the transparent water flea Daphnia, he saw ameboid cells ingesting the spores of a yeast, which otherwise multiplied and produced a fatal infection in the water flea. If all the spores were ingested, the host survived. Metchnikoff named this process phagocytosis and postulated that it is the basis for immunity from infectious disease. It soon became apparent that this is not the only mechanism of immunity, but it is a very important part.

Three years later, Pasteur discovered a method of weakening or attenuating the rabies virus so it did not kill but could be used to immunize humans. He infected rabbits with virus-containing material and then removed their spinal cords and dried them for varying periods of time. Daily injections of cord emulsions desiccated for progressively shorter intervals protected individuals bitten by rabid dogs from the virus infection. This was the first successful immunization procedure to be developed after Jenner's discovery, nearly a century earlier.

Behring and Kitasato introduced a different type of immunization in 1890. They developed tetanus and diphtheria antitoxins by injecting the corresponding toxins into animals. When serum from an immunized animal was injected into a nonimmune animal, the latter acquired temporary protection against the toxin. This is *passive immunization*. The success of the procedure demonstrated that immunity does not always require the direct participation of blood cells, but that soluble constituents of blood serum may also be effective. These are known collectively as *antibodies*.

In 1893, Buchner discovered complement, a complex of approximately a dozen proteins and other components in normal as well as immune serum that contributes to many of the visible or detectable results of immunologic reactions. For example, antibodies alone do not dissolve and may not kill bacteria, but they may do so with the aid of complement.

A different aspect of immunology was demonstrated in 1900–1902, when Landsteiner discovered the four major (ABO) human blood groups. These groups are defined according to the presence or absence of one or the other or both of two antigenic substances, A and B, on the erythrocytes. Natural antibodies, anti-A and anti-B, are always present in the sera of individuals whose cells lack the corresponding antigens. Blood groups were of relatively little significance until attempts were made to transfuse blood from one individual to another, when it was quickly found that transfusions often did more harm than good. Landsteiner's work revealed that the cause of harmful reactions in incompatible transfusions was the agglutination (clumping) or lysis (dissolving) of injected red cells sensitized by the natural anti-A or anti-B antibodies of the recipient.

Until this time, immunology had been concerned only with specific protection against infectious disease. With Landsteiner, the broader implications of the science became apparent. Recognition of the fact that individuals differ immunologically provided a rational basis for important developments in medical and surgical practice, and also started the train of thought that eventually led to understanding of the position of immunity in the overall field of animal physiology.

Another immunologic process not directly related to infectious disease was discovered in 1902 by Portier and Richet in their studies of *anaphylaxis* (Greek, *ana*, back + *phylaxis*, protection), one of the many forms of hypersensitivity. In attempting to immunize dogs with eel serum or sea anemone tentacle extract, they found that doses so small as normally to be harmless produced rapid and dramatic death when too great an interval elapsed between injections. Since then, several types and many examples of hypersensitivity have been described, including hay fever and asthma, food idiosyncrasies, and skin allergies.

After a period in which Landsteiner concentrated his attention on the chemical nature of the specificity of immunologic reactions, he returned to the study of blood in 1940, in collaboration with Wiener. They discovered that five out of six humans possess red blood cell antigens found also on rhesus monkey erythrocytes. These were designated Rh antigens. If blood from an Rh positive individual is transferred to an Rh negative individual, the recipient produces antibodies against the Rh factor. When he later receives another transfusion containing the same Rh antigen, he may have a serious reaction. This being an inheritable factor, an Rh negative mother may carry an Rh positive fetus, and occasionally she produces antibodies against the fetal Rh positive erythrocytes. In subsequent similar pregnancies, the fetal blood cells may be destroyed, producing the disease erythroblastosis fetalis.

In 1944–1945, Medawar laid the groundwork for understanding the problems associated with tissue and organ transplantation. Transplantation reactions are like transfusion reactions—they do not occur in Nature. Man learned the techniques for grafting skin from one part of the body to another or from one animal to another and thus created a situation in which an immunologic reaction might occur. The only comparable natural condition is pregnancy, but ordinarily the fetal and maternal tissues are physiologically separated from one another and do not interact immunologically.

It was discovered quite early that tissue can be transplanted successfully from one identical twin to another. With genetically nonidentical individuals, however, there is an initial period of about a week after transplantation during which vascularization of the graft occurs and the tissue seems to be accepted, but during the next week or two it dies and is completely rejected. Medawar worked with syngeneic mice, which had become essentially identical genetically by 20 or more generations of serial brother-sister matings. When skin from a pure brown line was transplanted to a pure white line, it was rejected, but transplants between pure brown mice or between pure white mice were accepted. Moreover, a mouse that had rejected one graft became immune to tissue from the donor and rejected a second graft more rapidly than the first.

Medawar also found that white mice injected just before birth (i.e., in utero) or just after birth with spleen cells from fetal brown mice became immunologically tolerant and later accepted grafts of brown adult skin. Tolerance persisted as long as spleen cells of brown mice were retained, but it could be terminated by injecting spleen cells from a nontolerant adult syngeneic white donor, whereupon a well-established brown graft died and sloughed off. This work pointed to the importance of lymphoid cells in transplantation immunity.

THE COMPOSITION OF BLOOD

It has been indicated that the immunologic mechanism comprises both cellular and soluble components. The cellular components include phagocytes of various kinds, which ingest bacteria and other particulate agents, and also lymphoid cells, some of which react directly with and destroy microbial or other cells against which they have been sensitized. Other lymphoid cells that may be present as transients in the blood participate in the production of antibodies, primarily in the spleen, lymph nodes, and other lymphoid tissues.

Blood, Plasma, and Serum

Blood consists of a fluid containing the red and white blood cells and the platelets. The fluid is an aqueous solution of salts, carbohydrates, and proteins. The total amount of blood in the animal body is normally one-twelfth of the body weight. The average man possesses 12 to 14 pints. The cells comprise slightly less than one-half the volume of whole blood.

Blood, plasma, and serum are related as follows:

Blood minus cells = plasma

Plasma minus fibrin = serum

Freshly drawn blood clots within a few minutes. Formation of the clot is a complex process in which a protein, fibrinogen, is converted into insoluble fibrin. Damaged tissue releases thromboplastin, a lipoprotein that reacts with Ca^{++} ions and blood proteins, such as proaccelerin and proconvertin, to form prothrombinase. This enzyme is also formed when platelets disintegrate and release constituents that react with Ca^{++} ions and other blood proteins, including antihemophilic factor. Prothrombinase catalyzes the partial hydrolysis of prothrombin, a protein from the liver. Ca^{++} ions are required in this step also. A proteolytic enzyme, thrombin, is formed, and this removes two peptides from fibrinogen, another blood protein, to produce fibrin monomers, which polymerize into long fibrils arranged in bundles. These steps are summarized in Figure 1–1.

Most of the blood cells are enmeshed in the fibrin clot (see Figure 1–2), which shrinks after a few hours at low temperature and expels the serum, a clear, straw-colored fluid. Clotting is prevented by mixing the blood with sodium citrate, potassium oxalate, heparin, or other chemicals. Sodium citrate and potassium oxalate interfere with the formation of thrombin by reacting with the available Ca^{++} ions and forming insoluble salts; heparin, a polysaccharide-sulfate derived from liver and certain blood cells, also interferes with thrombin formation. When blood treated with one of these anticoagulant chemicals is allowed to stand a few hours or is centrifuged, the cells settle and leave a clear supernate, plasma, which still contains fibrinogen.

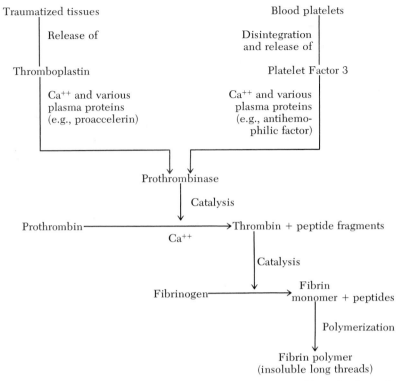

Figure 1–1. The series of reactions in the clotting of blood. Release of thromboplastin from damaged tissue or of a specific factor from platelets starts the enzymatic sequence that eventually leads to removal of two peptides from fibrinogen and formation of fibrin monomer, which polymerizes into long, insoluble threads in a network that traps red and white blood cells and platelets. (From Villee and Dethier, 1971. Biological Principles and Processes. Philadelphia, W. B. Saunders Company, p. 577.)

Serum Proteins

The serum proteins constitute 6 to 7 per cent of the weight of serum. Normal serum contains several proteins distinguishable by their electrophoretic properties, their molecular weights, and their solubilities in water, various electrolytes, and alcohol.

When serum is subjected to direct electric current, several fractions can be distinguished by their rates and direction of migration (see page 52). If the solution is maintained at approximately pH 8.5, the albumins migrate most rapidly toward the positive electrode, because they bear the strongest negative electric charge. After them come, in order, a series of globulins: alpha, beta, and gamma. The globulins account for about 50 per cent of the total protein of normal serum. The predominant globulin in most animals, such as man, monkey, and rabbit, has a molecular weight between 150,000 and 160,000, but other globulins with molecular weights of 200,000, 400,000, and 900,000 are also found in greater or lesser concentration. The molecular weight of human serum albumin is 69,000. Treatment of serum with sodium sulfate at a concentration of 21.5 per cent or with ammonium sulfate at half-saturation precipitates a crude fraction containing globulins, while albumins remain in solution.

Normal globulins assist in the maintenance of blood and tissue osmotic relations and take part in cell nutrition. Utilization of blood globulin in the manufacture of protoplasm is indicated by experiments with animals fed a protein-deficient diet, in

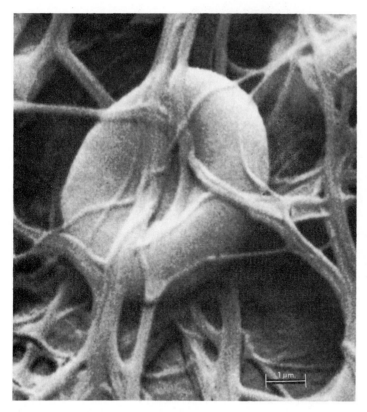

Figure 1–2. Fibrin threads enmeshing an erythrocyte. (Scanning electron micrograph courtesy of Emil Bernstein and Eila Kairinen, Gillette Company Research Institute, Rockville, Maryland, from (cover) *Science*, vol. 173, no. 3999, 27 August 1971. Copyright 1971 by the American Association for the Advancement of Science.)

which the circulating globulin decreased to a constant level. Furthermore, dogs from which plasma was regularly removed at short intervals replaced more than 20 times their normal blood protein content during a period of 16 weeks. It seems reasonable to assume that this high protein regenerating capacity is in fairly normal operation and that a certain percentage of the new protein consists of globulin, thus maintaining the customary balance of proteins in the plasma. The use of plasma protein in cell nutrition is confirmed by the observation that animals could be maintained in nitrogen equilibrium on a nitrogen-free diet when plasma from the same species was given intravenously as the only source of nitrogen.

Immune globulins or antibodies produced in response to infection or to injection of killed bacteria, foreign proteins, or various other substances differ from each other and from normal globulins in respect to the amino acid composition and sequence of a portion of each molecule, the physicochemical structure of which permits them to combine specifically with the substances that induced their formation.

Blood Cells

Normal human blood contains between 4,500,000 and 5,500,000 erythrocytes per cubic millimeter. These cells are about 7.5 μm in diameter and 2 μm in thickness. They are formed in the bone marrow and have an average life in the circulation of 100 to 120 days.

The white blood cells or leukocytes are an important defense against infection. Their total number varies between 5,000 and 8,000 per cubic millimeter. The several kinds of leukocytes are classified according to their size (7 μm to 22 μm), presence and type of granules, shape of nucleus, and character of cytoplasm, and are usually present in fairly constant percentages:

polymorphonuclear neutrophiles	50–70%
basophiles	0.5–1.0%
eosinophiles	1–5%
lymphocytes	20–30%
monocytes	2–6%

The mobile cells of the body, including all the blood cells, are believed to be derived ultimately from mesenchymal cells—unspecialized ameboid cells found between the epithelial layers in the early embryo. *Stem cells* or *blasts* in the marrow of the flat bones differentiate to produce the various blood cell series. Erythrocytes, granulocytes (polymorphonuclear neutrophiles, basophiles, and eosinophiles), and monocytes are formed in the bone marrow.

The bone marrow is also the source of the stem cells from which lymphocytes are derived. These stem cells are transported via the blood to primary lymphoid organs—the thymus, the bursa of Fabricius in birds (see page 12), and presumably mammalian organs or tissues corresponding in function to the bursa of Fabricius. In the primary lymphoid organs the stem cells differentiate and multiply extensively, and many migrate to the peripheral lymphoid system, which includes the spleen, lymph nodes, Peyer's patches, and other tissues. Lymphocytes are highly mobile and travel from region to region within a single organ and from one organ to another. The migration cycle from lymph node via the lymphatic circulation and the thoracic duct to the bloodstream and thence to the spleen and lymph nodes again may be repeated many times; these cells constitute the recirculating lymphocyte pool.

The average lifespan of granulocytes in the blood was formerly thought to be 2 to 3 days, but radioactive tracer studies indicate that it may be as long as 2 weeks. Lymphocytes, previously believed to live only a few hours, have been shown to be of two types: about 20 per cent live 2 to 3 days, and the other 80 per cent are very long-lived, some small lymphocytes even surviving a year or longer.

The principal function of the granulocytes, particularly the neutrophiles and eosinophiles, and of the monocytes appears to be phagocytosis. These cells can engulf particles, such as certain bacteria, and may eventually digest them by the action of intracellular proteases and other enzymes. A few bacteria, such as *Mycobacterium tuberculosis*, are ingested but not digested, the organisms often being transported by the phagocytic cells to other regions of the body, where they establish secondary sites of infection after the phagocytes have died and autolyzed.

Lymphoid cells, including leukocytes, comprise the major group of immunologically significant cells. Small lymphocytes are about the diameter of erythrocytes, composed almost entirely of nuclear material with a thin layer of cytoplasm. They are the principal lymphocytes of the blood and are also found in lymph and lymphoid tissues. Most of them are resting cells but are capable of responding to various stimuli by differentiating to diverse cell types. Multiplication of cells of the peripheral lymphoid system is usually triggered directly by antigenic stimulation, whereas cells of the primary lymphoid system multiply independently of the presence of antigen. Cells of the peripheral system are of several types, as indicated by their functions: (1) antigen-reactive or "memory" cells divide when stimulated but do not produce antibody; (2) antibody-forming cell precursors, perhaps identical with antigen-reactive cells, divide upon antigenic stimulation and yield antibody-forming progeny; (3) plasma cells release antibodies into the blood; (4) effector cells of cell-mediated immunity react with antigen and directly or indirectly damage tissue; and (5) other lymphocyte-like cells are postulated precursors of macrophages, normoblasts, and myeloblasts.

THE RETICULOENDOTHELIAL SYSTEM

An early step in evolution of the surveillance mechanism and in defense against infectious disease was based upon the primitive ameboid method of ingesting food in particulate form. Specialized cells developed that engulfed and destroyed dead tissue cells or their components and any other cells that might cause trouble, either because they were out of control or because they were foreign and not subject to the usual homeostatic mechanism. Phagocytic activity like that observed by Metchnikoff in the water flea is a major defense in invertebrates, whereas the type of defense represented by cellular and humoral (antibody) mechanisms, which depend on a lymphoid system, did not develop until vertebrates appeared. Present-day vertebrates possess both phagocytic and immunologic mechanisms, and their activities are somewhat coordinated and interdependent. The phagocytic process evolved to such an extent that elements are found in most parts of the body, and these comprise the reticuloendothelial system.

The reticuloendothelial system (R.E.S.) is composed principally of the network of reticular (supporting or structural) cells of the spleen, thymus, and other lymphoid tissues, together with cells lining the sinuses of the spleen, bone marrow, and lymph nodes, and the capillary endothelium of the liver (Kupffer's cells), brain, lungs, and the adrenal and pituitary glands. These comprise the sessile or *fixed* macrophages. In addition, *free* macrophages, such as the blood monocytes and other tissue macrophages, are transported by the body fluids or wander through the tissues.

The R.E.S. is best defined functionally by its ability to scavenge debris or other foreign matter. Inhaled particles are ingested by the pulmonary alveolar macrophages. Various dyes, carbon particles, or Thorotrast (thorium dioxide), injected intraperitoneally, are taken up by the peritoneal macrophages, and, if injected intravenously, they are deposited in the liver, spleen, bone marrow, lymph nodes, thymus, adrenals, and lungs, where they remain for several weeks. Their distribution serves to delineate the R.E.S.; this was, in fact, the approach used by Aschoff in 1924.

The reticuloendothelial cells perform two important functions. They remove worn out or damaged cells, such as erythrocytes and leukocytes, from the circulation, and they dispose of foreign organic matter that has penetrated the tissues. Removal from the blood of leukocytes damaged by the ingestion of bacteria simultaneously disposes of the ingested organisms. In addition, bacteria that escape leukocytic phagocytosis and enter the bloodstream may be ingested by reticuloendothelial cells in the various organs through which the blood passes.

The effectiveness of phagocytosis in removing microorganisms from the blood has often been demonstrated experimentally. Bull reported that the blood of dogs intravenously injected with typhoid bacteria contained 10,000,000 organisms per milliliter 1 minute after injection and only 40 per milliliter 14 minutes later. Noguiera found that *Streptococcus viridans* disappeared completely from the blood of rabbits within 6 hours after intravenous injection. The liver and spleen contained a large percentage of the organisms. Benacerraf and Miescher injected normal mice intravenously with heat-killed bacteria that had been labeled with ^{32}P and reported data indicating that 90 per cent of *Staphylococcus aureus* cells were removed from the blood in 7 minutes. Clearance of *Escherichia coli* was much slower, 61 minutes being required for 90 per cent removal. The difference was correlated with the gram reactions of the two species; phagocytosis of *E. coli* was greatly accelerated by the presence of antibody and complement and perhaps by properdin, as stated by Wardlaw and Howard.

There is no way of knowing how frequently infections terminate by phagocytosis of the pathogen. Probably many inapparent or mild infections progress to the stage at which some bacteria enter the bloodstream and are removed and destroyed, with the patient never realizing that anything spectacular has happened. It should be emphasized, however, that the eventual outcome of the infection depends upon many factors. The role of microbial virulence was strikingly illustrated in an experiment by Wright in 1927. Rabbits were injected with pneumococci of various grades of virulence, and the bacteria in the blood were counted at short intervals. After prompt partial removal from the blood, the virulent organism multiplied in the R.E.S. and soon "spilled over" again into the bloodstream, killing the animal (see Figure 1–3). It will be recalled that the natural course of typhoid fever in man is similar; an initial bacteremia is followed by a period of blood sterility during which the organisms multiply in the liver and finally produce secondary bacteremia.

IMMUNOLOGICALLY ACTIVE TISSUES

Immunologically active tissues are principally components of the lymphoid system, which consists of three major functional subdivisions: stem cells, primary lymphoid organs, and the peripheral (secondary) lymphoid system (see Figure 1–4).

Stem Cells

The bone marrow is the origin and principal pool of stem cells, although cells of similar function are also found in the spleen. Stem cells are multipotent; that is, under suitable conditions they can divide into a variety of cells—erythrocytes, granulocytes, lymphocytes—according to the hormonal and other influences that obtain in whatever body region they colonize. Stem cells migrate via the circulation from the bone marrow

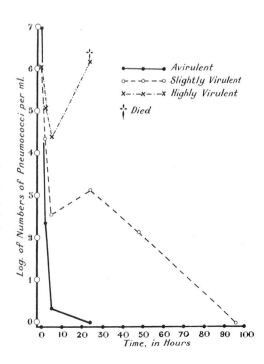

Figure 1–3. Avirulent pneumococci injected into rabbits are promptly removed from the blood by the reticuloendothelial system. Virulent organisms are only partially removed and then "spill over" again into the blood, producing fatal septicemia. (From Topley and Wilson, 1946. Principles of Bacteriology and Immunity, 3rd ed. Copyright 1946, The Williams & Wilkins Company, Baltimore.)

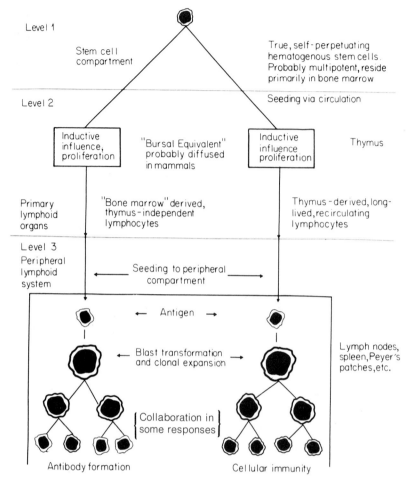

Figure 1–4. The three major subdivisions of the lymphoid system. (From Nossal and Ada, 1971. Antigens, Lymphoid Cells, and the Immune Response. New York, Academic Press, Inc.)

to nearly any location. It is of interest that injection of bone marrow, alone of all tissues, is able to "rescue" a lethally irradiated animal by providing the cells necessary to restore the structure and function of all the hematopoietic organs.

Primary Lymphoid Organs

THYMUS

The thymus in humans and many other mammals consists of a pair of lobes shaped like a pyramid, lying along the midline below the neck. The base rests upon the pericardium and the apex extends upward from the thoracic cage. Unlike other lymphatic organs, it is almost fully developed at birth and gradually atrophies with age.

The thymus is composed chiefly of epithelial cells infiltrated by lymphocytes (thymocytes). The central portion of each lobe is the medulla, consisting principally of epithelial cells. The outer portion of the thymus is the cortex; it contains many more lymphocytes than the medulla and relatively few epithelial cells. The latter remain firmly attached to one another at spots on their adjacent membranes by desmosomes, and are therefore greatly distorted into a stellate shape by the lymphocytes that wedge between them (Figure 1–5). Fingerlike processes of the medulla extend into the cortex

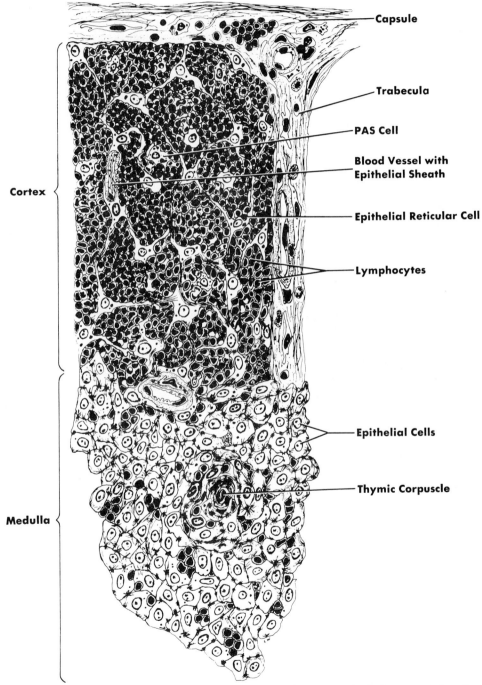

Figure 1–5. Part of a lobule of the thymus, an epithelial organ in which the cortex is heavily infiltrated by lymphocytes. (From Leon Weiss, ©1972. The Cells and Tissues of the Immune System: Structure, Functions, Interactions. Reproduced by permission of Prentice-Hall, Inc., Englewood Cliffs, N. J.)

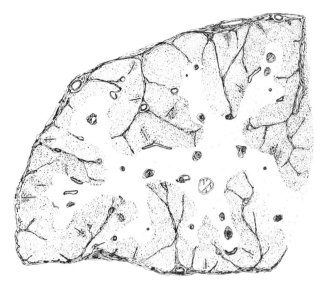

Figure 1-6. Several lobules of the thymus. The medulla is the central, lightly stippled area, and the radiating, fingerlike processes are capped by the densely stippled cortex. A thin capsule surrounds the entire organ, and vessel-bearing trabeculae extend from it into the cortex. Each lobule comprises a finger of medulla with its surrounding cortex. (From Leon Weiss, ©1972. The Cells and Tissues of the Immune System: Structure, Functions, Interactions. Reproduced by permission of Prentice-Hall, Inc., Englewood Cliffs, N. J.)

(Figure 1-6). Each lobe of the thymus consists of several lobules, a single lobule comprising one of the fingerlike medullary processes with its cortical cap.

The thymus possesses a moderately developed blood system. Afferent lymphatics are lacking, but small efferent lymphatics drain into nearby lymph nodes.

The thymus is remarkably constant from species to species in respect to its lobular pattern, its cell content, and its size in comparison to the total body weight. It is therefore not surprising that the functions of the thymus seem to be the same in all animals. There are minor differences in location, but these are not significant. One marsupial species, the quokka, found only on Rottnest Island off the southwest coast of Australia, possesses two thymus glands, one in the cervical region and the other in the thoracic cavity.

When stem cells from the bone marrow reach the thymus, they differentiate into lymphocytes. More than 95 per cent die within 3 to 5 days, not having left the organ or performed any known function except the production of more lymphocytes. The remainder have a life span of many months or years. These acquire a characteristic surface antigen, theta (in the mouse), and become the *T cells*, many of which are exported and colonize the thymic-dependent zones of the spleen and lymph nodes. Although the generation time of thymic lymphocytes is short—6.5 to 8.5 hours— maintenance of the population depends upon continuous immigration from the bone marrow. The dependence upon marrow has been demonstrated by attempting to restore to normal a thymus that has been irradiated to destroy its own lymphocytes; it cannot be restored by suspensions of thymic lymphocytes, but it can be repopulated by bone marrow cells.

THE BURSA OF FABRICIUS

The bursa of Fabricius, like the thymus, is a lymphoepithelial organ. It is found only in birds, however, in which it controls antibody production. A comparable organ in mammals has not been found, despite the fact that functions performed in birds by the bursa are known to be performed in mammals.

The bursa of Fabricius is a saclike structure weighing about 3 g. at maximal development in the chicken. It is connected to the posterior wall of the cloaca by a short duct (see Figure 1–7). The epithelial surface is thickly folded, and beneath is highly vascularized loose connective tissue, within which are lymphatic nodules in contact with the epithelium. These nodules have a central medulla and peripheral cortex. The epithelial cells of the medulla form a follicle that is filled with many cells: large lymphocytes, epithelial cells, reticular cells, macrophages, some granulocytes, and plasma cells. The cortex consists of a layer of small cells, including lymphocytes and plasma cells, and also some macrophages and granulocytes.

The bursa of Fabricius controls the development of plasmacytes and the production of antibody. As a primary lymphoid organ, epithelial cells are a prominent feature, mitosis is not stimulated by the presence of antigen, and it is not significant as a direct source of antibody. Some of the bone marrow stem cells that reach the bursa transform into lymphocytes bearing specifically reactive antibody-like sites (immunoglobulin determinants) on their plasma membranes, and possess the ability to divide continuously and to differentiate into plasmacytes. These lymphocytes are *B cells*. They are released by the bursa and colonize the secondary lymphoid organs: lymph nodes, spleen, and so forth.

A mammalian organ with characteristics comparable to those of the bursa has not yet been found. Many investigators believe that such properties occur in intestinal lymphoid tissue, the gut-associated lymphoid tissue (GALT), or even that the bone marrow itself may be the mammalian bursa equivalent.

Secondary Lymphoid Organs

LYMPH NODES

Lymph nodes are small, bean-shaped organs located along the lymphatic vessels in areas of lymphatic drainage. A lymph node is covered by a capsule of collagenous connective tissue and is divided into lobules by strands of connective tissue called trabeculae. The main mass of tissue comprising the organ is divided roughly into two areas: the cortex (outer) and the medulla (inner). The medulla is a supporting structure of reticular phagocytic cells and appears to serve as a drainage and collection system for cells and their products formed in the cortex.

Blood enters a lymph node through a single artery at the hilus, an indentation in the capsule. The artery and its branches extend through the trabeculae into the cortex and thence into the tissue of the organ. Venous drainage from the tissue passes out through trabecular veins to the central vein, which leaves the node at the hilus. A

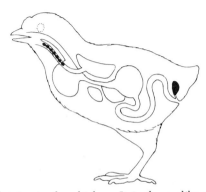

Figure 1–7. Bursa of Fabricius in the chicken. It is the saclike structure attached to the dorsal surface of the cloaca by a short duct. (From Good and Fisher, 1971. Immunobiology. Stamford, Conn., Sinauer Associates, Inc.)

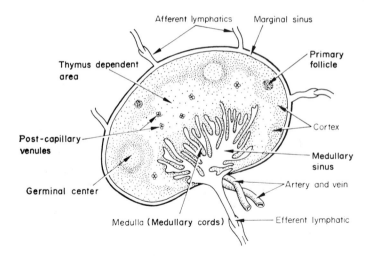

Figure 1–8. Structure of a lymph node. (From Herbert and Wilkinson, 1971. A Dictionary of Immunology. Oxford, Blackwell Scientific Publications.)

lymph node is well supplied with afferent lymphatic vessels at various points through the capsule, and the lymph collects in subcapsular sinuses. Some of it passes immediately to the efferent lymphatic, which leaves the organ at the hilus, but most of the lymph is filtered through the mass of lymphoid and reticular cells that comprise the major portion of the node (Figure 1–8).

The cortex contains tightly packed lymphocytes in nodules or primary follicles; secondary follicles or germinal centers, consisting of looser nodules enclosed within a shell of packed lymphocytes; and strips of lymphoid cells between germinal centers and making up the pericortical areas. The pericortical areas interdigitate irregularly into the medulla, a network of sinusoids that drain eventually into the efferent lymphatics. The cortex, especially the germinal centers, is the principal site of lymphocyte proliferation, which is greatly accelerated by antigenic stimulation.

SPLEEN

The spleen receives material only from the blood and hence has no direct connection with the lymphatic vessels. It is considerably larger than a lymph node, but like them it is enclosed in a capsule and subdivided into lobules by trabeculae (Figure 1–9). There is no demarcation into cortical and medullary areas, but the organ is composed of sinusoids, each with its arterial and venous system which connects to the main blood vessels at the hilus. The lobules contain "red pulp," largely red blood cells, surrounding islands of "white pulp," which consists of lymphoid cells located around the small arteries. Upon antigenic stimulation, germinal centers form in the white pulp and serve as sites for production of plasma cells. Lymphocyte multiplication also occurs in the white pulp outside the germinal centers.

PEYER'S PATCHES

Peyer's patches are found principally in the submucosa of the ileum. They are composed of lymphoid cells arranged in the form of germinal centers (Figure 1–10). Lymph from nearby intestinal villi drains into them via afferent lymphatics and travels from them to the thoracic duct. Histologically, they are considered to resemble secondary or peripheral lymphoid tissue more closely than primary lymphoid tissue. In addition to lymphocytes, the medullary tissue contains plasma cells and macrophages.

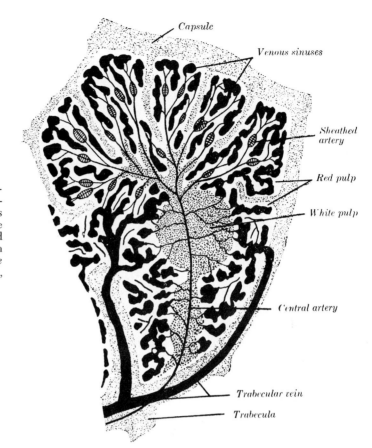

Figure 1-9. Diagrammatic section of part of the mammalian spleen. Venous sinuses and vessels are in black; white pulp is heavily stippled; red pulp is unstippled. (From Romer, 1970. *The Vertebrate Body,* 4th ed. Philadelphia, W. B. Saunders Company.)

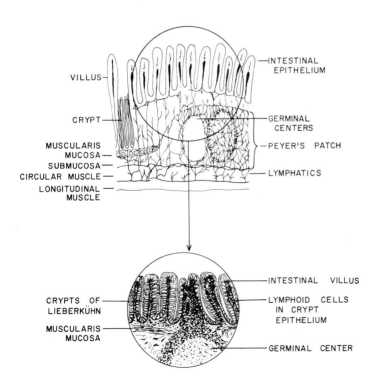

Figure 1-10. Section of a Peyer's patch, consisting of lymphoid cells arranged in the form of germinal centers along the ileum. (From Bloom and Fawcett, 1969. *A Textbook of Histology,* 9th ed. Philadelphia, W. B. Saunders Company.)

OMENTAL "MILK" SPOTS

The omental "milk" spots are aggregations of lymphocytes situated between the two layers of flattened cells comprising the omentum. They are very minute in an animal unstimulated by antigen, but following intraperitoneal administration of antigen, they enlarge greatly and also increase in number. They appear, therefore, to provide a rapid response to antigenic challenge in a large and vulnerable area of the body, the peritoneal cavity.

Distribution of T Cells, B Cells, and Plasma Cells

T cells comprise 75 to 85 per cent of the nucleated free cells of the lymph nodes in the mouse, 30 to 50 per cent of those of the spleen, and 85 to 90 per cent of thoracic duct cells; there are very few in bone marrow. They circulate in the blood and lymph and are found especially in localized regions—thymus-dependent areas—of the spleen and lymph nodes (see Figure 1–8).

B cells constitute 10 to 20 per cent of the nucleated free cells of the lymph nodes in mice, 20 to 35 per cent of those in the spleen, 5 per cent of thoracic duct cells, and are absent from the thymus. Like T cells, they tend to segregate in specific regions of the spleen and lymph nodes.

Plasma cells are conspicuous in the spleen, lymph nodes, bone marrow, and areas of chronic inflammation. They increase drastically in lymphatic organs regional to the site of antigen injection.

TYPES OF IMMUNE RESPONSE

Before discussing the types of immune response, which are often directed against noninfectious agents, it should be pointed out that there are three forms of protection against infectious disease. Two of these are nonimmunologic, but they will be discussed briefly at this point in order to assist in differentiating them from immunity.

1. *Nonsusceptibility* constitutes an absolute protection against particular diseases and is associated with species characteristics. It is dependent upon inherited physiologic and anatomic factors. Nonsusceptibility is illustrated by the fact that man is not subject to spontaneous infection by certain animal pathogens, such as chicken cholera, canine distemper, hog cholera, and cattle plague, nor do lower animals contract many human diseases, including dysentery, measles, gonorrhea, mumps, typhoid fever, and whooping cough.

Physiologic factors such as body temperature and diet contribute to nonsusceptibility. Classic early experiments with anthrax infections of frogs and chickens demonstrated the influence of body temperature. These animals are normally nonsusceptible to anthrax, but when frogs inoculated with *Bacillus anthracis* were warmed to 35° C., they succumbed to the infection, as did chickens when their body temperature was artificially reduced from its normal of about 41° C.

2. *Natural resistance* is relatively nonspecific and variable and is determined by physical or physiologic conditions that are subject to variation from time to time or between individuals.

The normal body possesses remarkable nonspecific resistance to infection. The first line of defense consists of the physical and chemical barriers presented by epithelial tissues. The relative impenetrability of the skin, the stickiness of mucous membranes, the ciliation of the upper respiratory tract, and the acidity or alkalinity of various parts of the digestive system are more or less effective against numerous pathogens or potential pathogens. Physiologic and pathologic characteristics of the host, such as its general state of nutrition, debilitation resulting from aging, fatigue, exposure to extreme temperatures, alcoholism, and concurrent disease, play an important part in determining the likelihood of infection and deciding the outcome of established disease. Animal tissues and body fluids contain various polypeptide and other chemical substances that have antibacterial activity (see Table 1-1). Other unknown factors, many presumably genetic in origin, participate in natural resistance.

Numerous examples can be cited of the evolution of resistance in human populations. For example, tuberculosis occurs in chronic form with frequent recovery in populations in which it has been present for many generations, but previously unexposed populations are nearly wiped out when the disease is first introduced. Syphilis was a highly fatal, epidemic disease in Europe in the fifteenth century but became milder and more chronic as resistance developed through the centuries.

3. In contrast to the foregoing, *immunity* is never absolute; it varies quantitatively from one individual to another and from time to time within the same individual. It is specific in the sense that it is directed against a given infectious agent; however, some degree of cross-protection may be afforded against chemically related infectious agents.

Immunity is attributed to specifically reactive cells or proteins (antibodies), either naturally occurring (i.e., without external stimulus), actively developed, or received from some outside source. Methods of inducing and acquiring immunity will be described later (see page 81 ff.).

Cell-Mediated Immunity

Cell-mediated immunity is a direct outgrowth of the postulated primitive surveillance mechanism for maintaining tissue integrity. It depends upon the activity of T cells possessing surface receptors, presumably globulins, complementary in structure to reactive determinant sites of antigenic cells or substances with which they come into direct contact. The antigenic agents may be cells transplanted from another individual, mutant cells of the same individual, or parasitic infectious agents, or under special

Table 1-1. *Antibacterial Substances from Animal Tissue or Fluid*[*]

Name	Common Source	Chemical Nature	Antibacterial Selectivity
Complement	Serum	Euglobulin-carbohydrate-lipoprotein (?)	Gram-negative
Properdin	Serum	Euglobulin	Gram-negative
Phagocytin	Leukocytes	Globulin	Gram-negative
Lysozyme	Ubiquitous	Small basic protein	Gram-positive (chiefly)
β-Lysin	Serum	Protein (?)	Gram-positive
Histone	Lymphatics	Small basic protein	Gram-positive
Protamine	Sperm	Small basic protein	Gram-positive
Tissue poly-peptides	Lymphatics	Linear basic peptides	Gram-positive
Leukin	Leukocytes	Basic peptides	Gram-positive
Plakin	Blood platelets	Peptide (?)	Gram-positive
Hematin, mesohematin	Red blood cells	Iron porphyrins	Gram-positive
Spermine, spermidine	Pancreas, prostate	Basic polyamines	Gram-positive

[*]Modified from Skarnes and Watson, 1957. Bacteriol. Rev., 21:273.

circumstances the inciting agent may be soluble material from any source (living or not) that chemically alters host cells or other constituents and in effect makes them "not self."

Contact between the antigen and a T cell bearing the corresponding specific surface receptor activates the cell membrane, and a signal is transmitted to the nucleus of the lymphocyte, which becomes derepressed. The cell transforms into a large blast cell, mitosis begins, and soluble mediator chemicals called *lymphokines* are released. Lymphokines induce various reactions, some of which presumably occur in vivo and are significant in immunologic responses. They include, among others, lymphocyte mitosis, cytotoxicity, chemotactic attraction of monocytes, activation of macrophages, inhibition of macrophage migration (and hence retention at the site of response), local skin reaction, and production of interferon, a protein that nonspecifically prevents the replication of viruses within susceptible host cells.

TRANSPLANTATION IMMUNITY

Medawar's observations on transplantation immunity have been described (page 3). It will be recalled that, when genetically nonidentical tissue is grafted, vascularization is initiated and the graft begins to "take," but within 7 to 10 days it is destroyed and rejected. This is the *first set reaction*. When another graft from the same or a genetically identical donor is later attempted, rejection occurs more quickly. This is the *second set reaction*. During the primary encounter with antigen, T cells of the recipient that can react with the transplanted tissue cells are specifically stimulated to proliferate. Blastlike "killer" cells form and destroy the transplanted cells. In the second set reaction, there is already a large population of specifically sensitive cells, so the second graft is destroyed more quickly.

GRAFT-VERSUS-HOST REACTION

The reverse of this phenomenon is the graft-versus-host reaction, in which transplanted lymphoid cells damage cells of the recipient. Lymphoid cells from a mature animal are introduced into an immature (i.e., immunologically incompetent) animal. The recipient soon develops symptoms of *runt disease*, a wasting diarrhea and anemia, with enlargement of the spleen and liver necrosis, and dies in a few weeks. The lymphoid cells from the mature animal include thymus-derived lymphocytes, some of which can be specifically activated by cells of the recipient. After a sufficient population has accumulated, physiologic damage and stunting become apparent. A similar disease occurs in mature recipients that have been X-irradiated to destroy their own lymphoid systems before receiving foreign lymphoid cells. The wasting disease in these animals is called *secondary* or *homologous disease*. In both instances, the injected lymphoid cells react immunologically against, and eventually destroy, vital host cells. If the recipient should be immunologically mature and not irradiated, its T cells would reject the donor lymphoid cells.

TUMOR IMMUNITY

An immunologic response to tumors occurs when the tumor tissue possesses antigens not present in the normal tissue of the individual. It may therefore incite a typical response, leading to eventual destruction of the tumor. However, humoral antibodies that are sometimes also produced may react with the tumor cells and shield them from the sensitized lymphocytes, so the tumor continues to grow. These antibodies are called *enhancing* or *blocking antibodies*. In some instances, the mass of tumor tissue is so great that it exhausts the supply of specifically reactive lymphocytes.

INTRACELLULAR PARASITIC INFECTIONS

The cell-mediated immune mechanism is operative in various infections caused by intracellular parasites, including certain bacteria, viruses, fungi, and protozoa. The cellular response is particularly characteristic of infections in which antibody is not produced or in which the parasite is protected from circulating antibody by its intracellular location. In some instances, as in poxvirus and herpesvirus infections, new antigens appear on the surface of infected cells. Populations of T lymphocytes specifically sensitive to these antigens develop in the same manner as to cells of a graft, with the result that infected cells are eventually destroyed. In addition, interferon released during the blast-cell transformation of T cells prevents replication of the virus.

Some bacteria, such as *Mycobacterium tuberculosis*, *Listeria monocytogenes*, and Brucella species, survive and even multiply within the cytoplasm of phagocytic cells, including macrophages. Animals that are infected with moderate doses of one of these bacteria may recover from the infection and thereafter be immune, as demonstrated by challenge with the infecting organism. However, this immunity is not strictly specific. If a recovered animal is challenged with a second intracellular parasite at the same time as with the first, resistance to both organisms is shown by the fact that ingested cells of both species are killed. This was demonstrated by Mackaness in the case of an animal infected with tuberculosis and later challenged with *L. monocytogenes* and *M. tuberculosis* simultaneously (Table 1–2). It is postulated that the specifically reactive cell is a T cell and that macrophages are effector cells in this situation. When a sensitive T lymphocyte encounters its specific antigen, *M. tuberculosis*, macrophage-activating lymphokine is released. It reacts with macrophages that have ingested either of the bacteria and activates intracellular enzymes that kill and/or digest the parasites. Macrophages that have reacted with activating lymphokine have been termed "angry" macrophages; they are very active metabolically and contain large numbers of intracellular granules (lysosomes) that possess potent hydrolytic enzymes.

DELAYED-TYPE HYPERSENSITIVITY

Delayed-type hypersensitivity is a cell-mediated response closely akin to the response to grafts, tumors, and chronic intracellular parasites. The classic example is the reaction to tuberculin by an individual who has had tuberculosis and developed cell-mediated immunity. Several hours after introduction of tuberculin into the skin, erythema and induration appear at the site of injection, reach a maximum at 24 to 48 hours, and subside gradually. The first histologic evidence of reaction is the passage of mononuclear cells through the walls of small blood vessels in the site and their local accumulation ("perivascular cuffing") and a more general accumulation of mononuclear and polynuclear cells. The latter soon leave the lesion, and a lymphocyte-macrophage infiltrate remains.

Table 1–2. *Nonspecific Immunity Caused by a Cell-Mediated Reaction*

Primary Infectious Agent	Mycobacterium tuberculosis			None	Listeria
Challenge	*M. tuber-culosis*	Listeria	*M. tuber-culosis* + Listeria	*M. tuber-culosis* + Listeria	*M. tuber-culosis* + Listeria
Result	Immunity	Infection	Immunity	Infection	Immunity

The delayed hypersensitivity response is elicited in many bacterial, viral, fungal, and parasitic infections upon intradermal injection of the appropriate antigenic test material (e.g., microbial extract). It occurs naturally as contact dermatitis in individuals sensitive to various chemicals (e.g., p-phenylenediamine used to treat furs), physical agents, or biologic products (e.g., urushiol from poison ivy), and can be demonstrated experimentally in animals rendered sensitive to simple chemicals such as chlorodinitrobenzene.

Humoral Immunity

Humoral immunity was doubtless a later evolutionary development than cellular immunity and was a refinement that made it possible to cope with toxic cell products and "indigestible" microorganisms. It depends upon the activity of antibodies, whose structure permits them to combine only with "mirror image" determinant sites or epitopes of homologous (i.e., corresponding) antigenic molecules or cells. The result of antigen-antibody union depends upon the nature of the antigen and the attendant circumstances (presence of phagocytic cells, serum components, etc.). In general, it results in destruction, removal, inactivation, or neutralization of the antigenic material.

Antibodies are produced principally by plasma cells, which are end cells formed when B cells are stimulated to replicate by contact with antigen. Antibody formation is the result of a complex series of processes in which T cells and macrophages may also participate (see page 100). An animal injected once with the antigen produces a moderate amount of antibody, detectable in the blood serum after a latent period of a few days, the exact interval depending upon the nature of the antigen, the animal, the dose and route of injection, and the test used to detect it. A second injection of antigen incites a more rapid response, which reaches a higher peak more quickly than occurred after the first injection. Infection with extracellularly parasitic bacteria often incites antibody production detectable within 2 or 3 weeks. The antibody content of the serum rises during a variable interval and then slowly drops after the patient recovers. In some diseases, antibody persists for several years, and in others it may disappear within a few months.

ANTIBACTERIAL IMMUNITY

The principal antimicrobial defense of mammals against infectious disease is the process of phagocytosis. As mentioned previously, this is apparently an adaptation of the primitive feeding mechanism. Bacteria adhere to macrophages, polymorphonuclear leukocytes of the blood, and other phagocytes by attaching to a "recognition site" on the phagocytic cell surface. Arms of cytoplasm then surround the microorganism, engulfing it and enclosing it in a phagocytic body, a *phagosome* (see Figure 1–11). A lysosomal granule in the phagocyte cytoplasm fuses with the phagosome and contributes a number of bactericidal basic polypeptides and hydrolytic enzymes, such as lysozyme, which kill and digest the ingested microorganism.

This process can occur to a limited extent in a nonimmune animal upon contact with a variety of microorganisms, but it is greatly improved or accelerated in an immune animal. Phagocytic cells apparently lack recognition sites specific for certain kinds of infectious agents, which are therefore only minimally susceptible to phagocytosis. One of the best examples of this situation is the behavior of virulent (encapsulated) pneumococci. As long as they possess the capsule, they do not adhere to phagocytic cells readily, but after being coated by specific antibody, they are rapidly

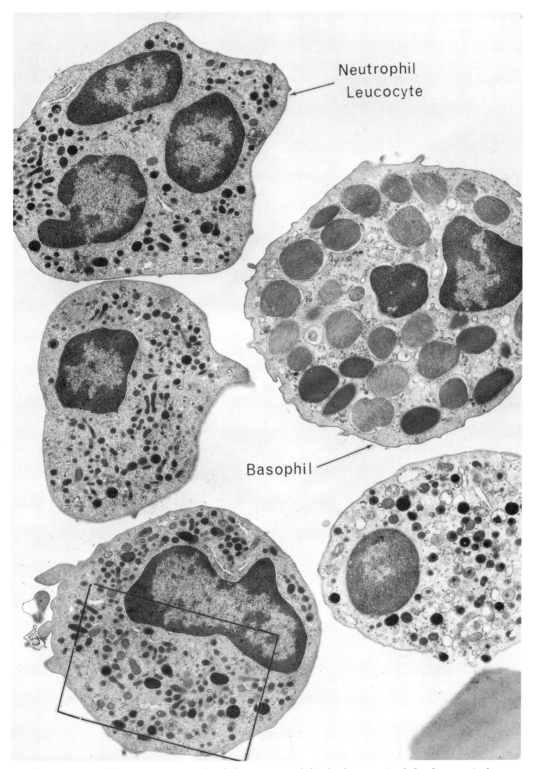

Figure 1–11. Electron micrograph of three neutrophilic leukocytes (at left of picture) showing numerous lysosomes, the densely staining cytoplasmic granules. They vary from about 0.1 to 0.7 μm in diameter (the cells are about 10 μm in diameter). (From Fawcett, 1966. An Atlas of Fine Structure. Philadelphia, W. B. Saunders Company.)

phagocytized and destroyed. This has been demonstrated experimentally in mice injected intravenously with pneumococci, either coated with antibody or uncoated (Figure 1–12). In normal animals injected with uncoated bacteria, approximately 40 per cent of the organisms remained in the bloodstream after 2 hours, whereas less than 0.02 per cent of antibody-coated bacteria remained in the circulation. Phagocytic cells, particularly macrophages, bear surface receptors with a high affinity for one region of an antibody molecule, and this portion of the pneumococcal antibody is exposed and accessible to phagocytic cells after reacting with the bacterial capsule.

Phagocytosis is promoted and accelerated by complement, a mixture of many serum components, largely protein, which are present in normal as well as immune serum. It participates in various in vitro as well as in vivo processes, but its activity is triggered only by the union of an antigen with its antibody. Phagocytic cells possess surface receptor sites with which complement can react, so its presence, together with that of antibody, increases the extent and rate of phagocytic action.

Another activity of specific antibacterial antibody is agglutination, the clumping together of bacterial cells due to simultaneous reaction of one antibody molecule with two bacterial cells. Aggregates containing many scores of bacteria may be formed, and these can be engulfed by phagocytes more efficiently than the same number of bacterial cells individually.

Some microorganisms are subject to bactericidal or bacteriolytic action by serum containing complement and antibody. Gram-negative bacteria that have a cell wall containing lipoprotein in the outer layer are particularly susceptible to this phenomenon. The outcome of a complicated series of reactions (see Chapter 8) involving antibody and the several components of complement is the production of "holes" in the

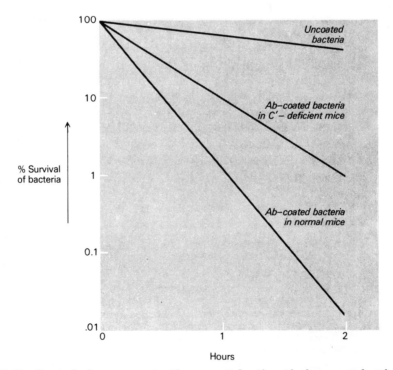

Figure 1–12. Survival of pneumococci, either uncoated with antibody or coated with antibody, in normal or complement(C′)-deficient mice. Antibody markedly increases adherence of bacteria to phagocytic cells, even in the absence of complement. (From Roitt, 1971. Essential Immunology. Oxford, Blackwell Scientific Publications.)

bacterial cell wall, which permit serum lysozyme to enter and digest the inner bacterial wall, leading to cell death. Some bacteria even appear to dissolve—hence the name "bacteriolysis" that is given to this process.

ANTITOXIC IMMUNITY

The vast majority of pathogenic bacteria produce disease by mechanisms that do not involve highly toxic products, but some score of bacteria do produce potent, soluble exotoxins, which are excreted into the medium and can produce specific destructive effects in the complete absence of the microorganism. Some of these exotoxins are among the most powerful poisons known (e.g., *C. botulinum* and tetanus toxins). The specific mode of action of many toxins has not yet been determined. Some are known to be enzymes or to be related to enzymes. For example, phospholipase C of *Clostridium perfringens* hydrolyzes lecithin, a vital component of mammalian cell walls.

Antibody (antitoxin) against an exotoxin combines with the toxin and neutralizes or destroys its toxic activity by means of allosteric changes in conformation. Additionally, when antitoxin reacts with toxin in suitable proportions, a precipitate of toxin and antitoxin forms, and this can be ingested and digested by phagocytic cells.

Immunologic Tolerance

Owen observed in 1945 that nonidentical (i.e., dizygotic) twin calves, which shared the same placental blood circulatory system, possessed erythrocytes of two different types; most of the erythrocytes were of their own type, but a few belonged to that of the twin. Both types persisted as the animals matured. Normally, foreign cells introduced into an adult would soon be eliminated by an immunologic mechanism. Each twin had therefore become tolerant of the red blood cells it had encountered in prenatal life.

Burnet (1949) deduced from this observation that an antigen present before birth suppresses any potential future immunologic response to that antigen that might be anticipated in a mature animal. This hypothesis explains why an animal distinguishes "self" components from "nonself" components and does not ordinarily produce antibodies against its own constituents.

Medawar and his colleagues then showed that foreign cells injected into a newborn mouse induced tolerance of cells of the same kind when the mouse became adult. Thus, A strain mice injected when newborn with spleen cells of CBA mice were able in adulthood to accept CBA skin grafts. It was also found that tolerance could be induced with soluble antigens. For example, rabbits injected at birth with bovine serum albumin (BSA) became tolerant and did not produce anti-BSA when later reinjected with this protein.

Subsequently it was learned that adult animals can be made tolerant by repeated injections of proper doses of certain antigens. Mitchison injected mature mice three times each week for intervals as long as 16 weeks with various doses of BSA and determined whether tolerance had been induced by challenging 10 days after the last injection with BSA emulsified in Freund's adjuvant, which markedly increases the antibody response of normal animals to BSA (see page 91). Surprisingly, he found that there were two dose ranges within which the animals became tolerant: a low dose range (0.001 to 0.010 mg.) and a high dose range (1.0 to 10.0 mg.). Intermediate doses (0.04 to 1.0 mg.) sensitized the animals so that they produced antibody in response to the challenge. It was noted also that high doses produced an initial short interval of immunity (1 to 2 weeks) before tolerance was established.

Substances that are highly antigenic, even at low doses, such as lysozyme, egg albumin, and diphtheria toxoid, do not induce low zone tolerance. However, simultaneous treatment with immunosuppressive agents (e.g., 6-mercaptopurine, sublethal X-irradiation, or antilymphocyte serum) to inhibit antibody formation aids in the establishment of tolerance in adult animals.

It appears that both T cells and B cells may become tolerant, and the nature of the tolerant state in a given animal depends upon which cells have been affected: in low zone tolerance T cells are unresponsive, and in high zone tolerance both T and B cells are unresponsive. Weigle and his colleagues found by kinetic studies that T cells readily and rapidly became tolerant and remained so, whereas B cells became unresponsive only after higher doses of antigen and following a longer induction period, and they soon regained their immunologic activity (Figure 1–13).

The physical state of the antigen influences the nature of the response. Proteins such as human gamma globulin (HGG) in the form of solutions containing polymeric aggregates of the protein tend to be immunogenic and induce antibody formation, whereas solutions from which the polymers have been removed by ultracentrifugation so that only the monomeric form remains are tolerogenic. It has been postulated that an aggregated antigen is first processed by macrophages, which then present it to lymphocytes, and the antibody-forming mechanism is called into play. A completely soluble antigen, on the other hand, encounters lymphocytes directly and turns them off. Whatever the explanation, it is evident that cellular and humoral immunity and immunologic tolerance are only different manifestations of the machinery that has evolved to maintain the physical and physiologic integrity of the body.

ACQUIRED IMMUNITY AGAINST INFECTIOUS DISEASE

Acquired immunity is that which an individual develops by exposure to a foreign (i.e., nonself) substance or organism or receives from some outside source. A person

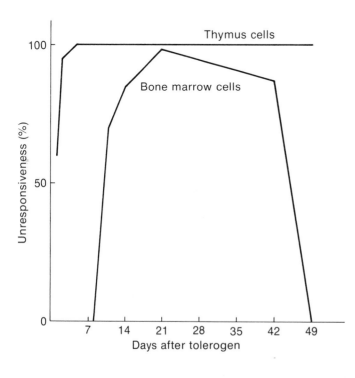

Figure 1–13. Development and loss of unresponsiveness in thymus (T) and bone marrow (B) cells of mice injected with deaggregated human gamma globulin as tolerogen.

who recovers from plague, cholera, yellow fever, or various other diseases is usually immune from second attacks of the same disease. Immunity against one infectious agent may contribute marked, little, or no immunity against other infectious agents, depending upon the chemical interrelationships of the causative organisms.

Immunity is quantitative rather than qualitative. The size of the infecting dose of organisms is important in determining whether or not a second attack occurs. An individual may possess sufficient immunity to protect against ordinary contact but not enough to overcome massive exposure. The immunity that develops from typhoid fever, smallpox, and mumps is often sufficient to protect against reinfection. On the other hand, little if any immunity is conferred by cases of gonorrhea, pneumonia, or influenza.

Active Immunity

Active immunity is that produced by the immunized individual in response to natural or artificial stimulation of the antibody-producing mechanism. In addition to obvious, clinical cases of disease, unrecognized or inapparent infections may also induce immunity. Many persons evidently suffer mild attacks of scarlet fever, poliomyelitis, diphtheria, or meningitis that are never diagnosed as such but nevertheless produce strong immunity.

Actual infection is not the only means of acquiring antibody or of stimulating the antibody-producing mechanism. The antibody-producing cells are stimulated artificially by introducing into the body the microorganisms that cause disease or some of their components or products. Microbial suspensions used for immunization are commonly called *bacterins* or *vaccines*, although the latter term is properly reserved for the specific immunizing agent of smallpox. Nearly all pathogenic agents produce fatal disease only when a susceptible individual receives a sufficiently large dose, usually by a particular route. Smaller amounts, or organisms introduced by unnatural routes, may cause illness of short duration or only local irritation without clinical disease. Sublethal doses of virulent microorganisms are not considered sufficiently safe for administration to man but are employed in veterinary practice.

Attenuated organisms are safer immunizing agents. The virulence of microorganisms may be reduced by many methods. Pasteur accidentally discovered one method when he inoculated fowl with old cultures of chicken cholera bacteria. The inoculated chickens survived later introduction of multiple lethal doses of the virulent bacteria. He also discovered that the anthrax bacillus cultivated at an unusually high temperature (42° to 43° C.) lost its ability to produce more than a transitory illness but induced immunity against virulent bacilli. A third method of attenuation was effective with the infectious agent of rabies. The virus in dried spinal cords of infected rabbits lost virulence in proportion to the duration of desiccation while retaining immunizing capacity. Another method of attenuating viruses consisted of cultivating them in unnatural hosts. The French neurotropic strain of yellow fever virus was attenuated for man by serial passage through mice and has been used for human immunization. A second yellow fever virus strain, after many transfers through tissue cultures, became sufficiently attenuated for human inoculation and is in wide use at present.

Injection of *killed microorganisms* is the most widely used means of stimulating active immunity. Much larger numbers of killed cells may be administered than is possible with viable organisms. Phenol, tricresol, formalin, acetone, and Merthiolate are widely employed killing agents. Heat is sometimes used but is likely to diminish the immunizing power of a bacterial suspension, even though the temperature is kept at the minimum consistent with sterilization (e.g., 56° C. for 1 hour). Chemical disinfectants must be carefully selected, because some chemicals combine with bacterial proteins to form complexes having different specificity from that of the living cells. Killed suspensions are always thoroughly tested for sterility before release for human use.

Chemical extraction has been employed in attempts to secure immunizing substances from the cells of dysentery, typhoid, and other bacteria. Some of these, such as the "somatic antigens" (see Chapter 5) or lipopolysaccharide complexes and the typhoid "Vi antigen," have given indication of considerable effectiveness.

Bacterial exotoxins are potent immunizing agents. The immunity produced is generally strong and relatively permanent. Sublethal amounts of unmodified toxins were originally employed but were soon found impractical because of their toxicity and the number of injections necessary for satisfactory immunization. These difficulties were largely overcome by combining antitoxin produced in horses with the toxin in such proportions that the toxin was nearly neutralized. The toxin was apparently released slowly within the body and stimulated active antibody formation over a considerable period. Toxin-antitoxin was a highly successful immunizing agent and is still employed, particularly to protect adults against diphtheria.

Heat or formaldehyde converts most toxins into nontoxic but antigenic *toxoids*. Toxoids are so harmless that comparatively large doses may be administered with no risk of tissue damage. They are commonly used in immunization of children against diphtheria and tetanus. Toxoid is employed in the natural fluid form or precipitated by alum. Alum-precipitated immunizing substances are released slowly from the subcutaneous tissues and thereby accomplish about the same results as multiple injections of unprecipitated materials.

Passive Immunity

Passive immunity is that form of immunity produced in an individual by antibodies derived from another individual, either by natural transfer or by injection. It is only temporary, lasting a few weeks to a few months, whereas active immunity is ordinarily more durable.

The first months of an animal's life are relatively free from certain infectious diseases. This is attributed to antibody acquired from the mother, either by passage through the placenta or by the first milk ingested after birth (colostrum). Antibody passage through the placenta occurs in animals such as man, in which a single layer of cells separates the maternal and fetal circulations. In ruminants, on the other hand, four layers of cells separate the two circulatory systems and prevent antibody from passing into the fetal blood. These animals secrete antibodies in the colostrum, which the young ingest within a few hours after birth, the antibodies being absorbed through the wall of the digestive tract. An animal soon loses the immunity it possessed at birth. This phenomenon is an interesting natural mechanism, because very young animals usually possess lower ability to produce antibody than do more mature animals.

Artificial passive immunization is accomplished by injection of antibodies produced actively in other individuals, either of the same or of other species. The widest use of artificial passive immunization is in the prevention of diphtheria, tetanus, gas gangrene, and botulism. Antitoxin is manufactured by inoculation of animals, often horses, with the respective toxins or toxoids. Serum of the immunized animals contains the antitoxins; it is often purified by chemical fractionation to get rid of extraneous, nonantibody proteins and other substances that might cause untoward reactions. Small prophylactic doses of antitoxin administered promptly to exposed persons prevent or modify the course of disease. The temporary protection afforded is usually fortified by active immunization as soon as possible. Antitoxins are also administered in larger doses to individuals with active cases of disease and, if given sufficiently early, bring about dramatically rapid recovery.

Passive protection is sometimes provided by transfusion of blood from a convalescent individual or by introduction of human immune globulin. This processed material, first prepared on a large scale during World War II, is one of the protein fractions obtained from blood and contains antibodies protective against measles, infectious hepatitis, poliomyelitis, and probably other diseases.

Antibacterial sera for treatment of pneumococcal pneumonia and cerebrospinal meningitis were formerly employed to help combat infection early in the disease, before the individual's antibody-producing mechanism had time to manufacture antibody. These antisera were also prepared in horses or other animals. Antipneumococcal serum was credited with reducing pneumonia mortality as much as 50 per cent. Antibacterial sera have now been superseded by sulfonamides and antibiotics.

Adoptive Immunity

Adoptive immunity is an immune state produced by the transfer of antigen-sensitive (primed) lymphocytes from an actively immunized donor to a nonimmune recipient. Primed lymphocytes are capable of reacting directly and specifically with antigen in a cell-mediated immunity response, or they may be stimulated to transform into antibody-producing plasma cells. They are derived from lymph nodes, bone marrow, and, to a lesser extent, from the spleen.

Adoptive immunization is an experimental procedure of considerable theoretic interest because of its bearing on the site and mechanism of antibody production and the roles of antibody and cells in immunity. It is not a practical means of inducing antimicrobial protection, but conceivably some immunologic change could follow bone marrow transplants in patients who have been accidentally exposed to lethal doses of radiation, in leukemia patients treated by whole-body irradiation, and in infants born without a thymus. In all these cases, there is a danger of homologous disease caused by the transplanted lymphoid cells, unless they are carefully matched genetically with cells of the recipient.

Additional Sources of Information

Alexander, J. W., and R. A. Good: Immunobiology for Surgeons. 1970. Philadelphia, W. B. Saunders Company.

Burnet, F. M.: Cellular Immunology. 1969. Carlton, Vic., Australia, Melbourne University Press.

Burnet, F. M.: Immunological Surveillance. 1970. Oxford, Pergamon Press.

Good, R. A., and D. W. Fisher (Eds.): Immunobiology. 1971. Stamford, Conn., Sinauer Associates, Inc.

Nossal, G. J. V., and G. L. Ada: Antigens, Lymphoid Cells, and the Immune Response. 1971. New York, Academic Press, Inc.

Roitt, I.: Essential Immunology. 1971. Oxford, Blackwell Scientific Publications.

Weigle, W. O.: Immunological unresponsiveness. In Dixon, F. J., and H. G. Kunkel (Eds.): Advances in Immunology, vol. 16, pp. 61–122. 1973. New York, Academic Press, Inc.

Weiss, L.: The Cells and Tissues of the Immune System. 1972. Englewood Cliffs, N.J. Prentice-Hall, Inc.

CHAPTER TWO

THE IMMUNE REACTIONS

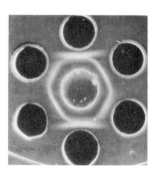

The normal function of antibodies and immunologically active cells is to assist in maintaining the integrity of body cells and tissues. Inasmuch as some of their surveillance activities are directed toward body components that are out of control, they are able to combat a variety of potentially harmful exogenous and endogenous agents, both infectious and noninfectious. Their presence can be detected and their concentrations can be assayed by numerous methods, some in vitro and some in vivo. The nature of the detection or assay procedure varies according to the nature of the antigen and the type of immunologic response under study.

THE REAGENTS IN IMMUNE REACTIONS

Antigens

An *antigen* is a substance that elicits a specific immune response when introduced into the tissues of an animal. The response may consist of antibody production, cell-mediated immunity, or immunologic tolerance.

Ordinarily, antigens are introduced *parenterally*—that is, by some route other than the alimentary tract. Otherwise, the antigen might be digested and lose its antigenicity before reaching the antibody-producing tissues. There is evidence that some antigenic materials pass undigested through the mucous membranes of certain individuals. Hypersensitivity to these substances often ensues, as in hay fever, food allergies, and similar disorders. The most effective antigenic stimuli, however, are obtained by injection into the skin or the underlying tissues, the body cavities, or the bloodstream, or by actual infection.

Most antigens are foreign to the animal in which they elicit an immune response; i.e., they are "nonself" substances. However, "self" components may be antigenic under some circumstances, or they may become antigenic as a result of changes (often minor) in composition or structure resulting from somatic mutation or chemical or physical agents that affect the host.

It is also characteristic of antigens that they can usually react with the antibodies or specifically sensitized cells they have called forth in some observable way. The word *antigenicity* is usually employed to indicate the ability of a substance to stimulate an immune response. The word *immunogenicity* is also used, particularly with reference to the development of specific protection against infectious disease. There is no single word to denote the ability of an antigen to react with antibody or sensitized cell. The term *in vitro antigenicity* may be employed for this purpose when the reaction has a visible result, such as formation of a precipitate, and *combining power* when the reaction can be detected only indirectly.

28

Haptens

A *hapten* is a simple chemical or a portion of an antigen that cannot induce an immune response, but that can react demonstrably and specifically with an appropriate antibody or cell. For example, the carbohydrate-like components of certain bacteria cannot by themselves stimulate antibody formation, but they yield a precipitate when mixed with antibodies produced against the whole organism. Haptens are also sometimes called *partial antigens* because they perform only one of the functions of an antigen.

Antibodies

An *antibody* is a modified blood globulin—an immunoglobulin—usually formed in response to an antigenic stimulus; it is capable of combining specifically with the homologous (i.e., corresponding) antigen. The word "specifically" implies that the antibody can react only with the substance that engendered its production. This is actually an oversimplification, because specificity depends upon the physicochemical structure of small surface regions of the reacting molecules or cells, called *determinant* or *receptor* sites, not upon their source. The same structure, or very similar structures, may be found in widely divergent forms of life; for example, human red blood cells of group A contain an antigen with a structure that appears to be identical to that of a substance in hog gastric mucin, horse saliva, pneumococci, and various plants. Antibody for the blood cell substance reacts equally well with the antigen from the various sources mentioned.

Cellular Immunity Effector Cells

Cellular immunity is a function of thymus-derived small lymphocytes that react specifically with antigen and directly or indirectly cause tissue damage; for example, they are responsible for graft rejection, delayed hypersensitivity, and tuberculin-type reactions, and are also important in immunity against infections caused by intracellular parasites, such as viruses and some bacteria. Their specificity depends upon receptor sites on their outer membranes analogous to the determinant sites of antibodies and, according to some investigators, composed of immunoglobulin. However, whereas an antibody determinant site is directed toward a small region equivalent in size to 3 to 5 amino acid residues, like a hapten, that of a lymphocyte active in cellular immunity is directed toward a larger site that serves as a carrier for the antibody-reactive or haptenic portion of an antigen.

These cells can apparently exert their effects in either of two ways (or perhaps there are two different kinds of cells): (a) by some unknown, directly cytotoxic mechanism, or (b) through the mediation of the low molecular weight substances, *lymphokines*, previously mentioned (page 18).

LABORATORY PRODUCTION OF ANTISERA AND CELLULAR IMMUNITY EFFECTOR CELLS

Antisera (i.e., sera containing antibodies) for experimental purposes are usually produced in laboratory animals, occasionally in humans. Rabbits are most often employed because they are inexpensive and easy to maintain, inject, and bleed. Guinea pigs are also used, as are chickens, rats, and mice to a lesser extent. Small animals possess the disadvantage that they yield little serum. Large animals such as horses, sheep, goats, and cattle are expensive but provide large quantities of serum. They are employed in the commercial production of antitoxins and antibacterial sera for prophylactic or therapeutic use.

Injections are usually made by the intravenous, intraperitoneal, or subcutaneous route. Material enters the bloodstream slowly from a subcutaneous depot but quite rapidly from the peritoneal cavity. Often a series of injections is given, varying from daily to weekly, the sizes of the doses depending upon the nature of the antigen. Highly toxic materials are given cautiously, beginning with small amounts that are increased gradually. The first injection of a tetanus culture filtrate into a rabbit might be 0.1 milliliter of 1:1000 dilution. Fairly large amounts of nontoxic agents may be given: 1.0 milliliter of 1 per cent protein solution or foreign blood serum diluted 1:5.

Periodic trial bleedings of a few milliliters permit titration of the antibody content of the serum. Final bleeding is performed when sufficient antibody has been produced, usually 3 to 5 days after the last injection. The serum is separated from the clotted blood, centrifuged if necessary until clear, and stored at a low temperature. Preservatives, such as phenol, tricresol, sodium azide, and Merthiolate, are customarily added to prevent growth of contaminants, especially if the bottle is to be entered frequently. Serum is often frozen and stored at $-20°$ C. Inasmuch as repeated freezing and thawing are somewhat deleterious to antibody, the entire quantity of antiserum is usually divided into smaller portions and frozen separately.

Parenteral injection of an organism into an animal stimulates production of antibodies in equal or greater concentration than is obtained in a naturally infected animal. The antibodies in a surviving susceptible animal protect against both natural infection and experimental injection; antibodies formed in an inoculated nonsusceptible animal protect only against parenteral injection of the organism. Mice, for example, are naturally susceptible to *Salmonella typhimurium,* and when immunized against this organism they develop antibodies that will protect against slight natural or parenteral exposure. On the other hand, mice and rabbits injected with *S. typhosa* acquire immunity only against parenteral inoculation of the same organism, because these species are not susceptible to typhoid fever.

Lymphocytes reactive in cellular immunity and other cell-mediated reactions are secured experimentally from the lymph nodes, spleen, thymus, peritoneal exudate, thoracic duct lymph, and blood of animals injected with protein suspended in Freund's complete adjuvant (a water-in-oil emulsion of the antigen plus killed mycobacteria) or with living B.C.G. *(Bacille Calmette-Guérin,* an attenuated bovine strain of *Mycobacterium tuberculosis* used to immunize man against tuberculosis). They are also formed in humans and animals infected naturally with various agents.

Organs and tissues are minced in a tissue culture medium and passed through nylon cloth or a fine stainless steel screen to suspend the cells individually. Peritoneal exudate is prepared by injecting the animal intraperitoneally with paraffin oil to induce an accumulation of cells, sacrificing after 3 to 5 days, and washing out the peritoneal cavity with tissue culture medium. Thoracic duct lymph is centrifuged lightly to sediment the cells, which consist largely of lymphocytes. The lymphocytes in blood may be concentrated by allowing defibrinated or heparinized blood to stand until the cells have settled, when they are found in the buffy coat, a grayish layer at the top of the sedimented red cells.

Macrophages can be removed from any of these suspensions by utilizing their ability to adhere to glass or plastic—the supernatant liquid after an hour contains nonadherent cells, largely lymphocytes. Phagocytic cells may also be removed from suspensions by adding carbonyl iron powder, mixing gently, and incubating a short time, after which excess iron and the iron-containing cells are collected with a magnet.

DEMONSTRATION OF ANTIBODIES

The techniques by which reactions between antigens and antibodies are studied in the laboratory constitute the methods of *serology* ("the study of sera"). Serology is a tool in the investigation of immunity. However, because of the ability of antibodies to react demonstrably with substances bearing specific chemical configurations, serology is also a tool in chemistry, biochemistry, physiology, taxonomy, and other fields. There are five or six major methods of demonstrating the reaction between an antibody and its antigen in vitro, and even more ways in which antigen-antibody reaction becomes apparent within the body.

Before discussing the various serologic reactions, it will help to describe a few basic ideas about the principal reagents and their mode of union. It is well established that the reactive or determinant site of an antigen may be a relatively simple structure at the surface of the molecule: for example, a substituted benzene ring with four or five adjacent amino acids in a protein or sugar molecules in a polysaccharide. This structure is repeated several times over the surface of the antigen. An antibody molecule capable of reacting with this antigen possesses a surface determinant site with a structural configuration complementary to that of the antigen, so the two can fit together as a key fits a lock. A normal antibody molecule has at least two such surface areas. During antigen-antibody reaction the two kinds of molecules join at their determinant sites, gradually forming a three-dimensional network or lattice in which antigen and antibody alternate.

An ideal antibody contains determinant sites whose structures conform closely to those of the antigenic determinant (haptenic) sites. When they interact, oppositely charged ionic groups and other attractive groups of the hapten and the antibody have close access to one another, and high affinity bonds form and hold the two molecules firmly together. However, many antibody molecules are not ideal. Kinetic studies with antibodies against antigens containing simple haptens, such as *p*-azobenzoate, demonstrate the formation of bonds with all grades of affinity from high to low. It must therefore be concluded that antibody determinant sites are heterogeneous in structure, varying in the extent to which they conform to the antigen haptenic sites. Figure 2–1 illustrates this situation in observations by Kitagawa et al. with the *p*-azobenzoate hapten.

Primary Antigen-Antibody Reactions

A primary antigen-antibody reaction occurs when the structure of an antibody determinant site conforms closely enough to that of an antigen so that union occurs:

$$Ag + Ab \rightarrow AgAb$$

Figure 2–1. Bottom center, Van der Waal's outline of the *p*-azobenzoate hapten with a small portion of the surface of the protein to which it is coupled. *A* to *G,* Outlines of combining sites of antibodies that could react with corresponding portions of the hapten. (From Kitagawa et al., 1965. J. Immunol., 95:455. Copyright 1965, The Williams and Wilkins Company, Baltimore.)

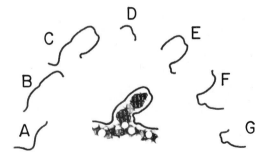

This reaction is not detected in the usual serologic procedures, because a simple complex containing only one antigen molecule and one antibody molecule is soluble. The fact that union has occurred can be shown only by indirect means and so far with only certain antigens.

ANTIGEN-BINDING CAPACITY

Using bovine serum albumin (BSA) as antigen, Farr capitalized upon the fact that albumins do not precipitate when their solutions are half-saturated with $(NH_4)_2SO_4$, whereas antibodies, being globulins, do. He coupled a radioactive tracer, ^{131}I, to BSA to provide a highly sensitive label (this treatment does not alter the reactivity of BSA with its antibody), and then mixed a large excess of ^{131}I-BSA with anti-BSA. There was no visible result. He then added $(NH_4)_2SO_4$ to one-half saturation and obtained a precipitate. This was washed to remove uncombined [131]I. The precipitate was found to contain radioactive iodine. Inasmuch as ^{131}I had been introduced only as ^{131}I-BSA, which is soluble in the $(NH_4)_2SO_4$, the presence of ^{131}I in the precipitate indicated that ^{131}I-BSA had combined with anti-BSA. From the amount of ^{131}I determined, the antigen-binding capacity of the antibody can readily be calculated.

IMMUNOFLUORESCENCE

The primary reaction between antibody and a particulate antigen can be demonstrated by use of fluorescent antibodies. Antibody molecules can be chemically combined with fluorescent dyes, such as fluorescein and rhodamine, without seriously interfering with their antibody function. They thus become microscopically observable labels, which can be used to detect the presence and location of specific antigenic fractions of cells when examined by ultraviolet microscopy. Simple union of the antigenic site with homologous antibody renders the antigen fluorescent (see Figure 2–2).

Secondary Antigen-Antibody Reactions

The visible result of an in vitro antigen-antibody reaction depends on the nature of the antigen (soluble or particulate) and the antibody, the presence of other blood

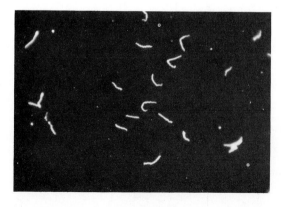

Figure 2–2. Fluorescence of syphilis spirochetes treated with serum of a syphilitic patient followed by fluorescent antihuman IgG. This is an indirect fluorescent antibody test. (From C. E. Miller, M.D., Fullerton, California, and the Scope® Publications, The Upjohn Company, Kalamazoo, Michigan.)

constituents (e.g., phagocytic cells, complement), the physical conditions, and other factors. The primary reaction—union of antigen and antibody—is rapid, but secondary reactions may require hours or even days to go to completion.

PRECIPITATION

Precipitation is the final visible result of a serologic reaction between a soluble antigen and its antiserum. Solutions of proteins or certain polysaccharides constitute the test antigens in precipitation tests with appropriate antisera. Antigens for these tests are derived from all forms of life: microorganisms, plants, and animals.

When a suitable amount of a protein such as egg albumin is mixed with 1 ml. of rabbit anti-egg albumin serum and incubated at 37° C., the mixture becomes cloudy within a few minutes, then flocculent, and a precipitate settles within an hour or two. If a series of mixtures is prepared with greater and lesser amounts of egg albumin combined with 1 ml. of antiserum, the amounts of precipitate will decrease progressively toward each end of the series, and some mixtures will contain little or no precipitate (see Table 2–1). Although largest precipitates are obtained by using undiluted antiserum, its cost may necessitate a twofold to fivefold dilution of the serum. Such a procedure should never be employed with weak antisera, as in attempts to determine normal antibodies.

The foregoing procedure can be made quantitative by analyzing the precipitate, usually by determining some distinctive element or elements in either the antigen, the antibody, or both. Simple nitrogen determinations by micro-Kjeldahl digestion of the washed precipitate and titration or colorimetric assay of the ammonia formed indicates the total amount of protein precipitated. The amount of antibody in the antiserum can be estimated by subtracting the amount of antigen in the mixture with the largest precipitate from the total amount of the precipitate, because this precipitate contains all or nearly all the antigen and antibody in the mixture. Mixtures prepared with less antigen yield precipitates containing less than the total available antibody, because there is insufficient antigen to form a complete, three-dimensional lattice; conversely, mixtures prepared with more than optimal antigen yield precipitates containing less than the total available antigen, because there is too little antibody to form a complete lattice. This is the *zone phenomenon;* it will be discussed further in Chapter 6.

Valuable antisera can be conserved and the precipitation reaction made very sensitive by use of the ring or interfacial test. A layer of antigen dilution is carefully placed over the antiserum in a very small test tube or a capillary tube. A fine line of

Table 2–1. Precipitation in Mixtures of Egg Albumin and Rabbit Anti-Egg Albumin Serum

Egg albumin (mg.)	0.0625	0.1250	0.2500	0.5000	1.0000	2.0000
Anti-egg albumin serum (undiluted)	1 ml.	1 ml.	1 ml.	1 ml.	1 ml.	1 ml.
Precipitation:						
Visual inspection*	+	+ +	+ + +	+ + + +	+ + +	±
Protein by analysis (mg.)†	1.13	1.94	3.32	5.25	3.26	0.56

*A heavy precipitate with clear supernatant liquid is graded + + + +, smaller precipitates are graded + + +, + +, etc.

†Nitrogen determined by micro-Kjeldahl method, multiplied by the factor 6.25.

precipitate appears at the interface within a few minutes and gradually increases in amount. If a series of dilutions of the antigen is used, this becomes a method for estimating the concentration of the antigen solution. It is employed in medicolegal work in the analysis of blood stains and other protein-containing materials.

The zone phenomenon illustrated in Table 2–1 indicates a characteristic of serologic precipitation that limits usefulness of the reaction: the fact that the reagents must be *in proper proportions* in order to obtain a visible result. Simple mixture of antigen and antibody in an unfavorable ratio produces no precipitate. In the ring test, diffusion of the reacting substances yields a point of optimal ratio, at which precipitation occurs. Addition of agar to one or both reagents retards the rate of diffusion (Oudin and Ouchterlony tests) and permits formation of multiple distinct lines of precipitate if several antigenic substances and their antibodies are present (see Figure 2–3). The gel diffusion technique is useful in studying the serologic identity of proteins from various sources and in determining the minimum number of antigenic substances in natural mixtures such as animal serum and tissue extracts.

AGGLUTINATION

Agglutination is the phenomenon observed when a particulate antigen, such as a saline suspension of bacteria or erythrocytes, is mixed with a small amount of homologous antiserum. The cells clump and gradually settle to the bottom of the fluid. Flocculent masses, compact granules, or thin sheets form in test tube mixtures and settle to the bottom, from which they may be dislodged by gentle agitation. In some instances microscopic examination reveals that the particles of antigen behave as though they are sticky and cling tenaciously together, whereas in other instances the clumps look similar but can be broken up by shaking.

Quantitative analyses to determine the agglutinating antibody content of an antiserum can be made by the micro-Kjeldahl procedure, as in precipitation, but for routine diagnostic and experimental work the antibody *titer* is determined by the "extinction dilution" method. Dilutions (1:40, 1:80, 1:160, etc.) of the serum are prepared in saline (0.85 per cent NaCl), and a suspension of the appropriate antigen is added. The test tubes are incubated in a waterbath at a suitable temperature (e.g., 37° C., 55° C.), and agglutination is read after a period determined by the nature of the antigen. A tube in which all cells have agglutinated is graded ++++. Absence of agglutination is designated −, and intermediate degrees of agglutination are indicated +, ++, or +++.

The results of a typical test might appear as recorded in Table 2–2. The titer of an antiserum is the reciprocal of the last dilution showing definite agglutination (+), so the

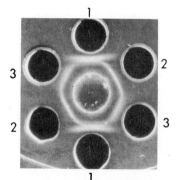

Figure 2–3. Ouchterlony gel diffusion precipitin test. Rabbit anti-*M. tuberculosis* serum in the center well tested against crude tuberculoprotein (1) and two purified fractions from tuberculoprotein (2, 3). (From Koga and Pearson, 1973. J. Immunol., 111:599. Copyright 1973, The Williams and Wilkins Company, Baltimore.)

Table 2–2. Results of an Agglutination Experiment

Antibacterial Serum Dilutions									Control (Saline)
1:40	1:80	1:160	1:320	1:640	1:1280	1:2560	1:5120	1:10240	
++++*	++++	++++	++++	++++	++++	+++	+	−	−

     *++++ = complete agglutination (all cells clumped)
          − = no agglutination

titer illustrated is 5120. The control tube, containing saline instead of antiserum dilution, is necessary because some cells clump spontaneously in physiologic saline.

The agglutination test is relatively easy to perform and is one of the most frequently employed diagnostic reactions. In its various modifications it is used to detect and assay antibodies in patients' sera, to identify bacteria, to determine blood groups and types, and for other purposes.

COMPLEMENT REACTIONS

Cytolysis. The reaction between certain cellular antigens and their antibodies in the presence of *complement* is followed by dissolution of the antigen. This phenomenon is known as *cytolysis. Bacteriolysis* and *hemolysis* are specific terms applied to the dissolving of bacteria and erythrocytes, respectively. The theoretic aspects of this reaction have been determined principally by study of hemolysis, in which a positive result is readily detected by macroscopic inspection.

Anti-erythrocyte serum is prepared by inoculating rabbits or other animals with foreign blood cells. The test antigen employed to demonstrate hemolysis is a saline suspension of erythrocytes washed several times with saline to remove normal serum proteins. Erythrocytes and complement (fresh guinea pig serum) are added to serial dilutions of antiserum. Hemolysis takes place within 15 to 60 minutes at 37° C. and is shown by complete laking of the cells, leaving a sparkling, clear, red solution. Unhemolyzed cells settle to the bottom of the tubes.

Bacteriolysis can best be demonstrated with *Salmonella typhosa, Vibrio cholerae,* and a few other gram-negative bacteria. Dissolution of the cells is sometimes macroscopically evident and can also be observed in stained preparations examined with the microscope in comparison with suitable controls.

Complement Fixation. Complement is "fixed" by specific precipitates. Egg albumin and anti-egg albumin serum, although reacting in proportions that do not yield a trace of precipitate, will nevertheless combine with complement to form a three-component complex (Figure 2–4). The complement is no longer able to react with other

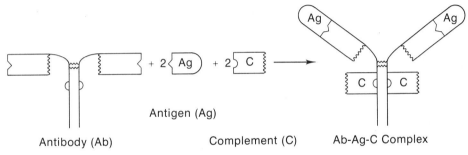

Antigen (Ag)

Antibody (Ab)   Complement (C)   Ab-Ag-C Complex

Figure 2–4. Diagrammatic representation of the formation of a complex of antibody, antigen, and complement. Only after union with antigen has caused change in shape of the antibody molecule can the latter combine with complement.

antigen-antibody systems subsequently added, such as red blood cells "sensitized" by contact with their homologous antibody (hemolysin). In the absence of antibody that can combine with the test antigen, egg albumin, complement hemolyzes the sensitized red cells.

An experiment illustrating *complement fixation* is shown in Table 2–3. Lack of hemolysis in mixtures containing low dilutions of egg albumin showed that no complement remained uncombined, whereas complete hemolysis in the mixture containing 1:1,000,000 egg albumin indicated insufficient antigen to fix complement in the presence of anti-egg albumin serum. The free complement lysed the erythrocytes sensitized by anti-erythrocyte serum, as also occurred in the saline control tube. The complement fixation titer of the anti-egg albumin is approximately 100,000, because this dilution of antigen with its antibody partially inhibited hemolysis.

The complement fixation test is exceedingly sensitive and can be used to detect traces of either antigen or antibody, depending upon the manner of setting up the test. It is the basis for the Wassermann test for syphilis, in which syphilis "antibody" or *reagin* is the unknown quantity.

Bactericidal Action and Immobilization.   The bactericidal action of antibodies in an antiserum is estimated by inactivating the normal complement in the serum at 56° C. for 30 minutes and then adding a known amount of guinea pig complement and a light suspension of the test organism. Plate counts of the surviving bacteria, when compared with suitable controls lacking the antiserum, indicate the bactericidal effectiveness of the antibodies. These experiments are often criticized because agglutination may be the factor that reduces the bacterial count, inasmuch as a clump of cells will produce only a single colony.

Certain motile organisms such as paramecia, trypanosomes, and *Treponema pallidum* lose their motility when incubated with their respective antibodies and complement. The *Treponema pallidum* immobilization (TPI) test was discovered in 1949 and, because of its accuracy, became established as a standard with which to compare other serologic tests for the diagnosis of syphilis. A suspension of the syphilis organisms prepared from infected rabbit testes is mixed with dilutions of the patient's serum and guinea pig complement. After anaerobic incubation at 35° C. for 18 hours, the percentage of immobilization is determined by darkfield microscopic examination. The immobilization titer is represented by the serum dilution that immobilizes 50 per cent of the treponemes. The test is more difficult than appears from this brief description, because *T. pallidum* is one of the most fastidious bacteria and can be kept alive in

Table 2–3.   Complement Fixation By a Soluble Antigen and Its Antibody

Egg albumin (0.1 ml.) Anti-egg albumin	1:100	1:1000	1:10,000	1:100,000	1:1,000,000	Saline
serum (ml. 1:5)	0.1	0.1	0.1	0.1	0.1	0.1
Complement (ml. 1:25)	0.1	0.1	0.1	0.1	0.1	0.1
Incubation at 37° C. for 30 minutes						
Anti-erythrocyte serum (ml. 1:500)	0.1	0.1	0.1	0.1	0.1	0.1
Erythrocytes (ml. 2%)	0.1	0.1	0.1	0.1	0.1	0.1
Incubation at 37° C. for 30 minutes						
Results: Hemolysis	–	–	–	+++	++++	++++
Complement fixation	++++	++++	++++	+	–	–

vitro only by exceedingly careful technique and constant attention to details. The test is used chiefly for reference rather than as a routine diagnostic procedure.

Immune Adherence. Immune adherence, sometimes called serologic adhesion, is the phenomenon of adhesion of microorganisms to certain nonphagocytic cells or "indicator particles," in the presence of homologous antimicrobial serum and complement. Dilutions of the antiserum are mixed with a constant amount of the microbial suspension and incubated 10 minutes at 37° C. Complement is added to each tube, followed by 30 minutes of incubation at 37° C. A suspension of the indicator cells or particles is then added, and after final incubation for 10 minutes the tubes are centrifuged sufficiently to sediment the particles and any microorganisms attached to them. Unattached organisms in the supernatant liquid are counted by direct microscopic examination. The percentage adherence is calculated by comparison with suitable controls, and the serum dilution that produces 50 per cent adherence is determined.

Cells or particles that give positive results include primate erythrocytes, yeast, bacteria, platelets, and leukocytes. The specific receptor site is assumed to be protein because it is inactivated by the proteolytic enzymes trypsin, chymotrypsin, and papain. A variety of incubation conditions have been used, as has direct microscopic examination of the uncentrifuged cells rather than enumeration of the unattached organisms. Immune adherence has been demonstrated with *T. pallidum, Diplococcus pneumoniae, S. typhosa, Staphylococcus aureus,* Leptospira, trypanosomes, and other organisms. Linscott and Boak found the test so sensitive that antibodies against Leptospira could be detected in rabbits within 40 hours after the first injection of an immunizing antigen.

Complement-Mediated Cytotoxicity. Cytotoxic reactions are the result of immunologic activity that damages tissue cells. The immunologic mechanism may be humoral or cell-mediated. Discussion of the latter will be deferred (see page 45).

Cell injury attributed to the humoral system begins with primary action of antibody on the cell membrane. Complement joins the antigen-antibody complex; phospholipase and other enzymes are produced or activated and damage the membrane, cytoplasmic matrix, mitochondria, and endoplasmic reticulum. There is first a rapid loss of intracellular potassium ions, amino acids, and ribonucleotides, with slower loss of protein and RNA. The cell membrane becomes permeable to sodium ions, which can enter from outside. "Holes" detectable by electron microscopy appear and permit exchange of cations and small molecules between the cell and the medium. The osmotic pressure of the cell increases, and rapid entrance of water stretches the membrane and the "holes" so much that macromolecules escape from the cell.

Cytotoxicity is studied in vivo by injecting antisera against tissues or organs into experimental animals, and in vitro by adding such antisera to tissue cultures. It is also investigated in vivo by injecting tissues or tissue extracts or components in an attempt to induce active anti-organ immunity.

Direct cytotoxicity can be demonstrated in vivo with antisera produced by injecting one animal species with blood cells or platelets of another species. When the antisera are injected into the species that donated the cells or platelets, various kinds of damage become apparent. Hemolysis of the circulating erythrocytes produces progressive anemia and death, destruction of the leukocytes permits bacterial invasion and fatal infection, and injury to the platelets disturbs the blood clotting mechanism.

It is obvious in the above example that the antibodies (anti-erythrocyte, anti-leukocyte, etc.) first combined with the corresponding antigenic cells and then damaged them directly. However, antibody localization is not necessarily followed by direct toxicity. *Indirect cytotoxicity* is shown by injecting rats with antiserum prepared by immunizing ducks with rat kidney. The duck anti-kidney antibodies localize within a few minutes in the vascular bed of the rat kidneys, as shown by use of radioactive tracers attached to the antibodies, but cytotoxicity and nephritis do not appear until a week later. The rat forms antibody to the injected duck proteins, and this antibody combines with the duck antibody attached to the kidney and damages the kidney cells, probably with the help of complement.

PHAGOCYTOSIS

Phagocytosis of bacteria is greatly accelerated by homologous antibacterial antibody. This can be demonstrated in vitro with *S. aureus*. Equal parts of whole blood, bacterial suspension, and antiserum are mixed and incubated at 37° C. for 30 minutes. A stained smear is prepared, and the average number of bacteria ingested by the polymorphonuclear leukocytes is determined. A similar preparation in which normal serum is substituted for antiserum indicates the "normal" phagocytosis by the leukocytes. The ratio obtained by dividing the number of bacteria ingested in the presence of antiserum by the number ingested in the presence of normal serum is called the *opsonic index*. This is a measure of antibody involved in phagocytosis.

Antibody appears to assist phagocytosis by altering the surface properties of the bacteria and by counteracting microbial products that paralyze or destroy leukocytes. The capsules of pneumococci and various other organisms resist phagocytosis except when the capsule has combined with antibody. *S. aureus* produces a potent leukocidin, which is antigenic and is neutralized by its antibody.

Lupus Erythematosus Phenomenon. Lupus erythematosus is a disease of connective tissue, occurring primarily in young females and having a strong hereditary tendency. Many organ systems of the body may be involved, including skin, blood-forming organs, joints, serous surfaces, and especially the kidneys, damage to which provides the greatest clinical problem. From a laboratory technician's standpoint, the most distinctive feature of the disease is formation of the lupus erythematosus (L.E.) cell in vitro when serum of a patient reacts with leukocytes. The nucleus of a polymorphonuclear neutrophile or a lymphocyte lyses first, becoming homogeneous and then swelling to as much as three or four times its normal size. It is then partially or completely extruded and is ingested by a normal polymorphonuclear leukocyte. The latter cell, with the lysed nucleus as an inclusion body, is an L.E. cell.

The fact that normal sera will not induce L.E. cell formation indicates that patients' sera contain a specific factor responsible for the phenomenon. This substance has been eluted from L.E. cells and found to be a γ-globulin with properties similar to those of antibodies. The isolated γ-globulin, when added to normal serum, promotes L.E. cell formation.

The L.E. factor is an antinuclear antibody. Tissue culture experiments have shown that in weak sera it reacts with the nuclear membrane and in stronger sera with the chromosomes as well. It has an affinity for intact DNA portions of the nucleoprotein. The L.E. factor behaves like an opsonizing antibody. Its specificity for nuclear matter is shown by the fact that cytoplasmic fragments are not phagocytized. There is strong indication that lupus sera contain a "family" of related antibodies with somewhat different properties and capabilities: precipitation of DNA, complement fixation with DNA, agglutination of RBC coated with DNA; moreover, they may react only with intact nuclei, with the nucleoprotein fraction, or with DNA and/or histone isolated from nuclei.

NEUTRALIZATION OF TOXINS

Exotoxins are neutralized by very small amounts of homologous antibodies (antitoxins). Neutralization is tested by inoculation of experimental animals, usually guinea pigs or mice. The potency of an antitoxic serum is assayed by comparison with a standard antitoxin. Antitoxin is very stable when stored under proper conditions, whereas most toxins are unstable and rapidly lose their toxicity. It is therefore necessary to titrate a batch of toxin with reference to antitoxin of known strength and then, using this "standardized" toxin, measure the protective power of the "unknown" antitoxin.

Various amounts of a toxin are mixed with a constant amount of standard antitoxin, incubated a short time to allow the reagents to combine, and injected. The end point of this titration is represented by death within a specified time interval or by some other response (e.g., skin necrosis) in a certain proportion (often 50 per cent or 100 per cent) of the animals inoculated with a given dose. Using this dose of toxin, mixtures with various amounts of the serum to be tested are prepared and injected, and the animals are observed as before. The dose of serum that produces the same end point as was obtained in the first titration contains the same number of protective "units" as the standard antitoxin.

PROTECTION TESTS

Protective antibodies are detected and titrated by "challenging" actively or passively immunized animals with multiple lethal doses of the pathogenic agent. Immune animals withstand a greater challenge dose than normal animals. The test is made more or less quantitative by varying the dosage of the immunizing agent or of the challenge; the virulence of the pathogenic agent is determined by simultaneous tests in nonimmune animals.

The protective power of anti-typhoid serum may be assayed by injecting groups of mice intraperitoneally with a constant amount (e.g., 0.5 ml.) of serum and challenging 1 hour later with graded doses of living typhoid bacteria suspended in mucin to enhance their virulence. Deaths are recorded for 6 days and the LD_{50} (lethal dose of organisms for 50 per cent of a group of animals) is then determined. Control animals, which receive normal instead of immune serum, are used to determine the LD_{50} of the culture in unprotected mice. Protection afforded by the antiserum is expressed as the ratio between the two LD_{50} values. For example:

$$\frac{LD_{50} \text{ (antiserum)}}{LD_{50} \text{ (normal serum)}} = \frac{120{,}000 \text{ bacteria}}{400 \text{ bacteria}} = 300$$

The antiserum was sufficiently potent to protect mice against 300 LD_{50} doses of typhoid bacteria.

The term *immunogenicity* is sometimes used to indicate the ability of an antigen to induce specific resistance demonstrable by an in vivo test. The effectiveness of a killed typhoid bacterin may be determined in mice injected intraperitoneally with constant doses of the bacterin. Seven days later they are challenged with graded doses of living typhoid bacteria in mucin, together with unimmunized controls, as described in the preceding paragraph. Similar results may be obtained:

$$\frac{LD_{50} \text{ (bacterin)}}{LD_{50} \text{ (control)}} = \frac{80{,}000 \text{ bacteria}}{400 \text{ bacteria}} = 200$$

This indicates that the bacterin induced formation of immunity that protected against 200 mouse LD_{50} doses of typhoid bacteria.

The methods employed in immunization and challenge must always be stated in describing the immunogenicity of a particular material.

IMMEDIATE-TYPE HYPERSENSITIVITY

Hypersensitivity is the exaggerated, specific responsiveness of an individual toward an antigenic substance, normally resulting from prior experience with the same or a chemically related substance. The essential feature of a hypersensitivity reaction is that the response to the inciting agent (allergen) involves body cells, which are usually damaged as a result.

There are two major kinds of hypersensitivity, the immediate type and the delayed type, formerly distinguished solely according to the speed with which the clinical manifestation followed exposure to the allergen. Later it appeared that immediate-type reactions are attributable to humoral antibodies and that sensitivity can be transferred passively from one individual to another via serum, whereas delayed-type sensitivity is entirely cell-mediated and can be transferred only by means of viable lymphoid cells from lymph nodes, spleen, and various exudates.

Formation of an antigen-antibody complex is the first step in an immediate-type hypersensitivity reaction. The reaction between antigen and antibody occurs on the surface of tissue cells, because (1) the antibody may be a special kind ("reagin") capable of attaching to cells (homocytotropic antibody); or (2) complement, which has some affinity for tissue cells, may participate in the reaction between antigen and antibody. The cells are injured and release several pharmacologically active substances, including histamine, serotonin, and bradykinin, which cause further local or general responses according to the nature and location of the tissues they affect. Muscles stimulated by histamine contract strongly; for example, increased peristaltic activity caused by contraction of the intestinal muscles produces cramps and diarrhea.

Damage to the vascular endothelium causes edema, and injured glandular epithelium secretes excess mucus.

Anaphylaxis. *Anaphylaxis* is one of the most dramatic examples of hypersensitivity. It is conveniently demonstrated in a guinea pig. The animal is given a small injection of a foreign protein, such as egg albumin or horse serum, and about 21 days later is reinjected intravenously with a larger dose of the same antigen. The animal begins to cough within a few moments, gasps for breath, has convulsions, and dies.

This reaction is attributed to an antibody produced in small amounts by the animal within 10 days to 3 weeks after the first injection. Thereafter the animal is hypersensitive to a second or "shocking" injection of the same antigen. A guinea pig can also be sensitized passively by injecting serum from a hypersensitive animal or by giving it a small amount of antiserum from an immunized animal, even of another species.

The antibody that reacts in anaphylaxis is associated with mast cells and circulating basophiles, and when it combines with its antigen the cells are injured, and some or all of the vasoactive substances mentioned above are released from cytoplasmic granules that are a prominent feature of these cells.

The anaphylactic reaction is a very sensitive indicator of antigenicity, particularly in the guinea pig. The ease of sensitization and severity of anaphylaxis differ in other animals. Anaphylactic manifestations vary in part with the distribution of smooth muscle, which contracts strongly in a typical reaction.

Toxic Complex Disease (Arthus Reaction). When a rabbit is given several weekly subcutaneous injections of a harmless protein, such as egg albumin or bovine serum albumin, the third or fourth and subsequent injections incite a local response consisting of redness and swelling. The reactions are increasingly violent, and the sites injected become progressively more hemorrhagic and necrotic. This is the Arthus reaction.

The first injections initiate production of antibody, which circulates in the blood. Antigen injected later reacts with some of the circulating antibody in the local (subcutaneous) site and forms precipitating complexes within the tissue and blood vessels injured in the process of injection. The reaction of complement with the antigen-antibody complexes starts a series of pathologic events, including degranulation of mast cells and agglutination of platelets, both of which release histamine, serotonin, and so forth, with consequent blood vessel dilatation and tissue edema. Leukocytes accumulate and release lysosomal enzymes, which cause inflammation of the vascular system.

The Arthus reaction is rarely encountered in man because it is not common to administer repeated doses of antigenic material into local sites. However, there are a number of situations in which antigen-antibody complexes accumulate, either locally or generally, and produce a pathologic condition. Serum sickness occurs in individuals who, for one reason or another, receive a large injection of foreign protein, such as an antitoxin or anti-lymphocyte serum. Six to ten days after the injection there is fever, with enlarged lymph nodes, painful and swollen joints, a general urticarial rash, and often albumin and/or blood in the urine. These symptoms gradually abate. They are attributed to antibody produced against the foreign serum protein while some of the latter still persists, so that for a time both antigen and antibody are present in considerable amounts. At first, there is an excess of antigen, and soluble complexes of antigen and antibody form throughout the vascular system, but particularly in the kidney glomeruli. These complexes induce most of the features of anaphylaxis, presumably through the release of vasoactive amines. However, the process is much more gradual, so detoxification mechanisms have a greater opportunity to operate; moreover, as antibody production continues, antigen is removed by precipitation and phagocytosis, as well as by metabolism.

The Unitarian Concept of Antibodies

The various antigen-antibody reactions were originally believed to be caused by different kinds of antibodies. The antibodies were named precipitin, agglutinin, lysin, opsonin, and antitoxin, corresponding to the respective phenomena of precipitation, agglutination, lysis, phagocytosis, and neutralization of toxins.

It soon became evident that two or more types of antigen-antibody reaction could be demonstrated with a single antigen and its antiserum. Antitoxins react with homologous exotoxins and neutralize their toxicity for animals; precipitates are also formed when the two reagents are combined in suitable proportions. Similarly, anti-protein serum precipitates the protein and fixes complement. Such observations led Dean in 1917 and Zinsser in 1921 to formulate the *unitarian hypothesis*, which stated that a single antigen induces the formation of only one kind of antibody. The antibody is capable of reacting with or sensitizing the corresponding antigen. A sensitized antigen may participate in various detectable reactions, depending upon the experimental conditions.

The variety of reactions obtainable is illustrated by the behavior of antibody against the specific capsular polysaccharide of pneumococci. This antibody sensitizes the intact cocci so that they agglutinate under appropriate conditions of electrolyte concentration and temperature. Phagocytosis of the sensitized cocci takes place when living leukocytes are present. The capsular polysaccharide itself, removed from the organisms and purified, is precipitated by the antibody, and the combination fixes complement. The polysaccharide can also be used to elicit allergic skin reactions or anaphylactic shock in sensitized animals and to induce active immunity against infection.

The pneumococcal polysaccharide-antibody system is perhaps an unfair illustration of the unitarian concept. Few other bacteria display as striking a parallel between the various demonstrations of antigen-antibody reaction. The hypothesis was useful, however, in directing attention to the essential similarities between the various antigen-antibody reactions.

It has been shown repeatedly since about 1935 that any antiserum usually contains a variety of antibodies for a given antigen. These antibodies possess a common immunologic specificity but have different physical, chemical, and biologic properties. The properties of an antibody are influenced by the nature of the cell in which it is produced. It may be presumed, for example, that a globulin synthesized in a cervical lymph node will differ in some respects from one produced in the spleen: its molecular weight, electric charge, and even its amino acid composition may be different. As will be discussed later (page 114), antibody-producing cells are the progeny of a comparatively small number of B cells. The antibody molecules formed by the progeny of a single B cell (i.e., a clone of antibody-producing cells) are presumably uniform in properties, but they may differ from those formed by other clones of antibody-producing cells. However, the stimulus that incited cell multiplication and antibody production by these various clones is the same—a single antigenic determinant site—so each molecule of antibody formed possesses corresponding determinant sites capable of reacting specifically with the antigen. Serologic specificity is now recognized as the principle that underlies the modern unitarian hypothesis.

DEMONSTRATION OF ANTIGEN-REACTIVE CELLS

Two types of T lymphocytes have been distinguished according to their functions: antigen-reactive cells (ARC) and helper cells. The latter are postulated to assist B cells in the process of antibody formation, and the former participate in cellular or cell-mediated immunity. There is good evidence that they bear an immunoglobulin or an immunoglobulin fragment on their outer membranes that serves as the receptor site to which a specific antigen is attracted. This event may lead to direct destruction of the antigen by some cytotoxic process, or it may stimulate the ARC to release lymphokines. It will be recalled that lymphokines are low molecular weight (20,000 to 80,000), nonantibody proteins whose activities include aggregation of macrophages, inhibition of migration and killing of macrophages, activation of macrophages, chemotactic attraction of mononuclear cells, and induction of lymphocyte mitosis and blast transformation.

Rosette Formation

T lymphocytes sensitized to foreign erythrocytes possess surface receptors with specific affinity for antigenic determinants of the red blood cell membranes. Therefore, when the two kinds of cells are mixed, the red cells attach to and form a rosette around the sensitive lymphocytes (Figure 2–5). It should be noted that, if the lymphocyte is a B cell that is *secreting* antibody, not only will a rosette of attached antigen cells form, but also there may be a cluster of cells surrounding the lymphocyte. Rosette formation can also be demonstrated with T cells sensitized to cells other than erythrocytes, including bacteria, and with T cells sensitized to a foreign protein that can be coated onto isologous erythrocytes.

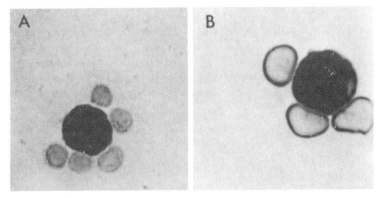

Figure 2–5. Rosettes of guinea pig lymph node cells with *(A)* sensitized sheep RBC and *(B)* rabbit RBC. (From Stadecker et al., 1973. J. Immunol., 111:1834. Copyright 1973, The Williams and Wilkins Company, Baltimore.)

Macrophage Migration Inhibition

The activity of macrophage migration inhibitory factor (MIF) is demonstrated by observing its effect on the migration of macrophages from capillary tubes, which are placed in small tissue culture chambers. In preparations lacking MIF, the macrophages grow out in a fan shape from the capillary on the glass surface of the chamber; when MIF is present, the fan of cell growth is inhibited (Figure 2–6). The extent of inhibition can be quantitated by photographing control and experimental preparations and

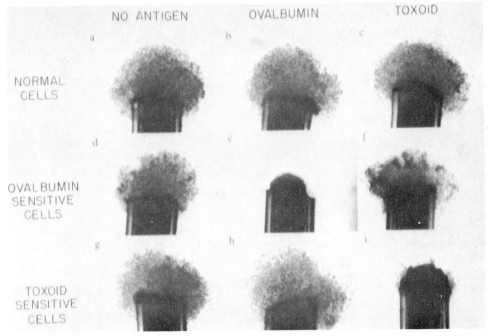

Figure 2–6. MIF test. Inhibition of migration of macrophages sensitive to ovalbumin or diphtheria toxoid when incubated 24 hours in the presence of homologous antigen (e and i). (From David et al., 1964. J. Immunol., 93:264. Copyright 1964, The Williams and Wilkins Company, Baltimore.)

measuring the areas of growth with a planimeter, or by using a prismatic projector on the microscope to trace the areas of growth on paper of uniform weight and then cutting out and weighing the tracings.

Laboratory animals are sensitized by intraperitoneal injections of antigen as a water-in-oil emulsion in Freund's complete adjuvant. Guinea pigs may require 8 weeks, and other animals require more or less time for the appearance of considerable numbers of sensitized lymphocytes in the lymph nodes, spleen, other lymphoid organs, and the alveolar and peritoneal exudates. For a simple demonstration of macrophage migration inhibition, a single animal can be used as a source of sensitive lymphocytes and macrophages.

To secure a large population of peritoneal cells, including both lymphocytes and macrophages, sterile paraffin oil is injected intraperitoneally, and 3 to 5 days later the animal is sacrificed and the peritoneal contents are washed out with tissue culture medium. Peritoneal cells are sedimented by centrifuging lightly, and they are washed repeatedly to remove oil and body fluids. Capillary tubes are then filled with the cells and packed by centrifugation.

Small lucite tissue culture chambers are prepared with a top and bottom consisting of 22-mm. microscope cover glasses. Duplicate pieces of the capillaries cut so that packed cells are flush with one end are placed in the bottom of each chamber and held firmly by droplets of Dow Corning silicone lubricant. The chamber is filled completely with tissue culture medium, with or without antigen. After incubation for 24 and 48 hours, each chamber is observed by microscope and the area of macrophage growth is measured. Percentage inhibition in the presence of antigen is calculated as follows:

$$\text{Per cent inhibition} = 100 - \left(100 \times \frac{\text{Ave. migration area with antigen}}{\text{Ave. migration area without antigen}} \right)$$

The MIF assay can be used to determine various parameters of the cell-mediated immunity or delayed-type hypersensitivity response:

1. In the "direct" assay, peritoneal cells from animals sensitized as just described are treated with various dilutions of antigen, and the end point is the least amount of antigen required to produce significant inhibition of migration.

2. Lymphocytes from the lymph nodes or other organs of a sensitized animal are mixed with peritoneal exudate cells from a *normal* animal to determine the presence and/or comparative activity of the various populations of lymphocytes.

3. In the "indirect" assay, MIF produced by incubation of lymphocytes with antigen is assayed by addition to the medium; the capillaries are filled with normal peritoneal exudate cells.

Inhibition of macrophage migration as demonstrated in vitro correlates reasonably well with the degree of delayed hypersensitivity demonstrable by skin test or by clinical experience. Søborg and Bendixen reported that an MIF test with buffy coat cells from the blood of a brucellosis patient and Brucella antigen agreed well with the results of a skin test.

MIF has been obtained in partially purified form. It is a protein, approximately 80,000 in molecular weight, rapidly inactivated by trypsin, and stable at 56° C. for 30 minutes.

MIF prepared from lymph node lymphocytes often displays skin reactive factor activity. Purified and concentrated material is tested by intradermal injection of guinea pigs. The diameter and degree of induration (thickening: flat, moderate, marked) are recorded hourly for 6 to 8 hours and at 18, 24, and 48 hours.

Lymphocyte Transformation

The cell-free liquid from sensitive T lymphocytes that have been treated with the homologous antigen may contain the *mitogenic* or *blastogenic* factor, a lymphokine that stimulates nonsensitized lymphocytes to undergo blast-cell transformation and mitotic proliferation. This process can be detected by microscopic examination of stained smears and enumeration of typical lymphoblasts: large cells with multiple nucleoli, basophilic cytoplasm, and a clear perinuclear zone. A more common and objective method is to measure the uptake of tritiated thymidine as evidence of DNA formation, which parallels cell division. Cell division and thymidine uptake do not occur during the first day or two (42 hours in a human lymphocyte system), but between 2 and 5 days they proceed exponentially, with a doubling time of approximately 12 hours. Incorporation of ^{3}H-thymidine into DNA occurs only during the first few hours after it is added to the mixture, which is routinely done when the cultures are 4 to 5 days old. Radioactivity counts in lymphocyte cultures with and without antigen provide quantitative indication of the amount of blastogenic factor produced.

The *mixed leukocyte reaction* is an application of the foregoing method that is highly significant in the selection of donors for tissue or organ transplantation. When blood lymphocytes from two genetically different individuals are mixed in tissue culture, some of the cells undergo blast transformation and mitosis. This occurs because some of the lymphocytes are or become sensitive to those of the other individual and mount a cellular immunologic response like that just described. The severity of the reaction varies directly with the histoincompatibility of the individuals.

A mixed leukocyte culture exhibits a two-way reaction, because cells of each individual react with those of the other. To match organ donors and recipients it is customary to inactivate (e.g., by irradiation) the cells of the prospective donor, so that only the reaction of the recipient's cells to the donor's tissue antigens is measured. This procedure is useful in cases in which there is no great urgency, because several days are required for the test: for example, when an organ can be stored satisfactorily before transplantation to the recipient, or when a selection is being made among a number of prospective donors.

Cell-Mediated Cytotoxicity

The cytotoxic effect of sensitized lymphocytes incubated in a mixture with the homologous cellular antigen can be demonstrated by various techniques: (1) viable cell counts (determined, for example, by vital staining); (2) total counts of intact cells measured with a Coulter counter; (3) protein synthesis assayed by measuring the uptake of ^{14}C amino acids; (4) release of DNA radiolabeled by ^{14}C-thymidine; (5) release of membrane-bound ^{51}Cr. Various kinds of immunizing and target cell antigens are used, including macrophages, fibroblasts, tumor cells, erythrocytes, and erythrocytes coated with soluble antigens.

Cytotoxic activity against standard mouse tumor cell lines is shown by lymphoid cells from the spleen, lymph nodes, blood, or thoracic duct of mice injected intraperitoneally 10 to 11 days previously with 30,000,000 cells. For the test, target tumor cells are incubated for 30 minutes with sodium chromate containing ^{51}Cr, which labels the cell membranes. Reaction mixtures are prepared containing the labeled tumor cells and varying numbers of lymphocytes from (a) immunized animals and (b) unimmunized animals (controls). After appropriate incubation the mixtures are centrifuged, and aliquots of the supernates are tested in a gamma radioactivity counter to determine the amount of ^{51}Cr released. A mixture lysed with distilled water is also counted to determine the maximum amount of ^{51}Cr that can be released, and the results of the assay are calculated as follows:

$$\text{Per cent lysis} = 100 \times \frac{\begin{array}{c}^{51}\text{Cr released by} \\ \text{immune cells}\end{array} - \begin{array}{c}^{51}\text{Cr released by} \\ \text{normal cells}\end{array}}{\begin{array}{c}\text{Maximum} \\ ^{51}\text{Cr released}\end{array} - \begin{array}{c}^{51}\text{Cr released by} \\ \text{normal cells}\end{array}}$$

Loewi and Temple used chicken red blood cells (CRBC) labeled with ^{51}Cr as target cells to study the cytotoxicity of spleen, lymph node, and peritoneal exudate cells of guinea pigs immunized with CRBC in Freund's complete adjuvant. Cells from all sources were active; cytotoxicity was usually maximal 2 weeks after immunization and persisted for 2 to 4 weeks, paralleling the intensity of delayed hypersensitivity reactions. Peritoneal exudate cells were somewhat more cytotoxic than spleen and lymph node cells; moreover, in peritoneal exudates both macrophages and lymphocytes were active.

Experimental Autoallergic Disease

Autoallergic disease, sometimes called autoimmune disease, can be induced by injection of tissues or tissue extracts emulsified in Freund's complete adjuvant. In some instances the disease is due to an immunologic response to "occult" antigens—tissue components that usually have little or no blood supply and hence do not encounter immunocompetent cells. In other instances tissue antigens are sufficiently altered by chemical, physical, or biologic events to become antigenic in the same species or individual, but the immunologically active cells or antibodies produced can cross-react with the native antigens. It has been suggested that the adjuvant may participate in this process, or it may break self-tolerance.

Some autoallergic diseases are caused by antibodies, and some are cell-mediated. The harmful effects induced experimentally in laboratory animals often resemble the damage that occurs naturally in human disease. However, there are many instances of autoallergic disease in animals for which no human counterpart has been discovered, and many human diseases for which an animal model has not been found. Two experimental autoallergic diseases due to sensitive lymphocytes will be described.

A form of allergic encephalitis is produced in various laboratory animals by injection of brain or spinal cord tissue in Freund's complete adjuvant. Two to 3 weeks after a single injection, a guinea pig's sense of balance and muscular coordination are impaired, paralysis soon occurs, and death follows within a few days or weeks. At autopsy, inflammatory areas are found in and near capillaries and veins throughout the brain and spinal cord. Experimental allergic encephalitis (EAE) can be transmitted serially from one animal to another by transfer of lymphocytes but not by serum; it is therefore clearly cell-mediated.

Injection of thyroid tissue or thyroglobulin emulsions in Freund's complete adjuvant induces thyroiditis and the production of sensitized lymphocytes and circulating antibodies in rabbits and various other species. In this case, homologous tissue (i.e., from the same species) is required, whereas in EAE heterologous tissue is also satisfactory. Pathologic changes include inflammation, disruption of colloid, sloughing of epithelial cells lining the follicles, eventual obliteration of their normal structure, and fibrosis. These changes are also seen in Hashimoto's disease or lymphadenoid goiter of man, a disease that has for some time been believed to be of immunologic origin.

Precipitating antibodies against human thyroglobulin are found in the sera of a large percentage of patients, but they are apparently not significant causes of damage.

Additional Sources of Information

Bloom, B. R.: *In vitro* approaches to the mechanism of cell-mediated immune reactions. *In* Dixon, F. J., and H. G. Kunkel, (Eds.): Advances in Immunology, Vol. 13, pp. 101–208, 1971.

Bloom, B. R., and P. R. Glade, (Eds.): *In vitro* Methods in Cell-Mediated Immunity. 1971. New York, Academic Press, Inc.

Roitt, L.: Essential Immunology. 1971. Oxford, Blackwell Scientific Publications.

Sternberger, L. A.: Immunocytochemistry. 1974. Englewood Cliffs, N.J., Prentice-Hall, Inc.

CHAPTER THREE

IMMUNOGLOBULINS

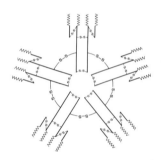

SERUM PROTEINS

Chemical Nature of Antibodies

As early as 1926, evidence that antibody is protein was obtained by Felton and Bailey in their study of the precipitate formed when pneumococcal polysaccharide reacts with homologous antiserum. They reported that 2.5 mg. of polysaccharide yielded a precipitate containing 37 mg. of protein, which could have come only from the serum and must have been antibody or so closely associated with antibody as to be inseparable from it.

Further evidence for the protein nature of antibody was derived by Dean, Taylor, and Adair from experiments with a polyvalent antiserum produced by immunizing a rabbit with two separate antigens simultaneously: egg albumin and horse serum albumin. They found that either antigen alone yielded the same amount of precipitate from equivalent amounts of antiserum, whether or not antibody corresponding to the other antigen had been previously removed by precipitation (Table 3–1). Moreover, the totals of the precipitates obtained with the individual antigens separately were the same as that formed when the antiserum was treated with the two antigens together. This experiment performed in the presence of heterologous antiserum or normal serum would have yielded the same result, because the amount of protein precipitated is completely uninfluenced by other proteins, including heterologous antibodies that may be present.

Treatment of antiserum with chemical or physical agents known to destroy or remove proteins also was found to decrease or eliminate antibody activity. Protein precipitants remove antibody from antiserum. The disappearance of antibodies from

Table 3–1   Precipitation of Two Different Antigens by a Polyvalent Rabbit Antiserum*

Tube	Antiserum vs. Egg Albumin + Serum Albumin	Antigen		Precipitate	Total Precipitate With Egg Albumin and Serum Albumin Antigens
		EGG ALBUMIN	SERUM ALBUMIN		
1	1 ml.	0.57 mg.	–	5.9 mg.	
2	Supernate from 1	–	1.14 mg.	9.9 mg.	15.8 mg.
3	1 ml.	–	1.14 mg.	9.7 mg.	
4	Supernate from 3	0.57 mg.	–	5.9 mg.	15.6 mg.
5	1 ml.	0.57 mg.	1.14 mg.	15.1 mg.	15.1 mg.

*Data from Dean, Taylor, and Adair, 1935. J. Hyg., 35:69; recalculated on the basis of 1 ml. antiserum. By permission of Cambridge University Press.

an immune serum acted upon by proteolytic enzymes depends upon the extent to which hydrolysis is allowed to proceed. For example, trypsin destroys partially purified pneumococcus type 1 antibody, and the rate of destruction is approximately the same as the rate of increase of amino nitrogen. Heat destroys antibody activity and denatures serum proteins at about the same rate. However, many years ago it was found that the heat resistance of all antibodies is not identical. Antibodies against the flagellar antigens of certain bacteria are more thermostable than somatic antibodies in the same antiserum; this observation foreshadowed the more recent discoveries of the physicochemical heterogeneity of antibody molecules.

Physical Properties of Serum Proteins

Before further consideration of the nature of antibodies, it will be helpful to review the physical characteristics of serum proteins.

ELECTROPHORETIC MOBILITY

Electrophoresis.   Electrophoresis is the migration of charged particles in an electric field. The rate of migration depends upon the magnitude of the charge upon the particles, the viscosity of the medium, the voltage of the electric field, and other factors. The particle charge is affected by pH and by the electrolyte and its concentration in the suspending medium. It is determined experimentally by measuring the rate of migration when all other factors are known. The direction and rate of migration of microscopic particles, such as bacteria and blood cells, are observed in a chamber mounted on the stage of a microscope. Electric current is applied through two electrodes, and the distance individual cells traverse per unit of time is noted. The net charge on the cells is calculated by means of a formula.

All proteins are amphoteric: that is, they contain radicals that dissociate to give positive and negative ions (e.g., $-COO^-$ and $-NH_3^+$). The relative and absolute numbers of positive and negative ions determine the sign and magnitude of the charge on the surface of the molecule or protein-containing particle. The charge is negative when negative ions predominate. A negatively charged particle migrates toward the positive electrode in an electric field. If such a suspension is made more acid, additional basic radicals dissociate, and their positive charges reduce the net negative charge on the protein. At a certain reaction (pH) known as the *isoelectric point* the protein is maximally ionized, although the net charge is zero because positive and negative charges are equal. The particle does not migrate in either direction in an electric field but may precipitate out of solution. The isoelectric points of serum proteins vary from pH 2.5 to 8.0. Below its isoelectric point a particle possesses a net positive charge and migrates toward the negative electrode.

Moving Boundary Electrophoresis.   The electrophoretic migration of submicroscopic or macromolecular particles such as proteins in solution is determined by the *moving boundary method* in a U-shaped cell (Figure 3–1). The solution is placed in the bottom half of the cell and covered with a buffer of proper pH. Electrical connections are made to the buffer in both arms of the cell. The protein migrates down one arm of the U-tube and up the other, through the buffer solution. The migrating faces of a pure protein form sharp boundaries, because each molecule of the protein moves at the same rate in the same direction. In a solution containing a mixture of proteins, the more highly charged molecules migrate faster and form separate boundaries. Slowly moving molecules are sorted out according to their respective rates of migration. The distance between boundaries constantly increases as long as the current is applied. Boundaries

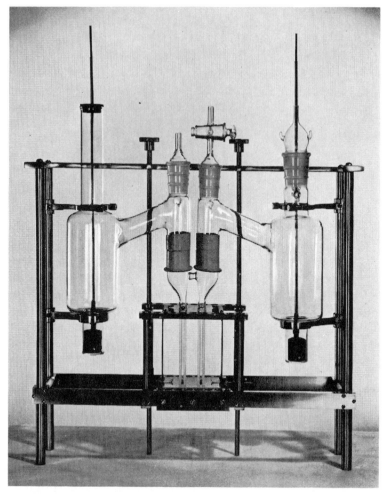

Figure 3–1. Electrophoresis cell. The U-tube is at bottom center, and electrodes are in glass columns at left and right. (From Gray, G. W., 1951. Electrophoresis. Sci. Amer., 185:45. Copyright © 1951 by Scientific American, Inc. All rights reserved. Photograph by Keturah Blakely.)

in solutions containing proteins of nearly the same charge are diffuse as a result of concentration gradients.

The various protein boundaries may be observed by their absorption of ultraviolet light or, more commonly, by special optical methods based upon the principle that a solution containing a substance such as protein has an index of refraction different from the pure solvent. A narrow beam of light passing through an electrophoretic U-tube containing a boundary or concentration gradient of protein is refracted at an angle dependent upon the protein concentration. Optical scanning of the entire contents of the U-tube yields a series of crests and troughs (see Figure 3–2). The number of crests corresponds to the number of electrically distinct proteins, and the areas under the crests are proportional to their concentrations. The most rapidly migrating fraction (i.e., that with the greatest net charge) forms the highest boundary in the so-called ascending limb of the U-tube and the lowest boundary in the descending limb; slower fractions form succeeding boundaries.

Zone Electrophoresis. Zone electrophoresis is the migration of a test material in an electric field through a supporting medium, such as paper, cellulose acetate, agar, or starch gel. The apparatus need not be expensive and may even be made in the

Figure 3-2. Electrophoretic diagram of normal pooled human serum diluted 1:1.5 in barbiturate buffer, pH 8.54, ionic strength 0.1. Total protein concentration, 3.3 per cent. The descending boundary after 121 minutes is shown, and direction of migration is toward the left. The concentrations of the protein fractions, determined from the areas under the respective peaks, were as follows: albumin, 59.1 per cent; α_1-globulin, 4.5 per cent; α_2-globulin, 8.6 per cent; β-globulin, 12.6 per cent; γ-globulin, 15.2 per cent. The so-called δ-anomaly at the extreme right does not represent another protein fraction. (Reproduced by permission of the American Instrument Company.)

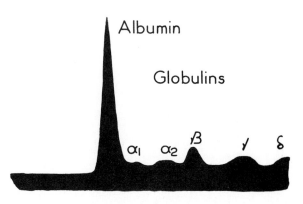

laboratory. Two electrode chambers that can be filled with buffer are necessary, together with a suitable power supply (Figure 3–3).

In paper electrophoresis of serum, strips of filter paper are moistened with buffer, commonly but not necessarily at pH 8.6, and the specimen is applied a little toward the cathode end from the center of the strip. The duration of electrophoresis depends upon the voltage, ionic strength of the buffer, and other factors; it is usually several hours. At the conclusion, the paper strip is dried at a constant temperature (105 to 120° C.), a procedure that coagulates the proteins, and stained with bromphenol blue, amido black, azocarmine, or some other dye with an affinity for protein. The result is a series of stained bands (see Figure 3–4). The stained and dried paper may be rendered translucent by treatment with oil, and the color intensity (and hence the relative protein concentration) in the various zones is measured by use of a photoelectric scanner. The plotted results give a curve similar to that shown in Figure 3–4. Instead of scanning, the strip may be cut into sections and the dye eluted and measured colorimetrically.

Agar, starch, and other gels are also used for electrophoresis. Agar gels, for example, are made in buffer solutions with Merthiolate or sodium azide as a preservative and poured in a 3- to 4-mm. layer on glass plates or microscope slides. When the agar is hard,

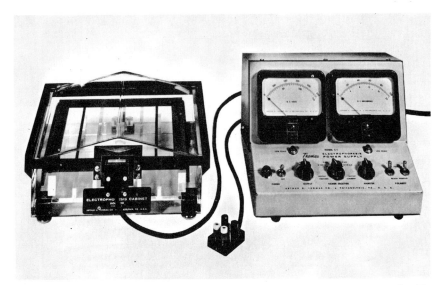

Figure 3-3. A form of apparatus used for electrophoresis on paper strips or on gels. (Courtesy of Arthur H. Thomas Company.)

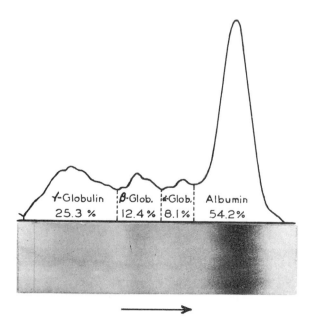

Figure 3-4. Electrophoretic separation of major rabbit serum proteins on a filter paper strip. The curve was plotted from points obtained with a photoelectric densitometer.

a circular or elliptical hole is cut and the agar removed from it. The hole is then filled with a mixture of the test solution in double strength agar. Electric contact is made with the electrode chambers via filter paper moistened with buffer, and electrophoresis is performed. Precautions are usually necessary to prevent heating or undue evaporation. After electrophoresis, the agar may be dried to a thin film and stained.

Preparative Zone Electrophoresis. Preparative zone electrophoresis is the use of zone electrophoresis to isolate purified fractions from mixtures of electrophoretically heterogeneous substances. Zone electrophoresis is more useful in preparative work than moving boundary electrophoresis because it is difficult to remove the intermediate fractions cleanly from the U-tube of the latter apparatus. A paper strip, on the other hand, can easily be cut into sections as desired, and each section eluted to secure the protein or other electrophoretic component it contains. A starch block can be used in a similar way; starch moistened with buffer and pressed into a mold constitutes the supporting medium in which electrophoresis is performed, and at its conclusion the block is cut and each section eluted. Paper curtain electrophoresis is a continuous process in which a protein solution in buffer flows vertically down a large sheet of filter paper while subjected to an electric potential horizontally from the sides (see Figure 3–5). As the proteins travel down the paper, they are separated into the various electrophoretic fractions. The bottom of the paper is cut into sawtooth points, and the proteins drip into a series of tubes.

Electrophoretic Fractions of Normal Serum. Electrophoretic analysis of normal serum reveals four major fractions (Table 3–2). At pH 6.02, the albumin in a normal specimen migrated toward the anode at a rate of 4.60×10^{-5} cm.^{2}/volt/second, and was followed in order by the alpha-, beta-, and gamma-globulins. The molecular charge and rate of migration of a protein clearly depend upon the pH of the solution. The four major components consist of many subfractions, which are detected by procedures of high resolving power, such as starch gel electrophoresis. The α-globulin subdivisions, α_1- and α_2-, are readily demonstrated by moving boundary electrophoresis (see Figure 3–2) and by zone electrophoresis on paper or in agar. Twenty to 30 separate proteins can be distinguished in starch gels: some of them are listed in Table 3–3 (see page 58).

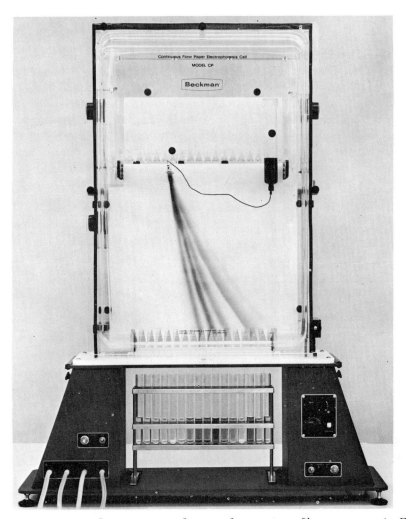

Figure 3–5. Continuous flow separation of protein fractions on a filter paper curtain. Electric current applied horizontally as the protein solution flows down the paper separates the various electrophoretic fractions, which collect in test tubes. (Reproduced by permission of the Beckman Company.)

Table 3–2 *Electrophoretic Mobility and Isoelectric Points of the Four Principal Protein Fractions of a Normal Serum**

pH	Mobility in Cm.²/Volt/Sec. × 10⁵			
	ALBUMIN	α-GLOBULIN	β-GLOBULIN	γ-GLOBULIN
6.02	−4.60	−3.34	−2.55	+0.01
8.03	−7.15	−6.16	−4.20	−1.51
Isoelectric point: pH	4.64	5.06	5.12	6.0

*From Tiselius, 1937. Biochem. J., 31:1464. By permission of Cambridge University Press.

The shape of a single crest or peak obtained by electrophoretic analysis reflects the homogeneity of the test substance or fraction. A narrow, steep peak is obtained with a highly homogeneous material. Most electrophoretic components of serum give broad curves, which indicate that the electric charges of the proteins grade into one another.

Electrophoretic Properties of Antibodies. Most antibodies migrate with the γ-globulin fraction of serum, or as a distinguishable component between the β- and γ-globulins. The electrophoretic properties of antibodies, as distinguished from other serum proteins, are clearly demonstrated by specific precipitation of antisera with homologous antigen. Removal of antibodies from an anti-egg albumin rabbit serum by precipitation with egg albumin did not greatly affect the α- and β-globulins (Figure 3–6) but decreased the γ-globulin approximately 75 per cent. This indicates that antibody is composed of γ-globulin, but that γ-globulin is not entirely antibody. Antitoxic

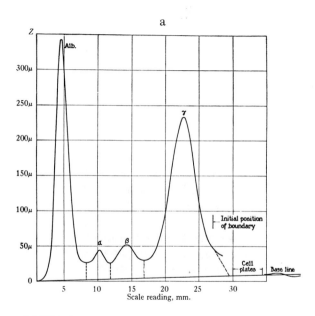

a

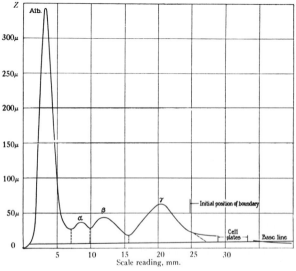

b

Figure 3–6. Electrophoretic scale diagrams of rabbit anti-egg albumin serum (A) before and (B) after absorption of the antibody. The γ-globulin decreased greatly. (From Tiselius and Kabat, 1939. J. Exp. Med., 69:119.)

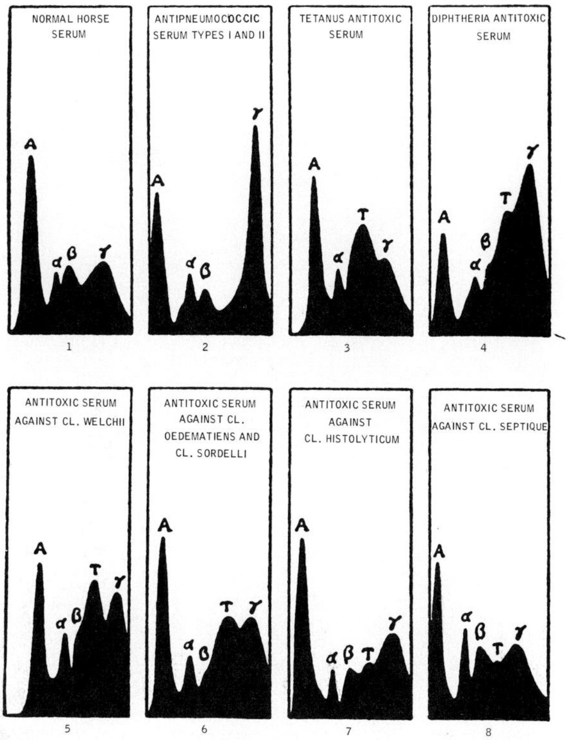

Figure 3–7. Electrophoretic diagrams of normal, antipneumococcal, and antitoxic horse sera: A = albumin; α, β, and γ refer to the respective globulins; T = "T" component. (From van der Scheer et al., 1940. J. Immunol., 39:65.)

antibodies produced by prolonged immunization of horses are found in a slow β or fast γ fraction, sometimes designated the "T" component (Fig. 3–7).

Immunoelectrophoresis. Immunoelectrophoresis is a combination of electrophoresis and specific precipitation by double gel diffusion. The various electrophoretic components of a protein mixture such as serum are first separated by electrophoresis in agar into a series of spots or bands. Troughs are then cut in the agar parallel with the line of migration of the proteins and a few millimeters away. The troughs are filled with antisera against one or more components of the original protein mixture. Antibody diffuses at a right angle from the troughs, and the various proteins diffuse radially from the points where they were left by electrophoresis. Lines of precipitate appear as in an Ouchterlony plate, usually in the form of arcs about the antigenic protein spots.

Immunoelectrophoresis is a powerful tool for resolving and identifying antigens or antibodies in a mixture. It demonstrates greater complexity in the protein composition of normal serum than does electrophoresis alone because it is determined by diffusibility as well as electric charge. Two proteins of identical charge can be distinguished if they diffuse at different rates. Figure 3–8 illustrates application of immunoelectrophoresis to human serum and furnishes several examples of proteins with the same electrophoretic character that are readily separated by their diffusion rates, e.g., haptoglobin and ceruloplasmin. Figure 3–8 also clearly shows the antigenic complexity of serum; 30 or more components have been identified. There are many distinct proteins of the α and β types, but the γ-globulins appear to be homogeneous. Actually, the γ-globulins comprise a family of antigenically related proteins that display such a continuously intergrading electrophoretic heterogeneity that their precipitation arc extends from the slower end of the serum protein range through the β zone and into the α_2 area.

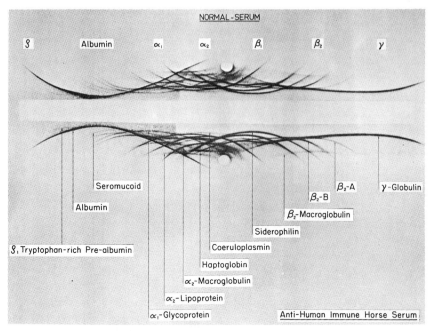

Figure 3–8. Immunoelectrophoresis of normal human serum. The serum specimen was placed in the two circular wells, and after electrophoresis the horizontal central trough was filled with horse anti-human serum. Lines of precipitate formed where antibodies, diffusing from the trough, reacted with serologically equivalent concentrations of antigens as they diffused from the spots to which they had migrated during electrophoresis. (By courtesy of National Instrument Laboratories, Inc., Washington D.C.)

MOLECULAR WEIGHT

Ultracentrifugation. Information concerning the molecular weights of proteins is obtained by centrifugation at speeds up to 70,000 revolutions per minute in special centrifuges driven by air, electric motors, or oil turbines. Sedimentation forces as high as 750,000 times gravity have been obtained. A transparent analytic cell (quartz or lucite) containing the protein solution is placed in a rotor so that a beam of light can pass through it every revolution. Molecules of different weights are sorted into layers or boundaries, the heaviest molecules falling the greatest distance from the center of rotation. Observation of the boundaries is made in the same manner as in electrophoresis. The sedimentation rate is determined from consecutive observations at short intervals by measuring the distance migrated per unit of time. The sedimentation constant is derived by dividing the observed velocity of migration by the acceleration caused by centrifugal force. The rate of sedimentation depends in part upon the temperature, so values are either determined at 20° C. or are corrected mathematically to this temperature, and the sedimentation constant is then designated s_{20}; it is expressed in Svedberg units (S). The sedimentation constant of the substance, its diffusion constant, its density and that of the suspending medium are used to calculate the molecular weight.

Figure 3–9 illustrates observations made in ultracentrifugal analysis of human sera. Row A consists of a series of photographs taken at 8-minute intervals during centrifugation of normal serum; rows B and C are studies of pathologic sera. The pictures in each row read from right to left. The right-hand picture in row A represents an early stage in centrifugation of normal serum and shows a small peak of heavy protein moving out from the right side. The next picture, 8 minutes later, shows this peak further advanced toward the left and now identified as 17S globulin, followed by a larger fraction of slightly less than 7S. This later resolves into a relatively minor 7S component and a major 4S component, the albumin. The heavy fraction eventually migrates out of the photographic field at the left. The pathologic sera show various abnormalities.

Molecular Weight of Serum Proteins.   The molecular weights of proteins vary, in general, with their sedimentation constants. Normal human serum contains two main components with sedimentation constants of approximately 4.5S and 7S, and a third, smaller fraction of heavy molecules (s_{20} = ca. 19S). The lightest (first) fraction consists of serum albumin, which has a molecular weight of about 69,000. The intermediate material is the principal globulin of normal serum; its molecular weight is 150,000 to 160,000. The heavy component is also globulin, frequently called macroglobulin. Its molecular weight is 800,000 to 950,000. Between the smallest and largest serum proteins is an almost continuous series of progressively larger molecules (see Table 3–3).

Gel Filtration.   The molecular weight of a protein can be estimated by making use of the molecular sieve effect of a hydrophilic colloid such as Sephadex. Sephadex is composed of cross-linked dextran macromolecules, and when it is hydrated it produces a gel consisting of "beads" or particles, which are more or less porous, depending upon the degree of cross-linking of the dextran. In use, a glass column is filled with the Sephadex gel, and a protein solution is applied to the top and washed through with an appropriate solvent. Protein molecules that are too large to enter the "bead" pores cannot penetrate the gel particles and therefore pass rapidly through the bed in the liquid phase and are quickly eluted. Smaller molecules penetrate the gel particles to a varying extent, depending upon their size and shape, and are eluted in order of decreasing molecular size. To determine the molecular weight of an unknown, the column is first standardized by running several proteins of known size, plotting the respective elution volumes against the molecular weights of the proteins. The unknown is then run through the column, and its elution volume is ascertained. This figure is used to read the molecular weight of the unknown from the curve (Figure 3–10).

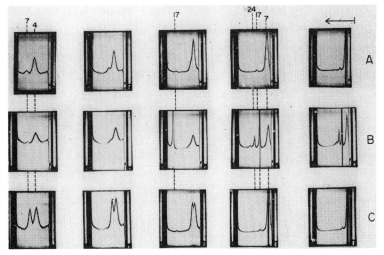

Figure 3–9.   Ultracentrifugal analysis of normal and pathologic human sera: *A*, normal; *B*, macroglobulinemic; *C*, hyperglobulinemic. Photographs in each row were taken at 8-minute intervals, reading from right to left. Sedimentation in each diagram is also from right to left. (From Putnam, 1959. Arch. Biochem., 79:67.)

Table 3–3   *Electrophoretic Fractions and Subfractions of Normal Human Serum and Their Sedimentation Coefficients**

Electrophoretic Fraction	Per Cent of Total Protein	Sedimentation Coefficients (S)
Albumin	55–64	4.0–4.6
α_1-Globulins	3.6–7.2	3.0
Glycoprotein		2.4–3.5
Lipoprotein		4.1–5.5
Ceruloplasmin		4.2 / 7.1 / 10.8–18 (trace)
α_2-Globulins	7.6–10.1	4.0 (55%) / 7.0 (15%) / 12 (trace) / 19 (30%)
Glycoproteins	1.2	6.0 / 9.0 / 14–19.5
Mucoproteins	0.5	4.5–5.5 (10%) / 6 / 9 (70%) / 12–20 (20%)
Haptoglobins		3.0–4.2 / 6 / 8–9 / 11
Macroglobulins	1.5–4.5	14–19.5
β-Globulins	11.6–15.2	5 (50%) / 7 (50%) / 12 (trace)
β_1-Globulins	3	5.0–5.5 / 7
Lipid-poor euglobulins	5	7 (66%) / 20 (33%)
Transferrin	3.0–6.5	5.0–5.3
Lipoproteins	4–14	2.9 / 5.9 / 7
Properdin	Trace	27
β_2-Globulins	3	7
$\beta_2{}_A$-Globulins		7 (81%) / 10–18 (19%)
γ-Globulins	10.1–17.2	7 (90%) / 12 (trace) / 19 (10%) / 28 (trace) / 44 (trace)

*Modified from Cooper. *In* Putnam, F. W. (Ed.): The Plasma Proteins, 1960, pp. 51–103. New York, Academic Press, Inc.

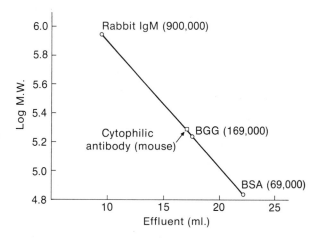

Figure 3–10. Molecular weight estimation by gel filtration. A Bio-Gel P-300 column was standardized with the known proteins (rabbit IgM, bovine gamma globulin, and bovine serum albumin), after which mouse cytophilic antibody was run through the column. Its elution volume indicated a molecular weight of about 195,000. (From data of G. L. Brown, Ph.D. thesis, University of Rhode Island, 1968.)

Solubilities of Serum Proteins

PRECIPITATION BY NEUTRAL SALTS

Ammonium and sodium sulfates have been used for many years to secure crude protein fractions from serum, and they are still useful for a partial purification of antibodies. Various globulin fractions are removed successively by increasing concentrations of these salts. "Euglobulin" is precipitated by 13.5 per cent sodium sulfate. Treatment of the filtrate with additional sodium sulfate in a final concentration of 17.4 per cent yields "pseudoglobulin 1," and a third fraction, "pseudoglobulin 2," separates at 21.5 per cent concentration of the salt. The albumin remains in solution. Cohn et al. reported that euglobulin precipitated from horse serum by ammonium sulfate consisted largely of protein with the electrophoretic mobility of γ-globulin and that pseudoglobulin was a mixture of α-, β-, and γ-globulins.

PRECIPITATION BY DIALYSIS

Precipitation of protein by dialysis is somewhat similar to precipitation by neutral salts, because both methods are based upon the relative solubilities of serum proteins in electrolyte solutions. Serum is placed in a bag of semipermeable material like thin cellophane and suspended in distilled water. The protein precipitate that appears when most of the electrolytes have dialyzed out of the serum is considered to be euglobulin. Pseudoglobulins are soluble in distilled water. The precipitated euglobulins dissolve in a dilute electrolyte, such as physiologic saline. Fractions obtained by dialysis are, in general, electrophoretically inhomogeneous.

PRECIPITATION BY ALCOHOL

A method of separating blood proteins that is adaptable to the large-scale concentration and partial purification of antibodies is based upon Felton's observation that antibody can be precipitated from antiserum by use of alcohol if precautions are taken to prevent denaturation of the protein. Denaturation is kept to a minimum by conducting all operations at temperatures very close to the freezing point of the serum-alcohol mixtures.

This method was further developed by Cohn and his co-workers during and after World War II. Several fractions were obtained by varying the protein and ethyl alcohol

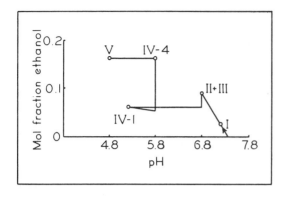

Figure 3–11. Flow sheet indicating the fractionation of plasma proteins by Cohn's Method 6. (Reprinted with permission from Cohn et al., 1946. J. Am. Chem. Soc., 68:459. Copyright 1946 by the American Chemical Society.)

concentrations, pH, and other factors. Some of these plasma fractions were purified for specific prophylactic or therapeutic uses.

The steps in one of Cohn's methods of separating plasma fractions are illustrated in Figure 3–11. Normal plasma, which has a reaction about pH 7.4, is chilled to $-2.5°$ C. A buffer solution containing alcohol is gradually added until pH 7.2 and a concentration of 8 per cent alcohol is reached, whereupon precipitate I forms. This contains most of the fibrinogen (Table 3–4) and is removed by centrifugation. The next precipitate is produced at $-5°$ C. by adding buffer and alcohol to pH 6.8 and 25 per cent alcohol concentration. This precipitate, II + III, consists of β- and γ-globulins with prothrombin, cholesterol, and other substances. The supernate is diluted with water to an alcohol concentration of 18 per cent and is acidified to pH 5.2. Precipitate IV-1 consists chiefly of γ-globulins, together with some lipoid material. The supernatant liquid is adjusted to pH 5.8 and the alcohol concentration to 40 per cent. Precipitate IV-4 separates and consists chiefly of α- and β-globulins. The supernate is brought to pH 4.8 and precipitate V forms. This contains most of the plasma albumin.

The major fractions can be further purified and subfractionated by alcohol precipitation. Fraction II + III contains at least seven components: II–1, II–2, II–3, III–0, III–1, III–2, and III–3. The subfractions of II are principally γ-globulin, whereas the subfractions of III include α-, β-, and γ-globulins.

The conditions employed in Cohn's method were selected to separate electrophoretic fractions. About 80 per cent of the fibrinogen is concentrated in fraction I; 97 per cent of the γ-globulin and 87 per cent of the β-globulin are in II + III; nearly 50 per cent of the α-globulin is in fraction IV-1 and 30 per cent in IV-4; and 83 per cent of the albumin is found in V. Antibodies, being largely γ-globulins, are confined to fractions II + III.

Table 3–4   *Protein Composition of the Principal Fractions Separated from Normal Human Plasma by Cohn's "Method 6"* *

Fraction	Albumin	α-Globulin	β-Globulin	γ-Globulin	Fibrinogen	Total
I	7%	8%	15%	9%	61%	100%
II + III	4	6	48	37	5	100
IV–1	—	89	10	1	0	100
IV–4	16	46	38	0	0	100
V	95	4	1	0	0	100

*Reprinted with permission from Cohn, et al., 1946. J. Am. Chem. Soc., 68:459. Copyright 1946 by the American Chemical Society.

Chromatography of Serum Proteins

Chromatography is a technique for separating the constituents of a mixture such as serum based upon differences in their strength of binding to an adsorbent like cellulose. The binding of a protein depends upon its possession of a sufficient number of electric charges of opposite sign to those of the adsorbent. Multiple bonds form between the protein and the adsorbent, and the strength of adsorption varies from one protein to another according to their sizes and net charges. The strength of adsorption is also affected by the nature of the adsorbent. Cellulose modified by addition of diethylaminoethyl radicals (DEAE-cellulose) binds anions, and when modified by addition of carboxymethyl radicals (CM-cellulose) it binds cations. CM-cellulose is therefore a better adsorbent for certain γ-globulins that have an alkaline isoelectric point and hence a net negative electric charge (i.e., an excess of cationic radicals).

The protein is removed from the adsorbent by elution, which is effected by washing with buffer to change the pH and reduce the number of charges on the protein or the adsorbent, or by washing with solutions of increased salt concentration to compete for the existing charges. The less firmly bound proteins are eluted first. If many bonds form between the protein and adsorbent, prolonged washing or a strong eluting agent is required. Often the pH and salt concentrations of the solution are changed at intervals during the washing process to elute progressively proteins that are bound more and more firmly and are therefore of increasing size or net charge.

Column chromatography is performed in glass tubes packed with the adsorbent and moistened with an appropriate buffer. The protein solution is added and the eluting fluid is then passed slowly through the column. Small fractions (e.g., a few milliliters) are collected and analyzed (chemically, physically, biologically) or used to prepare purified proteins. Chromatography of pooled sera from mice immunized with hemocyanin, pneumococcal polysaccharide, and sheep red cells is shown in Figure 3–12. Two antibodies were eluted with the first fraction of protein, whereas most of the sheep hemolysin came off the column with the last fractions.

Figure 3–13 illustrates the use of chromatography to study the homogeneity of antibodies in the γ-globulin of rabbits during immunization with ovalbumin. The rabbits were bled and their sera were fractionated by sodium sulfate precipitation. The product containing γ-globulin was passed through a chromatographic column, and the eluted fractions were examined for protein and antibody content. The protein curves were reasonably symmetrical, both from normal and immune animals. The antibody curves, however, showed two chromatographic types of molecules. The first

Figure 3–12. Chromatography of pooled mouse antisera against hemocyanin, pneumococcal type 3 polysaccharide, and sheep RBC. The sheep hemolysin was eluted from the DEAE-cellulose column with the last fractions of the protein. (From Fahey and Humphrey, 1962. Immunology, 5:104.)

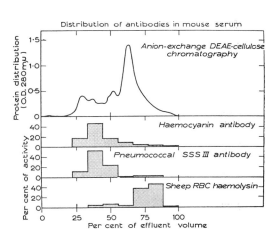

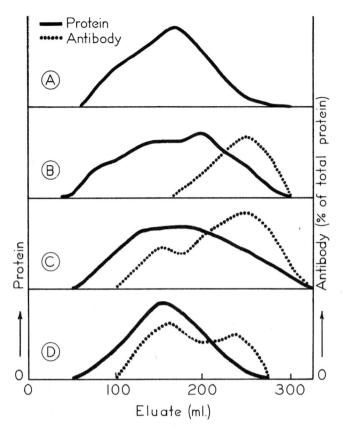

Figure 3–13. Chromatograms of normal and immune (anti-ovalbumin) rabbit γ-globulins: *A*, normal; *B*, immunized 4 weeks (nine injections); *C*, immunized 14 weeks (one course of nine injections and a second course of six injections 2 months later; *D*, same as *C* after an additional 10 days. (Redrawn from Porter, 1955. Biochem. J., 59:405.)

appeared promptly and was a "slowly running" variety; that is, considerable elution was required to remove it from the adsorbent. The second, a "more rapidly running" antibody, was found later. Humphrey·and Porter reported that pneumococcal and influenzal antibodies produced in response to intravenous injection also were of the same nature, whereas antibodies produced by intramuscular inoculation with ovalbumin in adjuvant were of the "slow" type throughout immunization. They concluded that a variety of cells capable of producing slightly different globulins participate in antibody formation, according to the route and duration of the antigenic stimulus. Lymph nodes and bone marrow seemed to produce the "slower" chromatographic type, whereas the spleen produced the "faster" antibodies.

Purification of Antibodies

For theoretic as well as practical reasons, there has long been an interest in purifying antibodies. Studies of their structure and mode of action are greatly facilitated by elimination of the nonreactive ingredients of serum, and fewer potentially dangerous (e.g., allergic) reactions attend the prophylactic or therapeutic injection of materials from which nonantibody constituents have been removed. Electrophoresis, gel filtration, precipitation, and chromatography can be used to concentrate antibody-containing fractions, but inasmuch as antibody is definable only in functional terms by its ability to combine specifically with antigen, it is apparent that pure preparations of antibody can be secured only by dissociation of antigen-antibody complexes. Antiserum is mixed with homologous antigen in proper proportions for maximum precipitation or agglutination. The aggregate, washed free from nonreacting serum constituents, is then dissociated by means that permit recovery of the antibodies.

Antibodies may be dissociated from agglutinated cells of certain Enterobacteriaceae by mild heating. Removal of the cells in a heated centrifuge leaves a supernatant liquid that contains the original concentration of antibody.

Heidelberger and his co-workers precipitated pneumococcal polysaccharide by homologous antiserum in physiologic saline. The washed precipitate was resuspended in 10 to 15 per cent sodium chloride and incubated for one hour at 37° C. Between 10 and 20 per cent of the bound antibody was released from the precipitate, which was then removed by centrifugation. Dialysis of the supernatant liquid against 0.9 per cent sodium chloride yielded antibody preparations from which 80 to 100 per cent of the nitrogen was specifically precipitable by pneumococcal polysaccharide. Antibody solutions were obtained that were homogeneous electrophoretically and ultracentrifugally. Satisfactory results were obtained with horse, cow, pig, rabbit, monkey, and human anti-pneumococcal sera. This procedure is applicable chiefly to carbohydrate-anticarbohydrate systems. Specific precipitates have also been dissociated with acids (hydrochloric, phosphoric, carbonic) and alkalies (sodium, calcium, and barium hydroxides), and with barium chloride and other substances.

Purification of antibodies against proteins by a method involving specific precipitation and dissociation is hampered by the necessity for separating two proteins after the antigen-antibody precipitate has been dissociated. Singer et al. devised a method to accomplish this and prepared antibodies against ovalbumin, bovine serum albumin, and ribonuclease that were at least 98 per cent pure and active. They treated the antigen with N-acetylhomocysteine thiolactone and thus coupled a small number (4 to 20) of —SH radicals to the surface of each protein molecule. This did not seriously impair its capacity to react with homologous antibody. The thiolated antigen was then used to precipitate the antibody, and the antigen-antibody precipitate was washed with buffer to remove nonspecific proteins and dissolved in glycine-H_2SO_4 buffer at pH 2.4. The thiolated antigen was removed from solution by precipitation with a bifunctional organic mercurial, 3,6-bis-(acetoxymercurimethyl)-dioxane (MMD), by cross-linking to form

$$\text{Antigen—S—Hg—Hg—S—Antigen}$$

bonds, leaving antibody in solution. The method was said to be convenient, simple, and reproducible. Only 1 gram of MMD was required for preparation of about 100 grams of pure antibody.

Some of the principles employed in the foregoing methods have been combined in the more sophisticated procedures of *immunoadsorption*. A specific immunoadsorbent may be made by capitalizing on the strong physical attraction between certain inorganic solids, such as glass, and various antigenic organic substances. For example, 40-μm glass beads are soaked overnight in a glass column with ovalbumin, washed with saline to remove free protein, and then used to adsorb anti-ovalbumin antibodies from diluted serum. The column is again washed thoroughly to remove nonantibody proteins, and finally the antibody is eluted from the beads by dissociation with glycine-HCl buffer at pH 3.0.

A soluble antigen can also be coupled to an immunologically inert, insoluble substance, such as CM-cellulose, agarose, or Sephadex. Treatment of CM-cellulose with cyanogen bromide yields a derivative that reacts with compounds containing a

free amino group, such as a protein. Dicyclohexylcarbodiimide joins protein antigens
to CM-cellulose through an amide linkage:

$$-\overset{\parallel}{\underset{O}{C}}-\overset{\mid}{\underset{H}{N}}-$$

The prepared immunoadsorbent, thoroughly washed, is mixed with antiserum in a
batch process, or it can be used in a column. After adsorbing antibody, the immunoadsorbent is again washed, and antibody is eluted. Hydrochloric acid at pH 2.3 is a
satisfactory eluting agent, and other agents are also available.

IMMUNOGLOBULINS

Immunoglobulins comprise a family of proteins consisting of light chains and
heavy chains linked together by disulfide bonds; all antibodies so far described are
immunoglobulins, but it is not known whether all immunoglobulins function as antibodies.

Tiselius and Kabat provided the first good evidence for the physicochemical
nature of antibodies in 1939 when they reported that antibodies migrated with the
slowest electrophoretic fractions of serum proteins, the gamma-globulins. Twenty
years later Porter digested rabbit immune γ-globulin with papain and obtained three
fractions, separable by chromatography on CM-cellulose; he demonstrated that two of
the fractions retained the antibody function of combining with antigen (although they
did not precipitate it) and that the third fraction lacked all antibody function but
possessed most of the antigenic specificity of the original, undigested γ-globulin.
Nisonoff et al. (1961) then showed that peptic digestion of antibody removed one-third
of the molecule, but the residual fraction retained its ability to precipitate antigen. This
function was lost upon reduction with 2-mercaptoethylamine, which split the fraction
into two components, each of which was still able to combine with antigen. Edelman
(1959) showed that antibodies are multichain structures, and Porter (1962) postulated
that they consist of four chains, held together by disulfide bonds. This basic structure is
now generally accepted.

Putnam (1965) and others then began reporting amino acid sequences of immunoglobulins. It quickly became apparent that it was impossible to prepare pure
antibody consisting of molecules with identical amino acid composition and sequence
by any technique then known. Even functionally pure antibody produced by methods
discussed above (page 62) from the serum of a single animal, although it reacted with
the homologous antigen, nevertheless was heterogeneous in its amino acid make-up.
However, protein similar in some respects to antibody was available in Bence Jones
protein, found in the urine of 50 per cent of patients with multiple myeloma, a disease
characterized by abnormal multiplication of plasma cells and lymphocytes. The
myeloma protein produced in a given individual is homogeneous in amino acid composition and sequence. A number of such proteins were secured in amounts sufficient
for complete study, which was conducted in several laboratories during a period of
about 10 years. The complete amino acid sequence of an entire myeloma protein was
reported by Edelman in 1969.

Immunoglobulin Nomenclature

Early studies demonstrated that antibodies are heterogeneous in physical as well
as chemical properties. Although the principal class of antibody in man and most

animals has a sedimentation coefficient of 7S and a molecular weight of about 150,000, there is another large class with a sedimentation coefficient of 19S and a molecular weight of about 900,000. The latter appears first in the sera of many animals under immunization and is eventually replaced by the former. Both react with the antigen that engendered their production, causing various readily demonstrated serologic reactions, including agglutination or precipitation, enhanced phagocytosis, and cytolysis. However, when they were studied as protein antigens rather than as antibodies, significant differences as well as likenesses were found. It therefore appeared that, although they possessed similar if not identical antibody determinant sites, they differed in some of the physicochemical features that determine antigenic specificity. Three additional classes of immunoglobulins with antibody activity were later discovered. Each of the five classes differs significantly in antigenic character from the other four but also displays antigenic similarities with the others. The nomenclature and some distinguishing features of the five classes of immunoglobulins are listed in Table 3–5.

Immunoglobulin Structure

The general structure of an immunoglobulin is illustrated diagrammatically in Figure 3–14. Two "light" chains comprising 214 amino acid residues are joined to two "heavy" chains of 440 amino acid residues by disulfide bonds, and the heavy chains are themselves joined by disulfide bonds. The results of amino acid sequence analyses have shown great variation between immunoglobulins in the arrangement of amino acids in the amino-terminal half of the light chains and the amino-terminal quarter of the heavy chains, and a high degree of constancy of arrangement in the remainder or carboxyl-terminal portion of each chain.

Papain digestion of an immunoglobulin splits the molecule into three fractions. Two fractions are identical and (if the immunoglobulin is an antibody) can react with homologous antigen but do not yield an agglutinating or precipitating aggregate; these are the Fab (antigen-binding) fragments. The third lacks antibody function, but it

Table 3–5   The Principal Classes of Human Immunoglobulins

Class	Sedimentation Coefficient	Molecular Weight	Concentration in Normal Sera (mg. per 100 ml.)	Physiologic Properties and Functions
IgG (γG)*	6.7S	143–149,000	700–1500	Placental transfer; precipitation, agglutination, opsonization, cytolysis
IgA (γA)	6.8S 11.4S	158–162,000 400,000	100–400 (Secretions)	Antibacterial and antiviral, especially in secretions
IgM (γM)	19.0S	800–950,000	50–200	Precipitation, agglutination, opsonization, cytolysis
IgD (γD)	6.6S	175–180,000	0.3–40	Unknown
IgE (γE)	8.0S	185–190,000	0.01–0.07	Reagin activity, mast cell fixation

*Alternate notation, no longer considered acceptable.

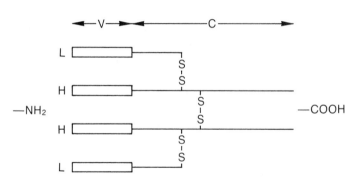

Figure 3–14. Diagrammatic sketch showing that the immunoglobulin molecule consists of four polypeptide chains: two heavy chains (H) and two light chains (L), joined as indicated by disulfide bonds. The amino-terminal (—NH₂) ends of the chains are at the left and the carboxyl-terminal (—COOH) ends at the right. The amino acid sequences of the amino-terminal ends of the chains are variable (V); those of the remainder of the chains are constant (C).

possesses most of the antigenic properties that distinguish the immunoglobulin class; this is the Fc (crystallizable) fragment.

Digestion with pepsin yields one large fragment, F(ab′)₂, which is capable of precipitating homologous antigen, and several smaller peptides. If the large fragment is reduced with mercaptoethylamine, it splits into two halves that can combine with but not precipitate the antigen. Each is slightly different from Fab in amino acid composition and molecular weight, and is designated Fab′.

Reduction of an intact immunoglobulin molecule splits it into two light (L) and two heavy (H) chains, with molecular weights of approximately 22,000 and 53,000 each, respectively. When papain digestion and reduction are combined, a fragment of the heavy chain known as Fd can be recovered; this comprises the amino-terminal half of the heavy chain, which includes the variable portion of the chain. Its immunologic function is to bind to antigen, and this process is enhanced by the presence of the light chain.

IMMUNOGLOBULIN CLASSES AND SUBCLASSES

The five classes of immunoglobulin are distinguished by the presence of heavy-chain antigenic determinants, which are designated by the lower case Greek characters corresponding to the Roman letters applied to the immunoglobulins:

Immunoglobulin	H-Chain Antigenic Determinant
IgG	γ (gamma)
IgA	α (alpha)
IgM	μ (mu)
IgD	δ (delta)
IgE	ε (epsilon)

There are also subclasses of IgG, IgA, and IgM, based upon other antigenic determinants, which are designated by numerals (e.g., γ1, α1, μ1). Four subclasses of IgG have been recognized, two of IgA, and two of IgM. All subclasses are found in the sera of all normal individuals. The class and subclass determinants are located in the constant region of the chain. The subclasses within a class have the common antigenic structure that defines the class (i.e., the heavy chain antigens γ, α, and μ), and they possess additional antigenic structural features that distinguish each subclass.

IMMUNOGLOBULIN TYPES AND SUBTYPES

The constant portion of the light chain of any immunoglobulin possesses an amino acid sequence characteristic of one or the other of two antigenic determinants, κ (kappa) or λ (lambda).

Both types of light chain are present in all human sera, but the kappa type normally is about twice as abundant as the lambda type. Subtypes of κ and λ determinants have been found. The classes, subclasses, and types of human immunoglobulins are listed in Table 3–6, which also includes molecular formulas indicating the antigenic components of each.

IMMUNOGLOBULIN GROUPS AND SUBGROUPS

Groups and subgroups are defined by antigenic variation based upon differences in amino acid sequence in the variable regions of kappa and lambda light chains and of heavy chains. The first 20 amino acids from the amino-terminal end of the chain are particularly concerned, a region that, according to some investigators, does not participate directly as an antigen-binding site.

AMINO ACID SEQUENCES

The first immunoglobulins for which amino acid sequences were determined were Bence Jones proteins, which are the light chains of proteins found in the urine of multiple myeloma patients, often in considerable amounts and readily secured in pure form. The amino acid sequences of a number of kappa-type proteins are presented in Table 3–7, and data obtained with three lambda proteins are shown graphically in Figure 3–15. It is readily apparent that amino acid variation occurred in approximately half of the positions in the amino-terminal portions of the chains, whereas there were few variations in the remaining portions of the chains. Similar studies of heavy chains

Table 3–6   Classes, Subclasses, and Types of Human Immunoglobulins

H-Chain Class	H-Chain Subclass	L-Chain Type	Molecular (Antigenic) Formula
IgG	IgG1	κ	$(\gamma 1)_2\kappa_2$
		λ	$(\gamma 1)_2\lambda_2$
	IgG2	κ	$(\gamma 2)_2\kappa_2$
		λ	$(\gamma 2)_2\lambda_2$
	IgG3	κ	$(\gamma 3)_2\kappa_2$
		λ	$(\gamma 3)_2\lambda_2$
	IgG4	κ	$(\gamma 4)_2\kappa_2$
		λ	$(\gamma 4)_2\lambda_2$
IgA	IgA1	κ	$(\alpha 1)_2\kappa_2$
		λ	$(\alpha 1)_2\lambda_2$
	IgA2	κ	$(\alpha 2)_2\kappa_2$
		λ	$(\alpha 2)_2\lambda_2$
IgM	IgM1	κ	$(\mu 1)_5\kappa_5$
		λ	$(\mu 1)_5\lambda_5$
	IgM2	κ	$(\mu 2)_5\kappa_5$
		λ	$(\mu 2)_5\lambda_5$
IgD		κ	$\delta_2\kappa_2$
		λ	$\delta_2\lambda_2$
IgE		κ	$\epsilon_2\kappa_2$
		λ	$\epsilon_2\lambda_2$

Table 3–7   *Amino Acid Sequences of Six Kappa-Type Light Chain Proteins, Showing Comparative Variability in Positions 0–108 and Constancy in Positions 109–214**

Region**	Protein	Sequence†	Residue Position (Eu Numbering)‡
(a)	Ag	-DIQM TQSPS SLSAS VGDRV TIT	0–22
	Roy	-DIQM TQSPS SLSAS VGDRV TIT	
	Eu	-DIQM TQSPS TLSAS VGDRV TIT	
	Ti	-EIVL TQSPG TLSLS PGERA TLS	
	Cum	EDIVM TQTPL SLPVT PGEPA SIS	
	Mil	-DIVL TQSPL SLPVT PGEPA SIS	
(b1)	Ag	CQASQ ----- -DINH YLNWY QQGPK KAPKI LIYDA S	23–52 (a-f insertion between 27 and 28)
	Roy	CQASQ ----- -DISI FLNWY QQKPG KAPKL LIYDA S	
	Eu	CRASQ ----- -SINT WLAWY QQKPG KAPKL LMYKA S	
	Ti	CRASQ S---- -VSNS FLAWY QQKPG QAPRL LIYVA S	
	Cum	CRSSQ SLLDS GDGNT YLNWY LQKAG QQPSL LIYTL S	
	Mil	CRSSQ NLLZ- -SBGB YLDWY LZKPG ZSPZL LIYLG S	
(b2)	Ag	NLETG VPSRF SGSGF GTDFT FTISG LQPED IATYY C	53–88
	Roy	KLEAG VPSRF SGTGS GTDFT FTISS LQPED IATYY C	
	Eu	SLESG VPSRF IGSGS GTEFT LTISS LQPDD FATYY C	
	Ti	SRATG IPDRF SGSGS GTDFT LTISR LEPED FAVYY C	
	Cum	YRASG VPDRF SGSGS GTDFT LKISR VQAED VGVYY C	
	Mil	NRASG VPNRF SGSGS GTBFT LKISR VZAZB VGVYY C	
(c)	Ag	QQYDT LPRTF GQGTK LEIKR TVAAP SVFIF PPSNE QLKSG TASVV	89–133
	Roy	QQFDN LPLTF GGGTK VDFKR TVAAP SVFIF PPSDE QLKSG TASVV	
	Eu	QQYNS DSKMF GQGTK VEVRQ TVAAP SVFIF PPSDE QLKSG TASVV	
	Ti	QQYGS SPSTF GQGTK VELKR TVAAP SVFIF PPSDE QLKSG TASVV	
	Cum	MQRLE IPYTF GQGTK LEIRR TVAAP SVFIF PPSDE QLKSG TASVV	
	Mil	MQALQ TPLTF GGGTN VEIKR TVAAP SVFIF PPSBZ ZLKSG TASVV	

Table continued on the opposite page

		134–164						
(d1)	Ag	CLLNN	FYPRE	AKVQW	KVDNA	LQSGN	SQESV	T
	Roy	CLLNN	FYPRE	AKVQW	KVDNA	LQSGN	SQESV	T
	Eu	CLLNN	FYPRE	AKVQW	KVDNA	LQSGN	SQESV	T
	Ti	CLLNN	FYPRE	AKVQW	KVDNA	LQSGN	SQESV	T
	Cum	CLLNN	FYPRE	AKVQW	KVDNA	LQSGN	SQESV	T
	Mil	CLLNN	FYPRE	AKVQW	KVBBA	LZSGB	SZZSV	

		165–194					
(d2)	Ag	EQDSK	DSTYS	LSSTL	TLSKA	DYEKH	KVYAC
	Roy	QQDSK	DSTYS	LSSTL	TLSKA	DYEKH	KLYAC
	Eu	EQDSK	DSTYS	LSSTL	TLSKA	DYEKH	KVYAC
	Ti	ZZBSK	DSTYS	LSSTL	TLSKA	DYEKH	KVYAC
	Cum	QQDSK	DSTYS	LSSTL	TLSKA	DYEKH	KVYAC
	Mil	ZZBSK	DSTYS	LSSTL	TLSKA	BYZKH	KVYAC

		195–214			
(e)	Ag	EVTHQ	GLSSP	VTKSF	NRGEC
	Roy	EVTHQ	GLSSP	VTKSF	NRGEC
	Eu	EVTHQ	GLSSP	VTKSF	NRGEC
	Ti	EVTHQ	GLSSP	VTKSF	NRGEC
	Cum	EVTHQ	GLSSP	VTKSF	NRGEC
	Mil	ZVTHZ	GLSSP	VTKSF	NRGEC

*From Day, 1972. Advanced Immunochemistry. Copyright 1972, The Williams and Wilkins Company, Baltimore.

**(a) N-terminal region of 23 residues; (b) variable loop region with insertion a–f; (c) switch region; (d) constant loop region; and (e) C-terminal region.

†Key to amino acids:

A	alanine	N	asparagine
C	cysteine	P	proline
D	aspartic	Q	glutamine
E	glutamic	R	arginine
F	phenylalanine	S	serine
G	glycine	T	threonine
H	histidine	V	valine
I	isoleucine	W	tryptophan
K	lysine	Y	tyrosine
L	leucine	B	asparaginyl, aspartic, or asparagine
M	methionine	Z	glutaminyl, glutamic, glutamine, or pyrrolidonyl

‡Amino acids aligned to provide maximum homology between proteins, aided by occasional blank (–) insertions. Residue positions numbered according to protein Eu.

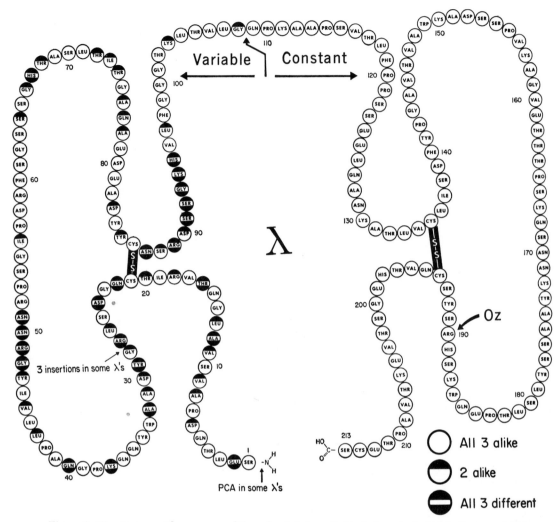

Figure 3–15. Amino acid sequence of three lambda-type light chains, shaded to indicate variability in sequence between two or all three proteins. Variation occurred in 53 of the first 108 amino acid residues from the amino-terminal end. (From Putnam, F. W., Immunoglobulin Structure: Variability and homology. Science, vol. 163, pp. 633–644, 14 Feb., 1969.) Copyright 1969 by the American Association for the Advancement of Science.)

demonstrate that the variable region consists of about the same number of amino acids as the variable region of a light chain; the constant region therefore comprises three-fourths of a heavy chain.

ISOTYPES AND ALLOTYPES

The various classes, subclasses, types, subtypes, and other groups of immunoglobulins that are differentiated by antigens found in all members of the species are known as *isotypes* (Greek, *isos*, equal, alike), and the variation between classes, for example, is called *isotypic* variation. All the antigenic determinants listed in Table 3–6 are isotypic determinants, because they are present in the sera of all normal humans.

Some antigens occur in the serum proteins of only certain normal individuals. These are under genetic control and are called *allotypic* (Greek, *allos*, other) antigens. Often the substitution of a single amino acid at a certain position in the chain, under the control of allelic genes, suffices to alter the antigenic specificity of a protein. Three principal human immunoglobulin allotypes have been described: Gm (IgG marker),

Am (IgA *m*arker), and Inv *(in*hibitor from patient *v* . . .). Three Inv groups have been discovered: Inv(1), Inv(2), and Inv(3). These are characterized by amino acid changes at position 191 of the kappa chain. For example, amino acid 191 is leucine in the Inv(2) allotype and valine in the Inv(3) allotype.

The Gm allotypes involve the human gamma chain in isotypes IgG1, IgG2, and IgG3, but apparently not in IgG4. They usually affect the Fc portion of the chain, occasionally the Fd portion. There are about 25 reported factors at the Gm locus, but only one seems to have been analyzed completely. Gm(1) is represented by the amino acid sequence asp-glu-leu (aspartic acid–glutamic acid–leucine) at positions 356–358, and Gm(−1) is represented by the amino acids glu-glu-met.

There are also two Am allotypes, Am(1) and Am(2), found in the alpha heavy chain of IgA.

Variation at position 190 of lambda light chains, characterized by lys-arg substitution, was originally thought to be allotypic, but instances were later found in which both types of chain were present in the same individual, so this seems to be isotypic variation. In some lambda chains, gly is substituted for ser at position 153.

Numerous allotypes have been found in laboratory animals. Allotypic antigens were detected early by the production in one rabbit of antibodies capable of precipitating serum proteins of other rabbits. Since then, allelic genes have been recognized at several loci, determining upwards of a score of antigenic specificities. For example, allelic forms a¹ and a³ control alanine, glutamic acid, phenylalanine, isoleucine, proline, arginine, threonine, and valine, in the corresponding antigenic sites a1 and a3, situated in the Fd fragment of the IgG heavy chain. Determinants a11 and a12 are methionine and threonine, respectively, located at position 225 in the Fc-Fd or hinge area (see page 73) of the IgA heavy chain. Some of the markers controlled by the a alleles are also present in heavy chains of rabbit IgM, IgA, and IgE. Other heavy-chain allotypic antigens are under the control of alleles of genes d and e, whereas light chain markers are regulated by various b and c allelic genes.

Allotypic antigens so far detected in mice are located exclusively in the heavy chains of subclasses IgG2a and in IgA, but not in IgG1 or in IgM.

Chemistry and Functions of Immunoglobulins

IgG

The structure of IgG is shown in Figure 3–16 in somewhat greater detail than was presented earlier to illustrate the basic structure of immunoglobulins. The intact molecule in its normal, relaxed configuration is represented as T-shaped. The two heavy chains are held together by two disulfide bridges, and the light chains are joined to their respective heavy chains by single disulfide bridges. Within each chain are disulfide bridges, which hold the chain in a loop configuration, the light chains containing two loops, the heavy chains containing four. This is shown more clearly in Figure 3–17, in which V designates the variable regions of the chains, L and H refer to light and heavy chains, respectively, and the entire molecule is divided into domains made up of variable (V_H and V_L) and constant (C_L, C_H1, C_H2, and C_H3) homology regions. Each domain is presumed to have a particular biologic function. The V domains serve the antigen-combining function, C_H2 is believed to provide the point of attachment for complement, and C_H3 probably attaches immunoglobulin to various cells, such as macrophages (cytophilic antibody) and lymphocytes.

The region in which the two heavy chains are joined by disulfide bonds is called the hinge region. Electron micrographs of antibody molecules indicate that the T shape of the relaxed molecule may change when the Fab portions attach to antigen, bending as much as 30 degrees toward a Y shape. It has been postulated that allosteric effects

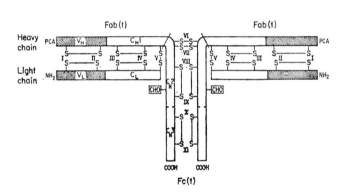

Figure 3–16. Structure of an IgG molecule (diagrammatic). Fab (t) and Fc (t) are fragments produced by tryptic digestion, which cleaves the heavy chains at the positions indicated by dashed lines. Numerals I to XI are cysteinyl residues, which participate in disulfide bond formation. Residues VI and VII join the heavy chains, and the two V residues join the light chains to the heavy chains. The remaining —S:S— bonds hold the chain in loops (two in the light chains, four in the heavy chains). (From Edelman, G. M. Antibody structure and molecular immunology. Science, vol. 180, pp. 830–840, 25 May 1973. Copyright 1973 by the American Association for the Advancement of Science.)

associated with distortion of the molecule make possible various effector functions of the Fc portion. For example, Figure 3–18 illustrates diagrammatically how the complement-combining site of C_H2 might be made accessible.

IgG is the most abundant immunoglobulin in the serum of normal humans (see Table 3–8). It is also found in the tissue fluids, and it can cross the placenta from the maternal to the fetal circulations. It has antibacterial, antiviral, and antitoxic activities in vivo, and in vitro it is moderately to strongly active in agglutination and precipitation, is moderately effective in complement fixation reactions (IgG1 and IgG3, principally), and has opsonic properties. IgG1 displays skin-sensitizing activity, and IgG2 is cytophilic—that is, its Fc region can combine with macrophages, which may then react with the antigen against which the antibody was raised.

IgA

IgA is the second most abundant immunoglobulin in human serum, and it is the chief immunoglobulin in exocrine secretions, including milk and colostrum, tears, nasal fluid, bronchial fluid, gastrointestinal secretions, bile, and urine.

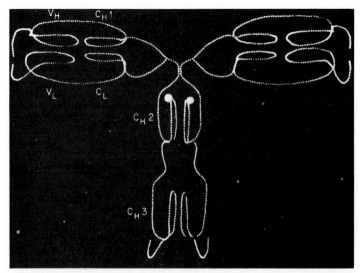

Figure 3–17. Poppit bead model of an IgG molecule, showing the loops that comprise the variable (V) and constant (C) domains of the heavy (H) and light (L) chains. Each bead represents one amino acid residue, and the two large balls represent the carbohydrate. (From Edelman, 1971. Ann. N. Y. Acad. Sci., 190:5.)

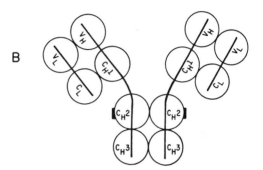

Figure 3–18. The domain hypothesis of the structure of an IgG molecule (A), showing distortion of the normal free immunoglobulin molecule after binding of antigen to the V domains (B). According to this hypothesis, the C domains then participate in effector functions, such as complement binding (at the black area on the C_{H_2} domain). (From Edelman, 1971. Ann. N. Y. Acad. of Sci., 190:5.)

In addition to the usual four-chain structure, IgA also is often associated with two small proteins, secretory component (SC) and J (junction) chain. The heavy chains are serologically distinctive of IgA, because they contain the α antigenic determinant. Two subclasses, IgA1 and IgA2, are found in all sera. IgA tends to polymerize into a dimer form, apparently because of some feature of the heavy chains, especially in secretions.

The secretory component, sometimes called "transport piece," is a glycoprotein, found both associated with dimeric secretory IgA and free in external secretions. It is not present in serum IgA. Its molecular weight is 50,000 to 90,000. It is a β-globulin and contains 9.5 to 15 per cent carbohydrate.

J chain is a small protein of molecular weight between 23,000 and 26,000, found in secretory IgA (and also in some IgM) but absent from normal serum IgA. It is apparently strongly attached to IgA by disulfide bridges; drastic reduction and alkylation are necessary to break the bonds, followed by dissociation with urea, guanidine, or sodium dodecyl sulfate.

Immunoglobulin serologically similar to human IgA has been found in many other animals: primates, dogs, cats, horses, cows, goats, sheep, pigs, and hedgehogs, and immunoglobulins that appear to be IgA are also found in mice, rats, rabbits, hamsters, guinea pigs, and chickens. In most animal species, serum IgA is mainly dimeric. Moreover, it comprises a much smaller fraction of total serum immunoglobulin than is the case in humans. As in man, however, secretory IgA is the principal immunoglobulin of external secretions in lower animals.

The half-life of IgA in man is much shorter than that of IgG (5 to 6 days vs. approximately 23 days).

Most of the secretory IgA is apparently produced by plasma cells beneath the epithelial surface of mucous membranes and exocrine glands. In this connection, it is of interest that IgA-producing cells are practically absent from germ-free animals but appear after a bacterial flora has been permitted to develop. It has also been found that local antigenic stimulation of a mucosal surface (e.g., by BSA injection) leads to appearance in the same site of plasma cells producing chiefly or exclusively IgA

Table 3–8　Physical and Biologic Properties of Human Immunoglobulins

	IgG1	IgG2	IgG3	IgG4	IgA SERUM	IgA SECRETORY	IgM	IgD	IgE
Electrophoretic mobility	α2–γ2				β2–γ1		β2–γ1	β2–γ1	γ1
Sedimentation coefficient	7S				7S, 9.6S	11S	19S (26S, 32S)	7S	7S
Molecular weight	150,000				160,000, 318,000	370,000–390,000	800,000–950,000	180,000	190,000
Heavy chain	γ				α		μ	δ	ε
Molecular weight	53,000				52,000–58,000		65,000–70,000	61,000–65,000	71,000–73,000
Light chains	κ, λ				κ, λ		κ, λ	κ, λ	κ, λ
Molecular weight	22,000 each				22,000 each		22,000 each	22,000 each	22,000 each
Carbohydrate (%)	2.9				7.5		11.8	12	10.7
Half-life (days)	23				5.8		5.1	2.8	2.4
Mean serum concentration (mg./ml.)	12				2.5		0.93	0.03	0.00003
Distribution (% of total in intravascular space)	45				42		76	75	51
Synthetic rate (mg./kg./day)	33				24		6.7	0.4	0.02
Per cent of total immunoglobulin	80				16		4	0.001	0.00003
Serologic properties (in vitro) Sensitivity to 2-mercaptoethanol	—				+		+	?	+
Agglutination	Moderate				Weak		Strong	?	?
Precipitation	Strong				Weak		Variable	?	–
Complement fixation	++	+	+++	–	–		Strong	?	?
Cytolysis	+				?		+	?	–
Opsonization	+						+	?	?
Immunologic properties (in vivo)	"Late" response to antigen; antibacterial, antitoxic, antiviral; blood group antibodies				Antibacterial, respiratory virus defense; blood group antibodies	Activity greater in secretions than in serum	"Early" response to antigen; antibacterial, antiviral; blood group antibodies	Unknown; antinuclear antibodies in some SLE and rheumatoid patients	Allergic reagin, possible respiratory tract defense
Cytophilic activity	+	+							
PCA activity (heterologous skin)	+		–	+					+ in monkey
Prausnitz-Küstner reaction									+ in man
Special biologic properties	Major immunoglobulin in serum Placental transfer (all subclasses)				Major immunoglobulin in human saliva, colostrum, nasal and bronchial fluids, intestinal tract, urine			Unknown	Fixation to skin

antibody against the homologous antigen. The functions of SC and J chain are not clear, but their presence in secretory IgA and not in serum IgA suggests that they have some role in the secretory process by which the immunoglobulin crosses the epithelial barrier separating the secretion from the interstitial fluid.

Serum IgA is synthesized both in the lymphoid tissues, such as the lymph nodes and spleen, and in the exocrine glands and mucosae. The digestive mucous membranes in particular contain great numbers of IgA-producing plasma cells, and some of the IgA produced in them finds its way in the mesenteric lymph to the blood. It is also of interest that oral immunization against certain antigens induces exclusively or predominantly IgA, and even though it may be found in the serum, its origin is apparently the gut.

The significance of secretory IgA is not clear. It appears to have protective functions, as shown by observations of spontaneously infected or artificially vaccinated humans, but the mechanism of protection is uncertain. Conflicting reports are found regarding the lytic, complement-fixing, and opsonic activities of IgA. A healthy individual may completely lack IgA, but this may be because IgM performs the same functions in secretions.

IgM

IgM is characterized by possession of heavy chains with the amino acid sequence that defines the antigenic determinant μ. It was at first thought to occur only as a macroglobulin with sedimentation coefficient 19S and molecular weight 900,000 to 1,000,000, but later it was found to comprise a spectrum of immunoglobulins ranging in size from 7S (M.W. ca. 174,000) to 26S and 32S. However, the 19S component is the most abundant, comprising about 85 per cent of IgM. It is a pentamer, each subunit of which consists of the usual two heavy and two light chains. Electron microscopic and other evidence indicates that the subunits are arranged in a pentagonal form, in which the Fc portions of each subunit are joined by disulfide bridges (Figure 3–19). Each subunit resembles an IgG molecule but possesses more carbohydrate residues.

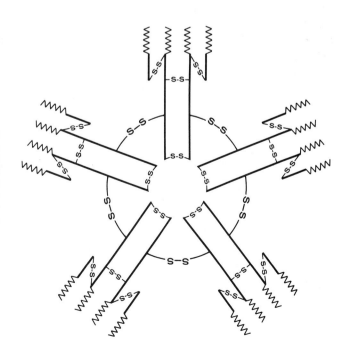

Figure 3–19. Diagrammatic representation of the pentameric form of IgM. Each monomer consists of two heavy chains and two light chains joined by —S:S—bonds, with the variable regions exposed, and the monomers are also joined by —S:S—bonds. (From Putnam et al., 1971. Ann. N. Y. Acad. Sci., 190:83.)

Whereas IgG has only one carbohydrate residue per heavy chain, IgM has five, as shown in Figure 3–20. C1, C2, and C3 are complex, containing fucose, mannose, galactose, N-acetylglucosamine, and possibly sialic acid, arranged in a highly branched structure. C4 and C5 are simple and contain only mannose and N-acetylglucosamine in an unbranched, linear array. The carbohydrate groups affect the conformation and general properties of the immunoglobulin but do not contribute to antibody specificity. They are probably located on the surface of the molecule.

Reduction with thiols breaks IgM into its constituent subunits, which can be stabilized by alkylation, with essentially the same results as are obtained with IgG, when allowance is made for the pentameric structure of IgM. The molecular weight of each of the five fractions obtained is about 180,000. A simple test that is commonly used to help distinguish IgM from IgG antibody (e.g., in studying the sequence of antibody classes produced following immunization) is to treat a portion of the antiserum with 2-mercaptoethanol (2-ME) before setting up antibody titration. If the titer obtained with treated antiserum is the same as that with untreated serum, the active antibody is considered to be IgG; if the titer obtained with treated antiserum is less, the difference represents IgM. It should be pointed out, however, that IgA is also sensitive to 2-ME.

Trypsin splits IgM into 5 F(ab')$_2\mu$ fragments, which can be converted to 10 Fabμ units by continued digestion. Each Fabμ fragment has only one antigen-binding site. Papain digestion of IgM yields F(c)$_5\mu$ with a molecular weight of 320,000.

Electron micrographs obtained by negative staining show star-shaped structures, usually with five arms radiating from a central ring or disc. The arms are sometimes seen to be branches (Figure 3–21). IgM combined with an antigen sometimes appears in cross-section like a staple (Figure 3–22). Feinstein et al. constructed a schematic model to represent their interpretation of the structure of the immunoglobulin (Figure 3–23).

The J piece of IgM is apparently present in the proportion of about one per entire pentamer. It seems to comprise part of the Fc fragment and is absent from the Fab portion. It is rich in cysteine and is probably attached by a disulfide bond to the bridge that holds the subunits together and acts in some way to stabilize the pentamer.

A distinguishing feature of the IgM function is its strong cytolytic and complement-fixing activity, which far exceeds that of IgG. A single molecule of IgM, attached to an antigenic cell surface, is sufficient to fix C1, the first component of complement, whereas two IgG antibody molecules side by side are apparently required for the same operation. This is the first step in any complement-mediated reaction (see Chap. 8). Moreover, Cl is activated more rapidly and completely by IgM

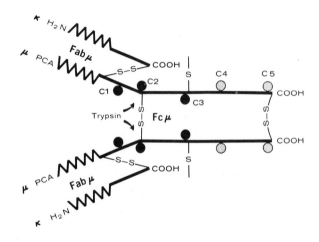

Figure 3–20. A more detailed diagram of an IgM monomer subunit than that shown in Figure 3–19. C1 to C5 are oligosaccharides associated with the Fc portion of the heavy chains. (From Shimizu et al., 1971. Nature [New Biol.] 231:73.)

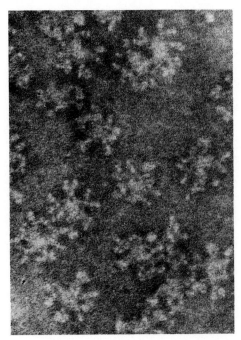

Figure 3–21. Electron micrograph of an IgM molecule. (Courtesy of Dr. R. Dourmashkin.)

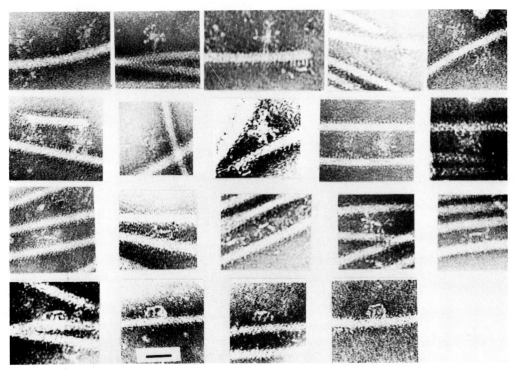

Figure 3–22. Electron micrograph showing IgM antibody molecules attached to bacterial flagella. Top row, simple attachment; second row, molecules cross-linked to two flagella; third row, "staplelike" forms linked to two flagella; bottom row, "staples" attached to single flagella. The bar in the bottom row is 250 Å. (From Feinstein et al., 1971. Ann. N. Y. Acad. Sci., 190:104.)

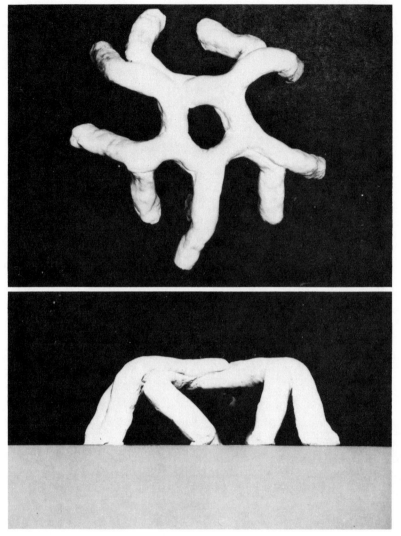

Figure 3–23. Model of IgM molecule by Feinstein and Munn, 1969. Nature (Lond.), 224:1307. (From A. Feinstein and E. A. Munn, Nature 224:1307, 1969.)

than by IgG antibody. It appears, however, that the effect of IgM is limited to the early steps in the reaction between antigen, antibody, and complement, because the final result of the reaction (cytolysis, cytocidal activity) is often as great with IgG as with IgM.

IgM is found predominantly in the intravascular pool rather than in the tissues or secretions, presumably because of its large molecular size. For the same reason, it does not tend to cross the placenta—the concentration in fetal blood is only about 10 per cent of that in maternal blood, and most of this may be accounted for by synthesis within the fetus, which in humans attains substantial proportions by the twentieth week of gestation.

IgM is usually the first antibody to appear in animals or humans following immunization. It is then gradually replaced by IgG. Overall, the daily production of IgM molecules in humans is only about one-twentieth that of IgG; moreover, it is catabolized at two to three times the rate of IgG, so the average concentration in the circulation is only 7 to 8 per cent that of IgG.

In that connection, it has been postulated that IgM molecules serve as antigen-receptor sites on lymphoid cells and that, being penta- to decavalent, they may more readily be triggered to respond to antigenic stimulation than lymphoid cells bearing IgG molecules as receptors. This might account for the more rapid initial IgM response to immunization.

IgD

Very little is known about the structure or functions of IgD. Its status as a separate class of immunoglobulin was established when myeloma patient sera were found that contained proteins precipitated by an antibody to a myeloma protein that lacked antigenic determinants for the other classes of human immunoglobulins. It comprises only about 0.2 per cent of immunoglobulins and, like IgM, is predominantly intravascular in distribution.

IgD has the typical four-chain structure, a sedimentation coefficient of about 7S, and a molecular weight of 170,000 to 180,000. It contains about 12 per cent carbohydrate.

It is present in all normal sera at very low levels. Its antibody activity has recently been established, but its specific biologic functions in vivo are not known. Antinuclear antibodies belonging to IgD have been found in 40 to 50 per cent of patients with systemic lupus erythematosus, and IgD antibodies to bovine serum albumin or bovine gamma-globulin or both were found in patients sensitive to cow's milk. The same patients also possessed antibodies of the other classes.

IgE

The discoverers and leading investigators of IgE are Ishizaka and Ishizaka. In studies of reaginic antibodies active in atopy (a familial tendency to develop immediate-type hypersensitivity disorders), they detected an immunoglobulin that proved to have skin-sensitizing properties and to be responsible for a variety of bronchial, gastrointestinal, skin, and other allergic reactions.

IgE does not appear to differ significantly from other immunoglobulins in molecular weight, amino acid composition, carbohydrate content, and electrophoretic mobility. Although at one time reagins were thought to be univalent antibodies, it was later found that they can agglutinate erythrocytes coated with homologous allergen, and comparison of IgE and IgG antibodies in the same serum showed approximately equal hemagglutinating activity. IgE is therefore bivalent. The molecule consists of the usual four chains, the heavy chains bearing the antigenic determinant ϵ. IgE differs from IgG and IgM in its failure to fix complement.

A feature that distinguishes IgE from most other antibodies is its ability to attach to and sensitize tissues from the same species (i.e., its homocytotropic property). The reactive site is in the Fc portion of the molecule. Skin and respiratory tissues are most readily sensitized by IgE. The immediate response is often the liberation of histamine and/or SRS-A (slow reacting substance of anaphylaxis), both of which are important chemical mediators of allergic reactions (see Chap. 9), and many of the symptoms of allergies are referable, at least in part, to their activities (e.g., mucus secretion by the nasal and bronchial passages in hay fever and asthma).

Important sources of these mediators are the metachromatic granules of the basophilic leukocytes and the mast cells of the tissues. The Ishizakas showed that reaction of an allergen with basophiles sensitized by homologous IgE results in degranulation of the cells and concomitant release of histamine, which then induces whatever effect is typical of other tissue cells it encounters. The same reaction occurs in tissues containing large numbers of mast cells.

Aside from their clinical effects, IgE reagins can be detected in vivo by direct skin test and by the Prausnitz-Küstner (P-K) test. In the former, the allergen is administered by a prick or scratch into the skin or is injected intradermally in very small amounts. A positive reaction appears rapidly, reaches maximum in 10 to 20 minutes, and resolves within 60 to 90 minutes. It consists of an urticarial wheal and erythematous flare, often with itching. The wheal is due to increased flow of blood serum through capillary walls made more permeable by histamine.

In the P-K test, serum from the hypersensitive individual is transferred to a normal recipient, whose skin is then tested with the suspected allergen. If the specific IgE is present in the serum, the recipient develops a positive wheal and flare reaction. This test is no longer used with humans because of the danger of transferring the serum hepatitis virus from an individual who may not realize he is infected.

IgE can also be detected by use of an antiserum against IgE (specifically, the ϵ heavy-chain antigenic determinants). The anti-IgE antibodies are radiolabeled with ^{125}I. The allergen is coated onto Sephadex or other particles, which are allowed to react with the IgE-containing serum, washed, and then treated with the radiolabeled anti-IgE. The amount of label on the particles is then counted, and the result indicates the amount of specific IgE in the serum specimen. A similar method can be used to determine total IgE—reaginic and nonreaginic.

Although IgE is the least abundant immunoglobulin in the blood and has the shortest half-life (2.3 days), it is probably produced continuously and fairly rapidly in atopic patients, because IgE levels in such patients may rise steeply during the allergen season (in cases of perennial allergy) or following exposure to other types of incitant. IgE-forming cells are widely distributed around the body, and they include the tonsils and adenoids, bronchial and peritoneal lymph nodes, respiratory mucosa (nasal, tracheal, and bronchial), and gastrointestinal mucosa. Plasma cells and even germinal centers are abundant in these various tissues, and it has been postulated that IgE antibody is formed locally in the organ and participates in causing allergic disease involving that organ.

Additional Sources of Information

Abramoff, P., and M. LaVia: Biology of the Immune Response. 1970. New York, McGraw-Hill Book Company.

Bellanti, J. A.: Immunology. 1971. Philadelphia, W. B. Saunders Company.

Bennich, H., and S. G. O. Johansson: Structure and function of human immunoglobulin E. In Dixon, F. J., and H. G. Kunkel (Eds.): Advances in Immunology, vol. 13, pp. 1–55, 1971. New York, Academic Press, Inc.

Day, E. D.: Advanced Immunochemistry. 1972. Baltimore, The Williams and Wilkins Company.

Dorrington, K. J., and C. Tanford: Molecular size and conformation of immunoglobulins. In Dixon, F. J., and H. G. Kunkel (Eds.): Advances in Immunology, vol. 12, pp. 333–381, 1970. New York, Academic Press, Inc.

Gordon, B. L., and D. K. Ford: Essentials of Immunology. 1971. Philadelphia, F. A. Davis Company.

Green, N. M.: Electron microscopy of the immunoglobulins. In Dixon, F. J., and H. G. Kunkel (Eds.): Advances in Immunology, vol. 11, pp. 1–30, 1969. New York, Academic Press, Inc.

Hopper, J. E., and A. Nisonoff: Individual antigenic specificity of immunoglobulins. In Dixon, F. J., and H. G. Kunkel (Eds.): Advances in Immunology, vol. 13, pp. 58–99, 1971. New York, Academic Press, Inc.

Inman, F. P. (Ed.): Contemporary Topics in Immunochemistry, vol. 1. 1972. New York, Plenum Press.

Kochwa, S., and H. G. Kunkel (Eds.): Immunoglobulins. In Annals of the New York Academy of Sciences, vol. 190, 1971.

Merler, E. (Ed.): Immunoglobulins. 1970. Washington, D.C., National Academy of Sciences.

Metzger, H.: Structure and function of γM macroglobulins. In Dixon, F. J., and H. G. Kunkel (Eds.): Advances in Immunology, vol. 12, pp. 57–116, 1970. New York, Academic Press, Inc.

Natvig, J. B., and H. G. Kunkel: Human immunoglobulins: classes, subclasses, genetic variants, and idiotypes. In Dixon, F. J., and H. G. Kunkel (Eds.): Advances in Immunology, vol. 16, pp. 1–59, 1973. New York, Academic Press, Inc.

Weiser, R. S., Q. N. Myrvik, and N. N. Pearsall: Fundamentals of Immunology. 1969. Philadelphia, Lea & Febiger.

CHAPTER FOUR

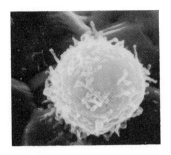

BIOLOGIC ASPECTS
OF THE
IMMUNE RESPONSES

Before discussing theories of the mechanisms of the immune responses, it will be necessary to describe the responses to antigenic stimuli and factors that affect them.

RESPONSES TO ANTIGENIC STIMULI

The immunologic responses to antigen vary with the chemical and physical nature of the antigen and any adjuvant substances that are present; the dosages, manner, frequency, and route of injection; and the genetic make-up of the animal.

The Responses to a Single Injection of Antigen

The gross response of the body to antigenic stimulation can best be observed with reference to a single injection of antigen: (1) it may be strictly cellular, detectable only by some type of cell-mediated immune or delayed hypersensitivity reaction; (2) it may be entirely humoral; (3) it may be both cellular and humoral; or (4) it may consist of specific immunologic unresponsiveness.

Certain antigens, such as glycoproteins on the cell membranes of skin grafted from another individual of the same species, incite a primarily cell-mediated response, which leads to rejection in 7 to 10 days. T cell proliferation can be detected as early as the third day after grafting, and the effector lymphoid cells that are produced interact directly with and destroy the graft cells. Similarly, tumor cells from one strain of mouse injected intraperitoneally into another strain incite the formation of cytotoxic lymphocytes with peak activity 10 to 11 days after injection.

Pneumococcal polysaccharide induces antibody formation in the mouse within 6 days after injection without evidence of a cell-mediated response. *Salmonella adelaide* flagellin, keyhole limpet hemocyanin, and ferritin also cause a purely or primarily humoral response in the mouse.

Other antigens, such as sheep red blood cells (SRBC), produce a combined cell-mediated and humoral response. The former can be demonstrated in mice 4 to 6 days after immunization by the rosette test, in which lymphocytes from the spleen or peritoneal exudate are mixed with SRBC and observed by microscope 2 hours later. The cell-mediated response is also shown by adherence of RBCs in a single layer around some lymphocytes (T cells) (see Figure 2–5). Antibody-producing cells, on the contrary, are surrounded by a cluster of RBCs several cells deep, held to each other by antibody. Moreover, serum from the same mice contains hemagglutinating and hemolytic antibodies demonstrable by separate test tube methods.

Induction of immunologic tolerance usually occurs only when certain conditions are met with respect to the animal, the nature of the antigen, or the dose of antigen. When an animal that is temporarily incompetent immunologically is injected with antigen, it may develop the tolerant state. In the case of a fetal or neonatal animal, tolerance persists indefinitely unless immunologically competent cells are recruited in the absence of the antigen. Inasmuch as thymectomized animals remain tolerant much longer than normal animals, it appears that the thymus is a significant source of immunologically competent cells (T lymphocytes).

As discussed previously (see page 23), induction of tolerance in an adult animal is more difficult than in the newborn. Repeated injections of either a low dose or a high dose of antigen are required in the case of moderately antigenic substances such as BSA; intermediate doses are immunogenic. Low doses of very antigenic substances also induce immunity, but tolerance can be induced if an immunosuppressive agent is used to prevent antibody formation.

ANTIBODY TITERS AFTER A SINGLE INJECTION OF ANTIGEN

The antibody titration curve observed following injection of antigen into a previously uninoculated animal shows four fairly distinct phases (Figure 4–1). There is often a latent or induction period after injection, during which antibody is not detectable or does not increase in the circulating blood. The latent period, which varies from a few hours to several days, is succeeded by a sharp rise in titer. Circulating antibodies increase to a peak or plateau of varying duration and then gradually decrease but may persist in detectable amounts for many months.

The apparent duration of the latent period depends upon the sensitivity of the method used to detect antibody. Complement fixation is 30 to 2000 times as sensitive as precipitation, and passive hemagglutination is even more sensitive. Among the most sensitive are tests for neutralization of viruses and bactericidal activity (see Table 4–1). Obviously, the latent period will appear longer if an antibacterial antibody is detected by precipitation of soluble bacterial components than if it is detected by agglutination of the intact cells, and it will appear much shorter if it can be assayed by a bactericidal test.

Antibodies against particulate antigens, such as bacteria and foreign erythrocytes, are demonstrable in the blood of rabbits within 2 to 5 days after a single intravenous

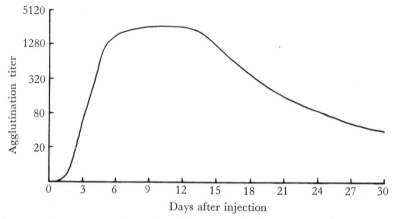

Figure 4–1. Agglutinating antibody in the serum of a rabbit injected once intravenously with approximately 500,000,000 killed Salmonella.

Table 4–1 *Sensitivity of Various Methods of Detecting Antibody*

Method	Lower Limit of Antibody-N Detectable (μg. per ml. or test)
Precipitation	3–20
Immunoelectrophoresis	3–20
Agar gel diffusion	0.2–1.0
Complement fixation	0.01–0.10
Bacterial agglutination	0.01
Hemolysis	0.001–0.03
Passive hemagglutination	0.005
Passive cutaneous anaphylaxis	0.003
Antitoxin neutralization	0.003
Antigen-combining globulin technique (Farr)	0.0001–0.001
Radioimmunoassay	0.0001–0.001
Virus neutralization	0.00001–0.0001
Bactericidal test	0.00001–0.0001

injection. The latent period following injection of protein or other soluble antigens is longer. Dean and Webb reported that 8 days elapsed after injecting horse serum into a rabbit before precipitating antibodies were detected (Figure 4–2). Diphtheria antitoxin appears within 2 to 3 weeks after administration of large doses of toxoid or toxin-antitoxin to guinea pigs or rabbits (Figure 4–3). Burnet found staphylococcal antitoxin in the sera of rabbits injected with antigen 8 to 13 days previously.

Maximum titers may be reached within 3 or 4 days or may be delayed a few weeks. Rabbits usually respond more rapidly than guinea pigs or humans, and horses appear to respond most slowly. Unfortunately, few comparable data are available that take into account the body weights of the respective animals. The persistence of high titers varies greatly and depends in part upon the immunizing material. Diphtheria antitoxin reaches a peak and starts to decrease sharply within 2 weeks in humans inoculated with a single dose of toxoid. It should be pointed out, however, that such individuals possess increased ability to respond to subsequent antigenic stimulation with toxoid and quickly produce high titers of antitoxin. Type-specific antibodies against pneumococcal polysaccharides are produced slowly in man but remain near maximum titer for 5 to 8 months.

The decrease in circulating antibody after the peak or plateau varies with the animal, the antigen, and other factors. Different individuals of the same species vary greatly with respect to the rate at which their antibody titers drop. Jensen reported that the diphtheria antitoxin in one child immunized with toxoid decreased 95 per cent in 3 months, whereas the same loss of antitoxin required 2 years in another child. There are

Figure 4-2. Precipitin titers in a rabbit injected with horse serum. (From Dean and Webb, 1928. J. Pathol. Bacteriol., 31:89.)

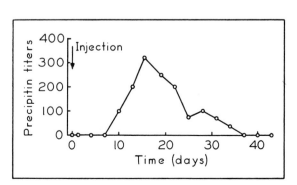

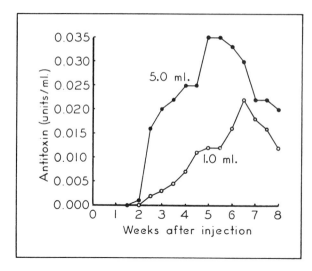

Figure 4–3. Antitoxin titers in rabbits injected intravenously with 1.0 or 5.0 ml. of diphtheria toxin-antitoxin. (Plotted from data in Glenny and Pope, 1925. J. Pathol. Bacteriol., 28:273.)

also wide differences between species, and it is often found that antibody titers diminish most rapidly in animals possessing a high metabolic rate.

Antibody formation is not demonstrable when the dosage of bacterial cells is below a certain minimum (Table 4–2). Topley noted that increasing amounts of antigen yielded greater antibody production but not in proportion to the increments of antigen. Topley and Wilson concluded that a maximum dosage is eventually reached, beyond which no further increase in antibody titer occurs.

PRIMARY VERSUS SECONDARY ANTIGENIC STIMULI

A second or subsequent injection of the same antigen at a considerable interval after the preceding injection usually causes a more rapid rise in titer than the first inoculation, the peak attained is greater, and antibody persists for a longer period. This is the secondary response. It is well illustrated by quantitative data of Dixon et al. obtained by immunizing a rabbit with bovine γ-globulin labeled with ^{131}I (Figure 4–4). In the same experiment the concentration of antigen in the blood was also determined; antibody was not detectable until antigen had disappeared. The latent period was 7 days after the first (primary) antigenic stimulus and 4 days after each of the other (secondary) stimuli. The greater persistence of antibody in man after a second injection of a bacterial antigen is shown by comparison of Figures 4–5 and 4–6.

Certain antigens do not appear to elicit a typical secondary response. Burnet and Freeman reported that Q fever rickettsiae produced no secondary response in rabbits injected intravenously. Heidelberger and co-workers immunized humans with killed

Table 4–2 *Effect of Dosage on the Maximum Titers of Flagellar Agglutinins for Salmonella schottmülleri in Rabbits Injected Intravenously* *

Bacteria Injected per Kilogram of Body Weight	Number of Rabbits	Highest Titer (Averages)
100,000,000	3	3540
10,000,000	3	2480
100,000	6	330
10,000	4	<4

*From Topley, 1930. J. Pathol. Bacteriol., 33:339.

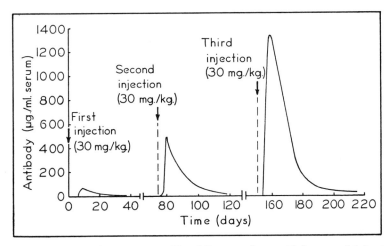

Figure 4–4. Antibody production in a rabbit following three widely spaced injections of bovine γ-globulin labeled with [131]I. (Redrawn from Dixon et al., 1954. J. Immunol., 72:179.)

pneumococci or purified pneumococcal polysaccharide and 2 years later reinjected the same antigen but obtained no rise in antibody. They suggested that the polysaccharide, which is extremely resistant to enzymatic digestion, may have persisted during this time in the antibody-producing cells. The second injection therefore did not provide a new antigenic stimulus. This phenomenon, originally called immunologic paralysis, is apparently an example of high-zone immunologic tolerance. The same phenomenon was demonstrated in mice by Felton. He found that a small dose of pneumococcal polysaccharide (e.g., 0.5 μg.) induced immunity to challenge with living pneumococci, but a dose 1000 times as large induced a state of tolerance that persisted at least 6 months.

The effect of repeated injections of antigen depends in part upon the immunologic condition of the animal at the time of the first injection. A rabbit that is injected with an

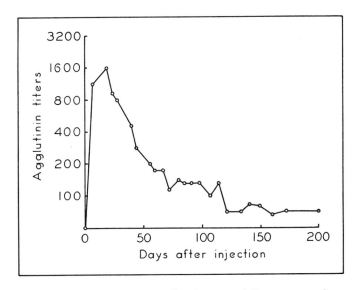

Figure 4–5. Agglutinin titers in an uninoculated person following a single injection of typhoid vaccine. (From Wilson and Miles, 1946. Topley and Wilson's Principles of Bacteriology and Immunity, 3rd ed. London, Edward Arnold and Company, Ltd.)

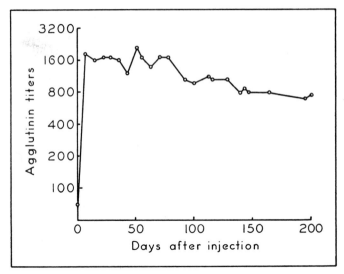

Figure 4–6. Agglutinin titers in a previously inoculated person following an injection of typhoid vaccine. (From Wilson and Miles, 1946. Topley and Wilson's Principles of Bacteriology and Immunity, 3rd ed. London, Edward Arnold and Company, Ltd.)

antigen such as BSA within its first 2 weeks of life may never produce antibody against that protein, whereas injections beginning after the animal has become immunologically competent incite typical primary and secondary antibody responses. Figure 4–7 illustrates this situation diagrammatically. The first animal received 100 mg. of BSA at 3 months of age. For about a week the concentration of antigen in its blood decreased at a fairly constant, moderate rate, owing to normal degradation and elimination, and then it

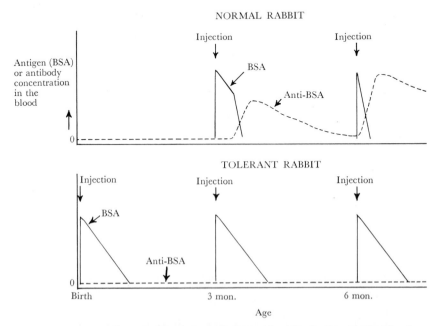

Figure 4–7. Antigen and antibody concentrations in the blood of normal and tolerant rabbits. The normal rabbit received its first injection of bovine serum albumin (BSA) at 3 months of age; the second animal became tolerant following its injection of BSA at birth. Each injection dose was 100 mg. (Redrawn from Burnet, 1962. The Integrity of the Body. Cambridge, Harvard University Press.)

abruptly decreased more rapidly as antibody formed and reacted with it. A later injection of BSA induced a secondary response with prompt formation of antibody and rapid *immune clearance* of antigen from the bloodstream. The second rabbit was injected with 100 mg. of BSA at birth. It became tolerant and produced no antibody; the antigen disappeared from its blood at the constant, moderate rate typical of normal elimination. The response to reinjection at 3-month intervals was essentially identical: no antibody was formed, and the antigen disappeared at the same normal rate.

The characteristic, sharp, secondary-type response to reinjection of antigen may be elicited months or years after the first injection, at a time when circulating antibody is not demonstrable. It was noted previously that 10,000 cells of *S. schottmülleri* per kilogram of body weight produced no detectable agglutinin in rabbits (Table 4–2). However, rabbits inoculated with this number of organisms and subsequently reinjected with the same dose produced a definite antibody response of the secondary type.

Cell-mediated immunity is enhanced by second contact with the antigen. This is illustrated by the accelerated second set rejection of transplanted tissue. The initial antigenic stimulus incites transformation of T cells to blast cells, and replication leads to a large population of cells specifically sensitive to the antigen. Rapid destruction therefore follows subsequent exposure to the same antigen.

Response to Reimmunization

Reimmunization of man is practiced for the purpose of increasing the antibody concentration when the titer has fallen below a protective level. It is illustrated by "booster" inoculations against diphtheria, tetanus, and typhoid fever. With certain antigens the usual course of injections is administered. Typhoid reimmunization may consist of a single intradermal injection of 0.1 ml. of killed bacteria. This procedure is said to give as good results as three weekly subcutaneous inoculations of 0.5 or 1.0 ml.

Antibody titers produced by reimmunization follow the general pattern of the secondary response. A high concentration of antibody is quickly reached and is maintained for many months or years.

THE ANAMNESTIC REACTION

The sudden secondary rise in antibody titer produced by reimmunization or by a second injection of the same antigen some time after the first will be called the *specific anamnestic reaction*. A similar increase in titer brought about by other stimuli will be referred to as the *nonspecific anamnestic reaction*. Specific anamnestic titers are maintained for long periods, but nonspecific anamnestic titers usually drop rapidly.

Typhus fever, lobar pneumonia, tuberculosis and, particularly, infectious mononucleosis have been found to stimulate reappearance of typhoid agglutinins in persons previously immunized against typhoid fever. However, the nonspecific anamnestic reaction is not limited to obvious prior experience with the corresponding antigen. Infectious mononucleosis frequently produces strongly positive Wassermann reactions in persons showing no history of syphilis. Normal isohemagglutinin titers often increase during febrile conditions. Injection of apparently unrelated antigens may also increase circulating antibodies against an earlier immunizing agent.

Other nonspecific anamnestic stimuli include injections of milk, casein, gelatin, and peptone. These and other substances were at one time employed to a considerable extent in *nonspecific protein therapy* of certain chronic infections, such as gonococcal arthritis and salpingitis, rheumatoid arthritis, and some focal infections. Foreign substances of this sort may induce fever, leukocytosis, and a general inflammatory reaction, together with renewed formation or release of antibodies. The possible beneficial effects of nonspecific protein treatment have been attributed to these factors.

The foregoing responses occur even in animals no longer possessing detectable antibody. Repeated bleeding stimulates continued formation or liberation of an antibody that is already present in high titer. Animal sera secured by large bleedings on successive or alternate days often contain a constant or even increasing amount of antibody. The maintenance of antibody titers in spite of bleeding may be caused by liberation of previously formed antibody from body cells or by continued production of antibody globulin in response to the decreased concentration of blood proteins.

White and Dougherty studied the effect of adrenal cortical hormones on previously immunized animals that no longer contained detectable circulating antibodies. A single injection of hormone or of adrenal cortical extract caused the appearance of antibodies in high titer within a very few hours, but these antibodies diminished rapidly and were hardly detectable after 24 hours. Adrenal cortical hormones are strongly lympholytic, so the sudden increase in titer may be due to dissolution of lymphoid cells and release of stored antibodies. The adrenal steroids are among the most powerful anti-inflammatory agents yet discovered, and this property can be expected to decrease the number of phagocytic and other cells available to react with and "process" antigen, and hence to reduce the immunologic response to antigenic stimulation. Use of these immunosuppressive agents in treatment of inflammatory conditions should be limited to diseases in which the immune response is not helpful (e.g., various noninfectious diseases).

IMMUNOLOGIC MEMORY

The rapid and exaggerated response to secondary antigenic stimulation betokens "memory" of previous experience with a given antigen. This is attributed to small lymphocytes, the activity of which can be demonstrated by cell transfer experiments. An animal is injected once with a specific antigen, and, after the usual primary response is detected, small lymphocytes from this animal are injected into a genetically identical animal (in which they will not incite a transplantation reaction). The recipient is then challenged with the same antigen, whereupon it displays a secondary type of antibody response to the antigen. Control animals that do not receive the small lymphocytes or that receive cells from unimmunized animals give a typical, slower, primary response of antibody in lower titer.

The first contact with antigen triggers division of a lymphocyte bearing an appropriate surface receptor, and differentiation leads to a series of plasma cells, some of which produce antibody in large amount, and also to a recirculating pool of long-lived small lymphocytes or memory cells (Figure 4–8). The latter possess the same surface receptors as those of the cell that was first stimulated. According to some investigators, the accelerated secondary response is attributable to an increased number of cells sensitive to the antigen, whereas others cite evidence that the new population includes cells that synthesize immunoglobulin at a greatly increased rate. It may be that both factors are significant.

The Response to a Series of Injections of Antigen

Prophylactic immunization of man or laboratory immunization of animals is almost always accomplished by a series of injections of antigen. Closely spaced injections provide constant presence of the antigenic material within the tissues without exces-

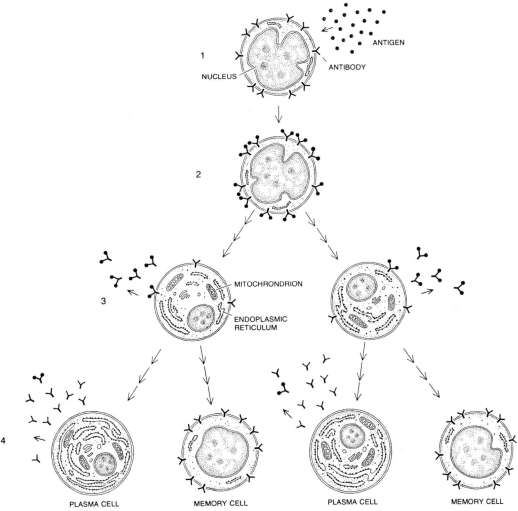

Figure 4–8. The immune response begins when an antigen encounters a small lymphocyte bearing appropriate receptor immunoglobulin molecules on its surface (1). Union of antigen with this cell-bound antibody (2) triggers division and differentiation of the small lymphocyte, with loss and replacement of the surface receptor antibodies (3). Further differentiation yields two kinds of cells (4): plasma cells that actively synthesize and secrete antibody, and memory cells with the same surface immunoglobulin receptors that can respond rapidly to further encounter with the same antigen. (From The human lymphocyte as an experimental animal. Sci. Amer., 228:82, 1973. Copyright © 1973 by Scientific American, Inc. All rights reserved.)

sive danger of toxic reactions that might follow introduction of the total quantity at one time. Moreover, even nontoxic antigens are often more effective antibody stimulants if given in divided doses.

The titer of circulating antibody increases more or less rapidly toward a maximum beyond which additional injections have no effect. Titers attained vary widely. It is not difficult to secure agglutinin titers of 40,000 in rabbits injected with members of the Enterobacteriaceae. Titers produced in man by the routine three weekly inoculations of killed typhoid bacteria are somewhat lower. Gram-positive bacteria induce relatively low antibody concentrations.

The steep rise in antibody that accompanies and follows immediately after the injections is succeeded by a plateau or interval of months or years during which high titer is maintained. Thereafter antibodies in the blood slowly diminish and may eventually (but not always) disappear completely. Antibody titers usually persist at a high level for a longer period following several immunizing injections. Barr and Glenny reported that serum taken from a horse 13 months after the last of 41 immunizations with tetanus toxoid and toxin still contained an antitoxic titer 88 per cent of the value when injections ceased. Two other horses that had been immunized only once or twice retained about 2 per cent of their highest antitoxic titers after 1 year.

The Response to Multiple Antigens

Simultaneous injection of several antigens usually induces antibodies for most if not all of the respective antigens. Hektoen and Boor immunized a rabbit with a mixture containing 35 albumins, pseudoglobulins, hemoglobins, and other proteins and detected precipitins against all except one in the antiserum.

Quantitative analyses of antisera obtained by simultaneous immunization of animals with more than one soluble antigen reveal decreased response to each antigen. Abramoff and Wolfe injected chickens with bovine serum albumin (BSA) and human gamma-globulin (HGG) simultaneously, and the combined antibody response to the two proteins was less than the sum of the responses to each protein administered singly to control birds. Similar results have been obtained with other combinations of proteins: BSA and bovine hemoglobin, ferritin and hemocyanin, ferritin and bovine gamma-globulin. This phenomenon, *competition of antigens*, has been noted in commercial attempts to produce polyvalent antisera for prophylactic or therapeutic use (e.g., horse antitoxins against the toxins of *Clostridium tetani*, *C. perfringens*, and *C. septicum*).

In man, however, combinations of three or four antigens are reported to yield as good antibody production as the respective single antigens. Children are regularly immunized with a mixture of diphtheria and tetanus toxoids and pertussis bacterin. There is evidence that the response to a combination such as this is better than that to the individual components of the mixture. This has been attributed to the fact that bacterial endotoxin in the pertussis bacterin exerts an adjuvant effect (see below).

It must be remembered that any immunizing agent consisting of bacterial or tissue cells is composed of many antigenic components, and that each such component incites formation of separate antibodies. These antibodies do not all necessarily appear simultaneously. Human erythrocytes of types A and B contain agglutinogens A and B, respectively, as well as species-specific and other antigens. A single injection of human A red cells into a rabbit frequently produces a high titer (5120) of A antibody before any human species antibodies appear. Subsequent injections cause the appearance of antibodies against the species antigens, and they may eventually equal or slightly exceed the type-specific A antibody. On the other hand, a single injection of human B red cells into a rabbit almost always induces formation of human species antibodies without any type-specific anti-B fraction. Several injections may be required to develop a satisfactory type-specific titer, which nevertheless seldom equals the titer of the human species antibodies.

Adjuvants

Numerous substances increase the formation and persistence of antibody when injected with the antigen. Kaolin, charcoal, tapioca, lanolin, magnesium and calcium salts, paraffin oil, and bacterial endotoxins are more or less effective. Toxoids adsorbed on aluminum phosphate or hydroxide are more efficient immunizing agents than fluid toxoids. Freund developed the technique of incorporating antigens in paraffin oil as a water-in-oil emulsion and found that one or two injections induced strong and persistent antibody formation. The antigenicity of such emulsions was sometimes further augmented by addition of a second adjuvant, killed mycobacteria (Figure 4–9). Acid-fast organisms improved typhoid agglutinin formation in rabbits but had little effect on production of diphtheria antitoxin. Antitoxin persisted longer following injection of diphtheria toxoid emulsified in oil than following injection of alum-precipitated toxoid.

Paraffin oil and mycobacteria enhance antibody formation, partly by inciting local inflammation; the oil also retards absorption, destruction, and elimination of the antigen and permits continuous antigenic stimulation for long periods. Herdegen, Halbert, and Mudd tested the retention of bacterial antigen in an oil deposit by aspirating material from the site of subcutaneous injection, inoculating it into normal mice, and determining the subsequent production of homologous antibodies in these recipient animals. *Shigella paradysenteriae* persisted in the oil depot as long as 24 weeks, the duration of the experiment.

Herbert made a thorough study of water-in-oil emulsions of ovalbumin in mice injected subcutaneously and concluded that the adjuvant effect of the emulsion was due to slow release of antigen from the inert depot over a long period of time. He reported that ovalbumin was detectable in an oil depot after 544 days.

Freund's complete adjuvant is also significant in the induction of cell-mediated immunity and delayed-type hypersensitivity. These immunologic responses are typical of various chronic infections of bacterial, viral, parasitic, and fungal etiology, and soluble antigens emulsified in Freund's adjuvant induce the same responses. It appears likely that the mycobacterial component of the adjuvant stimulates replication or activity of T lymphocytes, or both. Not only are T cells directly or indirectly responsible for cell-mediated immunity, but they may also participate as "helper" cells in antibody formation. The effectiveness of Freund's complete adjuvant is therefore due to its stimulation of an important cell population, as well as its depot effect.

Endotoxin administered with a toxoid or other soluble protein enhances antibody production against the protein. The adjuvant effect appears to be associated with its toxicity. The inflammatory response to endotoxin is accompanied by an increase in lymphoid cells and macrophages, so the induction period following stimulation is

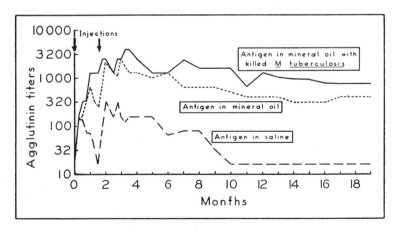

Figure 4–9.   Adjuvant effect of mineral oil and killed *Mycobacterium tuberculosis* on agglutinin titers (mean) in rabbits inoculated subcutaneously with formalin-killed *Salmonella typhosa*. (Redrawn from Freund and Bonanto, 1944. J. Immunol., 48:325.)

shorter, and there is a higher antibody titer, which is attained sooner than in animals injected with antigen alone. Histologic examination indicates rapid proliferation of tissue cells, and it can be shown that antibody-forming cells are more numerous in animals receiving endotoxin and antigen than in animals receiving only antigen. Endotoxin thus enhances the immune response by stimulating multiplication of antibody-forming cells.

Heterogeneity of Antibodies for a Single Antigen

Antibodies produced in response to what is usually considered an antigen are rarely, if ever, homogeneous, even when formed in response to only one immunizing injection. Heterogeneity increases with the lapse of time following immunization and may be more pronounced after repeated injections. The primary characteristics by which antibodies differ from one another are (1) *specificity*, which depends upon the chemical and spatial configuration of the antibody receptor sites; (2) *avidity* for antigen; (3) *physicochemical properties*, such as size, shape, electric charge, and amino acid and carbohydrate composition; and (4) *allotypic specificity*, dependent upon genetically determined differences in amino acid sequences. Secondarily, antibodies may differ in (5) aggregating capacity; (6) complement-fixing power; and (7) biologic activity, including cytophilic properties and cytotoxic and allergic consequences of antigen-antibody union.

It has long been observed that antisera produced early during the course of immunization are narrowly specific, reacting only with certain prominent determinant sites of their corresponding antigens, with which they form a comparatively loose union. Antisera produced later during the course of immunization are more broadly reactive, containing a variety of antibodies capable of combining with a more diverse population of determinant sites, and the antigen-antibody complexes formed are less readily dissociated. Heidelberger and co-workers reported quantitative antibody determinations in the sera of rabbits inoculated with several courses of crystalline egg albumin: antibody formed after later injections precipitated more antigen than that formed early and appeared to react with an increasing number of egg albumin determinant sites.

Numerous investigators, working either with pure proteins (e.g., HSA and BSA) or with azoproteins containing haptens, such as 2,4-dinitrophenol and 2,4,6-trinitrophenol, have found that the concentration of cross-reacting antibodies increases with the duration of immunization. Whereas a few days after the last antigenic stimulation most of the antibodies react with only one or the other pure antigen, in some cases as much as 40 per cent of the antibody present by the ninth or tenth day can react with both antigens. Cross-reacting antibody is obviously of much lower specificity than non–cross-reacting antibody. It is a common observation that the most narrowly specific antibodies are produced when adequate titers can be obtained with few injections. This is of practical diagnostic significance.

It should not be forgotten that the variety of different antibodies produced by injecting a pure culture of a bacterium such as S. *typhosa* reflects the multiplicity of antigens of which the organism is composed. The fact that antityphoid serum agglutinates certain paratyphoid and other bacteria is a consequence of the distribution of common antigens in the various bacteria and is not necessarily caused by variation in antibodies against particular antigenic fractions.

The increased avidity of antibody for antigen that develops during immunization affects both the rate and strength of union of antigen and antibody. It is particularly well demonstrated in the precipitation and agglutination reactions, in which rapid aggregation and low dissociability characterize the activity of highly avid antibody. The avidity of antitoxin was first defined in terms of the rate of neutralization of toxin, but emphasis was later placed upon firmness of union as a more important consideration in the prevention or treatment of disease.

THE IgM-IgG SHIFT

The physicochemical properties of the antibodies produced by a single animal against a given antigen vary during the course of immunization. The first antibody is usually high molecular weight IgM; it appears a few days after immunization, reaches a peak a few days later, and rapidly disappears. About the time that IgM reaches its maximum, IgG appears and increases to a higher maximum, which is maintained longer; it diminishes slowly. This is illustrated by the data of Uhr and Finkelstein. They injected guinea pigs intravenously with varying dosages of coliphage. The resulting 19S (IgM) and 7S (IgG) antibody curves are assembled diagrammatically in the composite graph of Figure 4–10. Following primary antigenic stimulation, 19S antibody appeared in about 3 days, reached a maximum at 7 to 9 days, and declined rapidly. Above a "threshold" dose of antigen, the relative rate of 19S antibody formation was independent of the amount of antigen injected. Figure 4–10 also shows that 7S antibody appeared 7 to 9 days after primary injection of antigen and increased exponentially for 4 to 5 days and more slowly thereafter. Without further antigenic stimulation, 7S antibody could be detected 10 to 12 months later. The rate of 7S antibody formation was directly dependent upon the amount of antigen administered.

Reinjection of antigen 1 month after the first injection produced a 19S response that was essentially the same as that elicited earlier—that is, a response of the primary type. The 7S antibody, however, rose sharply within 3 or 4 days in a characteristic secondary type of response.

Further injections of antigen induced the same primary 19S and 7S responses. Although it is generally believed that one cell produces only a single kind of antibody, Nossal and Lederberg obtained evidence from examination of individual cells isolated by micromanipulation during the early primary and secondary responses indicating that about 1.5 per cent of cells secrete both IgM and IgG simultaneously. Immunofluorescence studies have revealed occasional lymphocytes with IgM on the surface and IgG within. These might be cells in the process of shifting from production

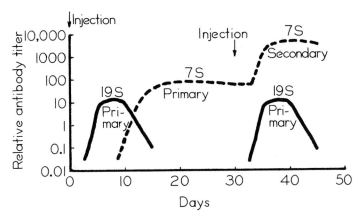

Figure 4–10. Primary and secondary antibody responses in guinea pigs injected intravenously with coliphage. (From data of Uhr and Finkelstein, 1963. J. Exp. Med., 117:457.)

of IgM to production of IgG. Nossal and Lederberg's observations can be explained in the same way.

Not all the factors responsible for the diversity of antibodies are known. The dosage, route, time, and number of injections are important. The route of injection may determine the particular organs within which antibody formation occurs. Minute amounts of antigen injected locally (i.e., subcutaneously) affect primarily regional lymph nodes, whereas antigen introduced intravenously reaches the spleen and bone marrow rapidly. Large or repeated subcutaneous injections eventually gain access to the spleen and bone marrow. All antibody globulins share the common property of combining with antigen, although to varying degrees according to the stereochemical "fit" between antibody and antigen determinant sites, but because of their varied tissue and cellular origins they do not necessarily possess identical physical characteristics. This may, in part, explain the heterogeneity of antibodies produced during continued administration of a single antigen.

ALLOTYPIC HETEROGENEITY

Allotypic heterogeneity of antibodies represents genetically controlled variation in the amino acid composition of immunoglobulin molecules and is shown in differences in their behavior as antigens rather than as antibodies. Most of these differences are found in the constant regions of the molecules, and they have been noted in various species, including man, rabbit, and mouse (see page 70). The occurrence of the Gm, Am, and Inv markers on human γ heavy chains, α heavy chains, and κ light chains, respectively, is controlled by allelic genes, which segregate and assort independently of each other following the usual mendelian pattern.

Most of these human genetic markers are detected by serologic tests with sera from rheumatoid arthritis patients who were accidentally discovered to contain antibodies that react with immunoglobulins of certain other individuals. Similar reagents for recognition of genetic markers in animals are prepared by injecting immunoglobulins into other animals of the same species. Since soluble proteins are poorly antigenic under these conditions, they are usually aggregated by means of homologous antigen. For example, a rabbit antibacterial serum may be used to agglutinate the homologous antigen, and the washed agglutinate is then injected into rabbits genetically different from the one that provided the antibacterial serum. Among the antibodies produced are some that react with allotypic genetic markers of the latter animal.

SITES OF IMMUNE RESPONSE

Sites of antibody formation were first investigated by determining the effect of removing various tissues or organs. As early as 1899, Deutsch found that if the spleen were removed from a guinea pig 3 to 5 days after immunization with typhoid bacteria, less antibody was produced than in control animals. However, splenectomy prior to immunization had no effect, from which it was concluded that antibody was produced both in the spleen and elsewhere.

Removal of the pancreas, stomach, and small intestine had no specific effect on the immune response. Although antibody appeared in the blood, it was not produced there, as Hektoen and Carlson demonstrated in 1910 by means of exchange transfusion experiments in dogs, one of which had received an injection of antigen. The immunized dog produced antibody, despite the fact that its blood was replaced by that of an unimmunized dog; the latter received the blood of the dog that had been injected with antigen, but it did not produce antibody.

Role of the Reticuloendothelial System

After delineation of the reticuloendothelial system by Aschoff in 1924, it was proposed that the phagocytic cells of these tissues constitute the major if not the sole antibody-producing sites. Animals whose R.E.S. was blocked by injection of carbon particles (India ink) or damaged by X-irradiation or benzene injection did not respond to antigen as well as normal animals. However, some of these experiments were rather drastic and undoubtedly caused severe general physiologic injury that might well have interfered with antibody formation.

Histologic studies that seemed to implicate cells of the R.E.S. in antibody formation were reported in 1939 by Sabin. She detected antigen that had been injected *intradermally* or *subcutaneously* within macrophages in the injected areas and in the regional lymph nodes. *Intravenously* injected antigen was seen in the Kupffer cells of the liver, in macrophages of the spleen, and to a lesser extent in the bone marrow. Shortly thereafter, antibody appeared in the blood.

Participation of Lymph Nodes

Evidence of the participation of lymphoid cells in antibody production was provided by McMaster and Hudack in 1935. They injected *Salmonella enteritidis* and *Serratia marcescens* intradermally into mice, one antigen being injected into each ear. The homologous antibody appeared first in the cervical lymph node of the injected side, preceding appearance of the same antibody in the serum. In similar experiments by Burnet and by Ehrich and Harris, antigen injected into the feet of rabbits induced marked hyperplasia of the lymph nodes draining the site of injection and a great increase in the number of lymphocytes in the efferent lymph; the antibody content of the efferent lymph was many times greater than that of the afferent lymph. These experiments were interpreted to indicate production of antibodies by lymphocytes.

This conclusion was supported by the observation of Wager and Chase that the antibody-producing function could be transferred from immunized to normal animals by means of lymph node cells. Rabbits inoculated with diphtheria toxoid were sacrificed 8 to 10 days later, before circulating antitoxin was present, and their lymph nodes were removed, washed, and injected into normal animals. Antitoxin appeared as early as 18 hours after introduction of the cells, increased until the fifth day, and decreased during the next 5 to 9 days. Antitoxin was not found in extracts obtained by grinding or by freezing and thawing the lymph node cells; moreover, transfer of damaged cells did not lead to antibody production.

Stavitsky also reported antitoxin formation in rabbits injected intravenously with cells from animals previously inoculated with diphtheria toxoid. Lymph node cells removed 6 days following *local* injection of toxoid were effective, as were spleen cells of rabbits inoculated *intravenously*. Stavitsky suggested that "the transferred cells either synthesize or cause the synthesis of antitoxin de novo in their new host."

Harris and Harris demonstrated that the cells producing antibody after a local injection of bacterial antigen are confined to the nearest regional lymph nodes, and also these cells continue to produce antibody after transfer to nonimmune animals. They injected typhoid bacteria into the front foot pads of rabbits and dysentery bacteria into the hind foot pads. Four days later the axillary, popliteal, and mesenteric lymph nodes were removed, and cell suspensions prepared from the tissues were transferred to normal recipient animals. The following day rabbits injected with axillary lymph node cells (regional to the injection of typhoid bacteria) contained demonstrable typhoid, but not dysentery antibodies; dysentery antibodies appeared in animals injected with cells from the popliteal lymph nodes (regional to the injection of dysentery bacteria).

Control animals that received mesenteric lymph nodes did not produce antibodies against either typhoid or dysentery bacteria. When dysentery bacteria were injected intravenously into the donor animal, dysentery antibodies appeared in recipients of transferred spleen cells, occasionally in recipients of popliteal lymph node cells, but not in recipients of mesenteric lymph node cells. It appears, therefore, that lymph node cells bear the principal burden of antibody production following local injection of antigen, and that spleen cells are important sources of antibody following intravenous injection of antigen. Both kinds of cells can continue to produce antibody when transferred to nonimmune recipients.

Antibody Production In Vitro

Attempts to produce antibody in vitro became feasible when tissue culture techniques were developed. Carrel and Ingebrigsten added goat erythrocytes as antigen to tissue cultures of guinea pig bone marrow or lymph gland cells and detected opsonizing and hemolytic antibodies on the third and fourth days, respectively. In tissue cultures of spleen, lymph glands, and omental milk spots taken from rabbits inoculated 3 to 5 days previously with typhoid bacteria, Meyer and Loewenthal reported agglutinin titers of 320, a fourfold increase above serum titers in the animals from which the tissues were secured.

Stavitsky injected diphtheria toxoid into the left foot pads of rabbits and tetanus toxoid into the right foot pads. After 1 month the same antigens were reinjected into the same sites, and 3 days later the popliteal lymph nodes were removed and cultivated in vitro. Diphtheria antitoxin appeared in tissue cultures made from the left lymph nodes only, and tetanus antitoxin appeared in the right lymph node cultures. Wolf and Stavitsky later showed that diphtheria antitoxin was formed in tissue cultures of bone marrow, spleen, and lymph node cells in synthetic media containing amino acids. Actual incorporation of amino acids was demonstrated by use of radioactive tracers.

Plasma Cells

The participation of plasma cells in antibody formation was suggested by Bjørneboe and Gormsen (1943) in their report of serologic and histologic investigations of rabbits strongly immunized with a mixture of eight types of pneumococcus. These animals exhibited marked hyperglobulinemia, due to very high concentrations of antibody, and showed evidence of pronounced multiplication of plasma cells in nearly all organs. The number of plasma cells appeared proportional to the concentration of antibody protein. Further observation indicated that plasma cells produced mainly antibody globulin.

Plasma cells do not usually appear in peripheral blood but are found in the spleen, lymph nodes, adipose tissue of the renal pelvis, and other organs, particularly following antigenic stimulation. Their extensive cytoplasm contains a well-developed rough endoplasmic reticulum, consisting of coiled, paired, parallel membranes, which are attached to the nuclear membrane (see Figures 4–11 and 4–12). The roughness of its surface is due to the numerous ribosomes attached to it. The RNA associated with the latter gives the cytoplasm a basophilic character. One of the stains commonly used to detect plasma cells, because of its affinity for RNA, is pyronine, which colors the cytoplasm deep red. The presence of large amounts of RNA, ribosomes, and rough endoplasmic reticulum is typical of cells that produce and secrete protein.

Fagraeus (1948) observed a great increase in the number of plasma cells in the rabbit spleen during the secondary response to intravenously injected antigen at a time

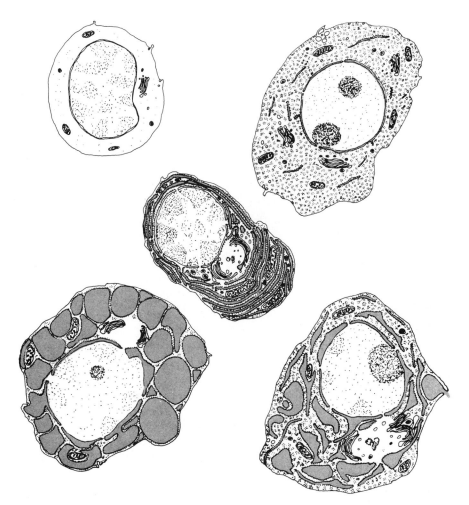

Figure 4–11. Sketches of several stages in the life cycle of plasma cells. *Top left,* A lymphocyte that may be a plasma cell precursor. *Top right,* A plasmablast showing organelles and other structures indicating active protein synthesis: polysomes, rough endoplasmic reticulum (RER), nucleoli. *Bottom,* Intermediate plasma cells with dilated perinuclear spaces and ER, both containing antibody; the outer nuclear membrane is continuous with the ER; these cells are most active in antibody production. *Center,* A classic plasma cell, past the peak of antibody manufacture, with excentric nucleus, deeply basophilic and pyroninophilic (RNA-containing) cytoplasm. (From Leon Weiss, © 1972. The Cells and Tissues of the Immune System: Structure, Functions, Interactions. Reproduced by permission of Prentice-Hall, Inc., Englewood Cliffs, N. J.

when there was also a great increase in circulating antibody. The plasma cells were confined almost exclusively to the red pulp.

Coons, Leduc, and Connolly demonstrated the cellular localization of antibody in animal tissues during immunization with protein antigens by use of the fluorescent antibody technique. Frozen tissue sections of immunized rabbits were treated with a dilute solution of the protein. Antibody present in the tissue, presumably because it was produced there, reacted with the antigen, which in turn combined with the fluorescent antibody. When examined by ultraviolet microscopy, the yellow-green fluorescence of fluorescein appeared in those areas where a cellular antibody-antigen-fluorescent antibody reaction had occurred.

After antigenic stimulation, antibody was first demonstrable in the cytoplasm of large, immature cells in the medulla of lymph nodes draining the site of injection.

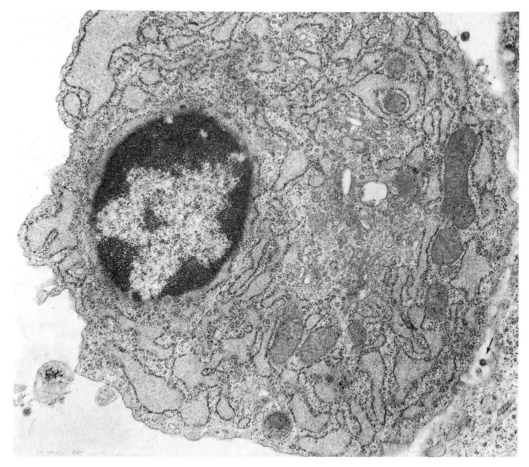

Figure 4-12.   Electron micrograph of mouse tissue culture plasma cell, intermediate size, showing excentric nucleus with marginated heterochromatin, and with much RER in the cytoplasm. (From Weiss, 1968. J. Immunol., 101:1346. Copyright 1968, The Williams and Wilkins Company, Baltimore.)

These cells later multiplied and differentiated into colonies of typical mature plasma cells, and concurrently the concentration of antibody in their cytoplasm increased. The response to primary injection consisted of the development of only a few antibody-containing cells; hundreds of antibody-containing cells appeared in a similar area after a secondary injection. In both cases the morphology of the cells was the same.

Ortega and Mellors concluded from fluorescent antibody studies that γ-globulin is formed in the cytoplasm of plasma cells in the germinal centers of lymphatic nodules. The germinal center cells were arranged in a systematic, discrete aggregation, which seemed to constitute a miniature organ of internal secretion of γ-globulin. Cells that formed γ-globulin in normal animals were of the types shown previously by Coons and Leduc to contain specific antibody in immunized animals.

Antibody Production by Single Cells

The development of highly sensitive techniques for detecting antibody permitted the study of antibody production by single cells in microdroplets or micropipettes. Attardi et al. (1959) immunized rabbits by injecting two serologically unrelated coliphages, T2 and T5, into the foot pad of a hind leg. The popliteal lymph node was later removed, and washed cell suspensions were placed in microdrops or micropipettes with the two phages and a third coliphage, T1, unrelated to the others. Forty-eight hours later the fluid was plated on *Escherichia coli* strains to test for phage inhibition by antibody produced by the lymph node cells; T1 phage served as a control. Fifty-eight of 300 cells tested produced antibody. Phase microscopy indicated that nearly one-third of the positive cells were lymphocytes and over two-thirds were plasma cells.

Nossal studied the primary and secondary responses of rats to flagellar antigens of Salmonella. Following primary stimulation with antigen, 601 cells were placed in microdroplets with motile Salmonella cells; 93 produced antibodies that immobilized the bacteria. All but two of the antibody-producing tissue cells were plasmablasts. These observations support the conclusion that cells of the plasmacyte series are the principal producers of antibody.

Role of the Thymus and Gut-Associated Lymphoid Tissue in the Immune Mechanism

A source from which immunologically competent cells may be directly or indirectly derived was suggested by the observations of Miller (1962) on the effects of removing the thymus before immunization. He thymectomized mice at birth and at various intervals thereafter and found that, when the operation was performed on neonatal animals, there was marked depletion of lymphocytes and serious impairment of the immune response, both to injected cellular antigens (foreign RBCs, bacteria, etc.) and to skin allografts. Thymectomy of older animals had little direct effect, but it did interfere with the ability of lethally irradiated adult mice to regain their lymphocyte-forming and immunologic functions following injection of bone marrow cells. Control animals that were irradiated and given marrow but not thymectomized regained normal lymphocyte populations and immune functions 4 to 10 weeks after irradiation. Miller concluded that the thymus plays an important role in the maturation of immunologic powers in the newborn mouse, and in the adult it may be essential for reestablishing immunologic activity under circumstances in which it is depleted or destroyed.

A few years later, Di George (1965) described a congenital disease in human infants characterized by complete or nearly complete absence of the thymus. The cell-mediated immune responses of these infants were severely impaired, but their humoral immune mechanism was well developed. They produced normal amounts of the immunoglobulins, including serum antibodies, but they did not display delayed hypersensitivity, and they retained skin allografts permanently or much longer than normal. They had a severe but not total lack of circulating lymphocytes, and their lymph nodes and spleens contained greatly decreased numbers of small to medium lymphocytes but normal numbers of plasma cells and germinal centers. Patients with this disease have severe viral, fungal, and chronic bacterial infections. One patient was reconstituted immunologically by a thymus graft from a fetus aborted at 13 weeks, and another, who received a 20-week fetal thymus, displayed normal T cell activity within 48 hours and was vaccinated successfully against smallpox 1 month later.

The Di George syndrome is one of several examples of "immunologic experiments of Nature." Another is congenital agammaglobulinemia, reported in 1952 by Bruton. This disease has been described as an inborn error of metabolism transmitted as a sex-linked recessive trait. Found only in males, it is characterized by the absence of marked deficiency of gamma-globulin in the serum and tissues. Patients therefore usually possess little if any antibody, nor can they produce it in response to infection or attempted active immunization. They also lack normal isohemagglutinins. Plasma cells are absent from bone marrow and lymphatic tissue, even after intense antigenic stimulation. Most cases are now recognized within the first year or two of life by the prevalence of severe bacterial infections.

An early observation of great importance was that many agammaglobulinemic patients had viral diseases, such as mumps, measles, chickenpox, poliomyelitis, and Asian influenza, and recovered with no more or less difficulty than other persons. Moreover, after recovery they appeared to possess a normal degree of immunity to reinfection. It was then found that these individuals responded in an essentially normal manner to immunization and reimmunization with smallpox vaccine. They did not produce circulating antibodies against smallpox, nor against any other viral immunizing agent, but they did acquire specific, active immunity against these and certain other viral diseases.

The likelihood that the response to these viruses is cellular rather than humoral was supported by the response of agammaglobulinemic children to BCG immunization: they developed typical delayed skin reactivity to tuberculoprotein. Moreover, such patients could be sensitized by dermal contact with 2,4-dinitrofluorobenzene and by intradermal injection of diphtheria toxoid or horse serum precipitated with horse antitoxin or rabbit anti-horse serum. The delayed sensitivity could be transferred to normal individuals by subcutaneous injection of the agammaglobulinemic patient's leukocytes, but not by even large doses of serum.

The participation of the bursa of Fabricius in the immunologic response of chickens was discovered accidentally by Glick, an Ohio State University graduate student, in 1954. He had removed this organ from several chicks in the course of experiments on its role in sexual development, since it had been observed to atrophy as the birds matured. Later, a friend borrowed some of the bursectomized chickens to demonstrate antibody production for a class. The demonstration was a failure—the chickens did not produce antibody. Glick and his colleagues reported in 1956 that bursectomy destroyed the ability of chickens to develop humoral immunity. Their paper was published in a poultry journal that was not widely seen by immunologists, so their observations were overlooked for several years.

Between 1960 and 1962 several groups of investigators became interested in the immunology of birds and the role of the bursa of Fabricius and confirmed Glick's findings (Mueller et al., 1960; Warner et al., 1962; Papermaster et al., 1962). It turned out that the bursa of Fabricius is one of the two lymphoid organs in birds, the thymus being the other. As mentioned previously, neonatal thymectomy deprives an animal of the cell-mediated immune response, and bursectomy deprives birds of the humoral immune response. The analogue of the bursa of Fabricius in mammals is still unknown, although it is strongly suspected to be associated with the gut. Bruton's agammaglobulinemia accomplishes naturally in man what bursectomy does artificially in birds.

It is apparent at this point that these experiments of Nature, when finally recognized and understood, confirm what had begun to be suspected; namely, that there are two types of immunologic systems, each of which is equipped to respond to certain antigenic stimuli. The two systems are interrelated, and the humoral system depends in part upon the cellular system for its expression. The cellular system is called into activity by chronic bacterial infections, certain viruses, and various contacts with foreign tissue cells and soluble materials (as in organ transplants, ivy poisoning, etc.). The humoral system responds to acute infections, some viruses, and parenteral experience with foreign cells and substances.

T Cells and B Cells

It will be recalled that the principal cells of the immunologic system are lymphocytes derived from stem cells of the bone marrow. They migrate via the blood and colonize various organs, where they come under the influence of different hormones and other local conditions. Those that develop in the thymus become T lymphocytes, and those that develop in the avian bursa of Fabricius or the mammalian equivalent become B lymphocytes.

Most of the T lymphocytes die quickly in the thymus, but a small percentage survive many months or years, recirculating continuously through the thoracic duct and the bloodstream. Some of these become established in peripheral lymphoid tissues, such as the cortex of the lymph nodes and the periarterial lymphatic sheaths, in the white pulp of the spleen, and in Peyer's patches and other tissues. They are very numerous in germinal centers, especially after antigenic stimulation.

T cells and B cells are indistinguishable by ordinary microscopic examination, but scanning electron microscopy shows numerous surface projections on B cells, which are almost completely lacking from T cells (see Figure 4–13). The surface membranes of B cells possess many immunoglobulin receptors that can react with antigenic determinants, also receptors for the complement component, C3, and for aggregated immunoglobulin. According to most investigators, T cells have fewer surface immunoglobulin receptors and lack receptors for C3 and aggregated immunoglobulin, but they may possess binding sites that attach to heterologous red blood cells, forming rosettes (see page 42). Lymphocyte membranes also have receptor sites for various natural substances, such as streptolysin, phytohemagglutinin, and other mitogens, and in addition they possess antigenic determinants characteristic of the species, the allotype, and the individual.

A normal, small lymphocyte is comparatively inactive. Its nucleus occupies most

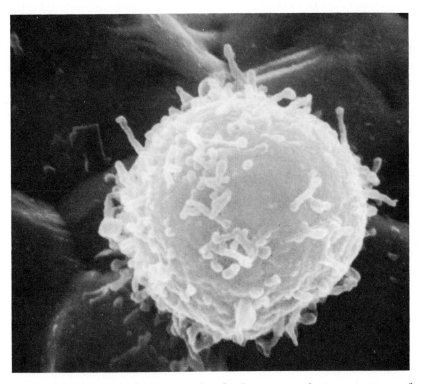

Figure 4–13. Normal human leukocyte viewed under the scanning electron microscope after fixation with glutaraldehyde, critical point dried, and metal coating. Surface microvilli are prominent. The number of these surface structures is generally larger among B lymphocyte populations than among T lymphocytes. Ca. × 13,000. (From Polliack et al., 1973. J. Exp. Med., 138:607.)

of the cell contents, and its small amount of cytoplasm contains few structures active in protein sythesis. It is essentially a resting or nonreplicating cell until stimulated by some agency that causes "perturbations" of the cell surface. These are presumably distortions or disturbances (e.g., alterations in permeability) of the cell membrane that induce allosteric or other changes in more deeply situated organelles and derepress the protein synthesizing machinery, which is normally repressed in a resting cell. The cell then undergoes blast transformation; ribosomes accumulate in the cytoplasm; the rough endoplasmic reticulum, Golgi apparatus, and other structures necessary for protein synthesis develop; DNA replicates, and the cell multiplies. A variety of agents can induce this process. They comprise three principal groups.

(1) Mitogenic agents include phytohemagglutinin (PHA), pokeweed extract, milkweed extract, concanavallin A (Con A), streptolysin, and lipopolysaccharide (LPS) from the cell walls of gram-negative bacteria. These are nonspecific; that is, they induce blast transformation and replication of most lymphocytes without regard to their immunologic properties. Some, such as Con A and PHA in soluble form, transform T cells only, but when attached to Sephadex beads they transform B cells. LPS stimulates transformation of B cells only. Low doses of pokeweed mitogen in soluble form stimulate both T cells and B cells.

(2) Immune or natural antibodies in the serum or body fluids react with homologous lymphocyte cell surface antigenic determinants and incite blast transformation. The antigenic sites include the histocompatability antigens and the immunoglobulin antigens characteristic of the κ and λ light chains, the γ, α, μ, and other heavy chains, and the allotype markers. The antibodies are found in anti-lymphocyte serum (ALS); anti-IgG, anti-Fab, and anti-Fc sera; anti-γ, anti-α, and anti-μ sera; anti-allotype sera; and others. These reactions are highly specific, in contrast to those involving the mitogenic agents just described, but their specificity is determined by and limited to the respective lymphocyte membrane antigens.

(3) The typical immunologic response is induced by the union of extrinsic antigens with antibody-like receptors on the surface membranes of lymphocytes. In an embryonic or newborn animal, each immunologically different receptor may be present on one or at most a few lymphocytes. B cell receptors apparently are complete immunoglobulin molecules, estimated to number about 100,000 per cell. They have been demonstrated microscopically by use of fluorescent anti-Fab and anti-Fc and by autoradiography. T cells seem to have much less immunoglobulin on their membranes—perhaps 100 to 1,000 molecules. There are indications that it consists of only a light chain and/or that most of it is submerged in the cell membrane, only the hypervariable region being accessible as a receptor site. However, Marchalonis and his colleagues at the Walter and Eliza Hall Institute in Australia obtained evidence that T cell surface membranes contain as much immunoglobulin as B cell membranes; it is a 7S IgM, and it appears to be released rapidly from the cells.

The response of lymphocytes to contact with antigen is highly specific, inasmuch as the immunoglobulin receptors on each cell can react with only a single antigenic determinant or with closely related determinants. The response to primary union of antigen with the lymphocytic receptor is blast transformation and multiplication, yielding a clone of cells with the same immunologic specificity as the cell initially stimulated.

The cellular response to antigen varies with (1) the animal (its species and state of immunologic maturity or competence); (2) the antigen (its identity, dosage, living or nonliving condition, soluble or aggregated physical state); and (3) other circumstances attending antigenic stimulation (route of administration, presence of adjuvants, etc.). These and other factors determine whether the observed response is cell-mediated immunity, humoral immunity, or immunologic tolerance. As yet no clear picture of the interaction of all these factors has emerged. Antigens that are immunologic in one animal may be tolerogenic in another, and antigens that incite T cell activity in one species may incite B cell responses in another.

The cells active in cell-mediated immunity and delayed hypersensitivity are solely thymus-dependent, and it has been shown that they do not secrete antibody. However, T cells often cooperate in antibody production and greatly increase the effectiveness of B cells. Claman et al. demonstrated this in mice lethally irradiated to destroy their lymphocytes and restored with either T cells or B cells or both from syngeneic mice. Sheep RBCs were then injected as an antigenic challenge. Animals that had been reconstituted with bone marrow cells alone (principally B cells) or with thymus cells alone (T cells) did not produce significant amounts of antibody, but those that received both kinds of cells produced more antibody than the total produced by the other two groups together. This suggested synergistic cooperation between T and B cell populations.

The cooperative activity of T cells is significant principally when the concentration of antigen is low; injected bone marrow cells alone yield a good antibody response to high concentrations of antigen.

The specificity of T cell receptors is of a lower order than that of B cell receptors, as can be demonstrated by injection of Salmonella flagellar proteins into suitable animals. T cells stimulated by the flagellins of S. *typhimurium* and S. *adelaide* induce delayed hypersensitivity, but the skin reactions produced by intradermal injection of antigen into a sensitized animal are almost identical, no matter which of the two proteins is injected. However, the circulating antibodies formed by B lymphocytes or plasma cells are highly specific and sharply distinguish the two proteins.

Synthetic antigens consisting of a protein to which haptenic groups have been coupled induce both delayed hypersensitivity and humoral immunity. The protein carrier activates T cells, which incite the cell-mediated reaction, while B cells respond to the hapten. T cells are therefore said to be carrier-specific and B cells to be hapten-specific.

Mitchison and Rajevsky reported that a secondary B cell response to a hapten bound to a protein carrier was obtained only when T cells sensitized to the carrier were also present. This is illustrated in Figure 4–14. An explanation offered by this observation is that the T cell receptor site binds carrier determinants and thus concentrates the hapten groups in one area, so that when presented to B memory cell receptors, they constitute a significant stimulus.

When a soluble antigen is introduced into an immunologically competent animal, the nature of the antigen may determine which lymphoid cells are activated. Antigens that consist of repeating identical units, such as pneumococcal polysaccharide, polymerized flagellin, and polyvinylpyrrolidone, are thymus-independent; they stimulate B cells directly and induce the formation of antibody-producing plasmacytes. Thymus-dependent antigens include soluble proteins in general—human gamma-globulin, bovine serum albumin, and so forth. They react with T cells, inducing blast transformation, replication, and development of a clone of cells responsible for delayed hypersensitivity or other manifestations of cell-mediated immunity. Many antigens can react with both T cells and B cells, but the antigenic determinants that react with T cell receptors usually differ from those that react with B cell receptors. Both must be present on the same molecule or cell, the former being the carrier protein and the latter being the haptenic portion.

Although it is not known how the reaction of an antigen with its homologous immunoglobulin receptor triggers the observed response, it seems likely to result from a conformational change in the receptor and hence presumably in the lymphocyte membrane. Either stress produced by this interaction alters the lymphocyte directly, or

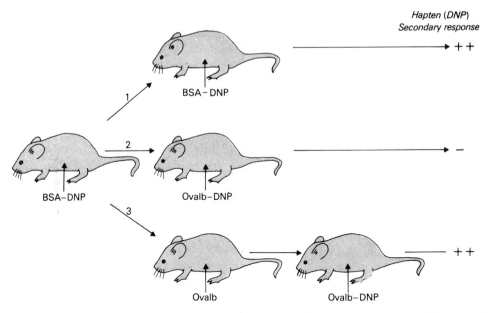

Figure 4–14. An experiment showing that priming with both carrier protein and hapten—dinitrophenol (DNP)—is necessary to elicit a secondary response to the hapten. *1,* A mouse primed with BSA-DNP gives a typical secondary response to another injection of BSA-DNP. *2,* Secondary injection of the hapten coupled to a different carrier (ovalbumin-DNP) does not elicit a response to the hapten. *3,* If the animal is also primed with ovalbumin, it can then respond to secondary stimulation with ovalbumin-DNP. (From Roitt, 1971. Essential Immunology. Oxford, Blackwell Scientific Publications.)

else the antigen, serving as a specific bridge, brings the lymphocyte into intimate contact with another cell, and this changes the membrane or some more deeply situated structure or both. In either case, the primary reaction induces some other event, which causes the lymphocyte to replicate, and eventually it or its progeny cells produce characteristic proteins, such as immunoglobulins or lymphokines.

In order to induce "perturbation" of the surface membrane of a lymphocyte, it is probable that a certain minimal area must be affected. This necessitates an antigen of sufficient size or the presence of several reactive sites distributed in such a way as to involve an adequate proportion of the membrane. The spatial requirement may be fulfilled by aggregation (e.g., polymerization) of the antigen, by use of an antigen containing many repeating units, or by attachment of the antigen to other cells, such as macrophages or T cells, which then "present" a suitable number of antigenic determinants to the antigen-sensitive lymphocyte. This process has been called *antigen focusing.*

CELL-MEDIATED IMMUNE REACTIONS

Features common to cell-mediated immune reactions that distinguish them from humoral reactions include (1) the delayed evidence of response of a previously sensitized individual to a second experience with the same antigen (one or more days vs. minutes or hours); (2) the predominance of mononuclear cells in inflammatory lesions; (3) passive transfer of sensitivity by lymphocytes instead of by antibodies; and (4) the larger size of the inciting agent (i.e., protein "carriers," especially on cell surfaces, rather than small oligopeptide or oligosaccharide determinants).

The essential steps leading to a cell-mediated immune response are illustrated in Figure 4–15. When a thymus-derived lymphocyte is activated by contact with the antigenic protein for which it bears receptors, it transforms into a blast cell and replicates, producing a clone of cells with the same immunologic specificity. The clone includes both long-lived memory cells and effector cells; it is not certain whether they are the same or not. Reexposure to the same antigen causes further blast transformation and replication and also the release of soluble products (lymphokines and "helper" substance) that are responsible for most of the observed cell-mediated reactions.

Macrophages are more abundant than lymphocytes at the site of a reaction of the delayed hypersensitivity type and participate obligately in many cell-mediated immune responses. They may be attracted and/or aggregated by lymphokines and prevented from leaving a site where they have accumulated by migration inhibitory factor (MIF). Macrophages act nonspecifically and presumably are the "angry" cells that kill antigenically diverse bacteria and other microorganisms and participate in graft rejection, tumor immunity, and various drug allergies and autoimmune diseases.

Some of the soluble products released by activated lymphocytes upon specific antigenic stimulation are listed in Table 4–3. In addition to those that act particularly upon macrophages, other lymphokines induce or enhance blast transformation in lymphocytes and promote differentiation in antibody-forming cell precursors. One may kill cultured cells or inhibit their proliferation or clone formation; another inhibits virus replication in cultured cells; and still another produces an indurated lesion when injected into the skin of a guinea pig.

In addition to these indirectly mediated effects, activated lymphocytes may participate directly in the destruction of target cells, such as allograft and tumor cells. The lymphocytes possess specific receptors for transplantation, organ-specific, tumor, and other membrane-associated antigens of various body cells. Sensitized lymphocytes

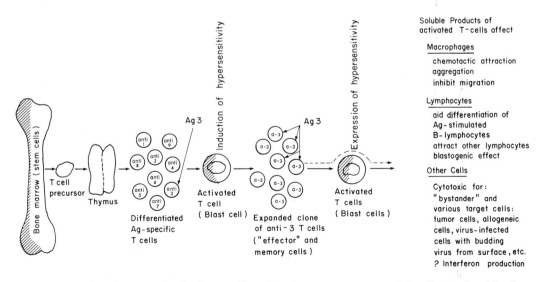

Figure 4–15. The steps that lead to a cell-mediated immune response. A T cell stimulated by the antigen for which it bears a specific receptor proliferates into an expanded clone, presumably including both memory and effector cells. Antigenic stimulation of the latter causes them to release soluble products that are responsible for most of the observed reactions. (From Davis et al., 1973. Microbiology, 2nd ed. Hagerstown, Md., Harper and Row, Publishers, Inc.)

Table 4–3   Soluble Mediators From Lymphocytes

Mediator	Cells or Tissues Affected	Activity
CF	Macrophages	Chemotactic migration toward the factor
AF		Aggregation (agglutination) of suspended macrophages
MIF		Inhibits migration of normal macrophages
BF (MF)	Lymphocytes	Blastogenic (mitogenic) factor: induces blast formation
PF		Potentiates (enhances) blast formation in cultures stimulated by antigen
HF		Helper factor: enhances differentiation of cultured antibody-forming cells
PIF	Cultured cells	Proliferation inhibition
ClIF		Cloning inhibition
LT		Lymphotoxin: damages various cultured cell lines
IF		Interferon: inhibits virus multiplication in cultured cells
MDF	Peritoneum	Macrophage disappearance factor: IP injection causes adherence to peritoneum
SRF	Skin	Skin reaction: indurated lesion in normal guinea pigs

from the spleen, lymph nodes, thoracic duct, and peripheral blood have been found effective. T lymphocytes may be cytotoxic in the absence of B cells and macrophages. Direct contact is established between the lymphocyte and the target cell by a tail-like organelle or "uropod." To be effective, lymphocytes must be viable and metabolically active—cytotoxicity is reduced by agents that suppress RNA and protein synthesis, decrease the rate of replication, or inhibit respiration and electron transport.

HUMORAL IMMUNITY

Humoral immunity is the result of a more complicated process than cell-mediated immunity. The latter is a primitive, relatively crude mechanism for dealing with cells or with cellular constituents or products that are incompatible with the rest of the body—whether they are foreign or are "self" components that are out of control or in the wrong place. Direct cytotoxicity—i.e., hand-to-hand combat—was an early form of defense, partially replaced by indirectly cytotoxic chemical mediators or lymphokines. The antibody mechanism evolved later: it utilized some aspects of the cellular mechanism but added refinements that made it much more subtle. By their presence in the bloodstream and tissue fluids, antibodies protect body cells from direct complicity in surveillance and defense. The T cell system, aided by macrophages, provides cell-mediated immunity; addition of the B cell system with its active protein synthesizing machinery affords an extra level of defense.

Inasmuch as antibody production is a direct function only of B cells, humoral immunity depends upon activation of them. Activation requires the presence of antigen but, as Dutton reasonably assumed, the only thing an antigen can do is to bind to an antibody receptor site. Activation of B cells therefore must be a consequence of this interaction. It might be caused by a direct conformational change in the receptor molecule or, more indirectly, as a result of the joining of two separate receptor molecules by way of an antigen bridge.

B cells possess many surface immunoglobulin receptors. It is uncertain whether a particular number of these receptors must react or whether those that react must be arranged in a definite pattern in order to activate the cell. Possibly both conditions are required. As mentioned previously, substances with many identical repeating groups, such as pneumococcal polysaccharide, polymerized Salmonella flagellin, and gram-negative bacterial lipopolysaccharide, are highly immunogenic and induce antibody formation, even in the absence of T cells. These materials provide a distinctive pattern of antigenic determinants. Antigens that lack this degree of repetition and regularity are thymus-dependent. Soluble plasma proteins, such as serum albumin and gamma-globulin, are poorly immunogenic and do not activate B cells directly. After reacting with carrier-specific receptor sites on T cells, they are presumably concentrated in large enough numbers and in a suitable array to react with hapten-specific receptors of B cells. The resulting conformational change or allosteric effect activates the cells.

There is some evidence that the helper effect of T cells includes or consists of the release of a low molecular weight, diffusible, chemical mediator similar to the lymphokines released in cell-mediated immune reactions, and that this substance activates any B cell within reach that has been sensitized by contact of its receptors with homologous hapten. There is also evidence that the mediator liberated by T cells is a special "carrier" antibody that is cytophilic for macrophages. The antibody reacts with the carrier portion of its antigen, and the antigen-antibody complex then attaches to a macrophage. When the macrophage bears a suitable number of antigen molecules, it provides a stimulus adequate to activate a B cell.

It was mentioned earlier that the first antibody produced after antigenic stimulation is IgM, and that there is a shift after a few days to IgG production. IgM is produced prior to the period of cellular multiplication, and the shift to IgG occurs at about the time when cell multiplication gets well under way. IgM titers are not great, and this antibody is apparently produced by a small population of B lymphocytes. The thymus-independent antigens are especially likely to induce formation of IgM, even in the absence of T cell activity. However, contact with carrier protein stimulates T cells to undergo blast transformation and replication and, according to Katz and Benacerraf, to release the lymphokine-like substance that stimulates proliferation of B lymphocytes and differentiation into antibody-forming cell precursors and eventually into plasma cells. The function of T cells is regulatory, according to this hypothesis. Selective forces triggered by T cells and mediated by the soluble, diffusible substance they release stimulate B cells whose surface receptors have reacted with haptenic determinant groups. Evidence supporting this hypothesis has been derived from experiments in which T cells and B cells were separated by a membrane that permitted passage of such a low molecular weight substance but not of the antigen or the cells themselves.

If the antigen inducing an immune response is a transplantation antigen situated on a cell surface, as is the case when mouse tumor cells are injected into mice of a different genetic strain, both humoral and cell-mediated immunity are produced. Brunner et al. observed that intraperitoneal injection of 30,000,000 viable tumor cells of a DBA/2 mouse line into C57BL mice yielded cytotoxic lymphocytes with peak activity 10 to 11 days later. At the same time circulating antibody appeared, following the usual 19S–7S sequence: 19S antibody reached its maximum at 10 to 11 days, and 7S antibody at 24 days.

IMMUNOLOGIC TOLERANCE

The induction, intensity, and duration of immunologic tolerance vary with the species and strain of animal, its immunologic competence, and with the nature, dosage, and route of administration of the antigen.

In general, rabbits can be made strongly and solidly tolerant to poorly immunogenic antigens, such as serum proteins; mice and guinea pigs can be made tolerant, but the unresponsive state is shorter; and chickens cannot be made completely tolerant, although their responsiveness is reduced. There is often considerable variation between strains of animals. For example, doses of deaggregated (i.e., monomeric) human gamma-globulin required to produce tolerance in three highly inbred strains of mice vary more than 100-fold:

C57BL	0.1 mg.
A/J	0.5–1.0 mg.
BALB/cJ	>10 mg.

The less immunocompetent an animal is, the more easily it is made tolerant. Embryonic or neonatal animals therefore usually become tolerant more readily than adults. Newborn rabbits acquire the ability to produce antibody to BSA at 8 to 21 days, and tolerance is best induced before the age of 9 days. Adult animals can often be made tolerant when antigen is administered concurrently with immunosuppressive agents or measures, such as irradiation, anti-lymphocyte globulin (ALG), 6-mercaptoethanol, amethopterin, cyclophosphamide, and thoracic duct drainage, which reduces the lymphocyte population to a very low level.

Native (serum) protein solutions contain two physical forms of antigen, which can be separated by ultracentrifugation or by other methods. The high molecular weight form (aggregated, polymeric) is strongly immunogenic, whereas the low molecular weight form (deaggregated, monomeric) is tolerogenic. The latter is found in the supernate after high-speed centrifugation; the former is concentrated in the sediment. The aggregated form can also be prepared by mildly heating the native protein.

Some haptens or hapten-protein conjugates that normally incite both antibody formation and delayed hypersensitivity when injected intradermally into guinea pigs induce a tolerant state when administered orally or intravenously, as shown by subsequent intradermal challenge.

Whereas most serum proteins are poorly immunogenic and tend to be highly tolerogenic, bacterial and viral antigens tend to be immunogenic rather than tolerogenic. They may induce a hyporesponsive condition, which can be maintained only by repeated injections. Pneumococcal polysaccharide is an unusual microbial constituent in that it is markedly tolerogenic; it is highly resistant to tissue or phagocytic enzymes and persists in undigested form for many months or years in the animal or human body. Heterologous erythrocytes are good antigens and are poorly tolerogenic.

The dosage of antigen is important. Usually, the greater the dose, the greater are the degree and duration of tolerance, but some exceptional situations have been noted. Weigle found that 95 per cent of rabbits injected with 100 mg. of BSA on the day of birth were tolerant when challenged 3 months later, whereas all rabbits injected twice a week for 10 weeks with 0.01 mg. were tolerant when tested at the same age. The latter animals had received a total dose of only 0.2 mg.

Some species of animals become tolerant when given very low or very high doses of certain antigens, whereas intermediate doses produce immunity. Mice respond in this way to the poorly antigenic substances, BSA and HSA. More highly antigenic proteins—lysozyme, ovalbumin, diphtheria toxoid, and RNase—produce high zone tolerance but not low zone tolerance. As stated by Weigle, the high zone–low zone tolerance phenomenon seems to be demonstrable only when two conditions are met: (1) the animal is able to respond to the immunogenic form of the antigen, and (2) the injected material contains both immunogenic and tolerogenic forms of the antigen. The occurrence of the two-zone phenomenon may then be attributed to competition between the two forms and depends to a greater extent upon the absolute amount of each form of antigen introduced than upon the ratio of one to the other. Only one zone occurs when the animal cannot produce antibody or when only the tolerogenic form is present. The two forms apparently compete for receptor sites, and, if the immunogenic form is present in sufficient amount, an immune response results before tolerance can be produced. Moreover, if the animal cannot respond because of immunologic immaturity or immunosuppression, it displays high zone tolerance only.

Lymphoid cells transferred from a tolerant animal to a lethally irradiated syngeneic animal (which they will "rescue" from death) usually remain specifically tolerant, leaving the recipient unresponsive to the antigen in question. The reverse is not true; that is, it is difficult to transfer a responsive state from a normal donor to a tolerant recipient.

According to one hypothesis, tolerance is the result of damage to the cells that are concerned in the immunologic response, i.e., T cells and B cells. Inasmuch as T cells possess relatively few surface receptor sites, only a low dose of a poorly immunogenic antigen is required to combine with all of them. The result of this union in an immunologically competent animal is blast transformation, the production of more T cells of the same immunologic specificity, and cell-mediated immunity. In immunologically immature, incompetent, or immunosuppressed animals, union of antigen with T cell receptors damages the latter instead of triggering blast transformation. Whether the cell is killed is not known, but in any event it can no longer react with and/or respond to the same antigenic determinant.

Whereas low doses of poorly immunogenic substances incite immunologic tolerance by reacting with T cells, large doses induce tolerance by reacting with both T cells and B cells. It is not necessary that both T and B cells be affected in order to produce the tolerant state: either cell suffices.

Serum proteins lack repeating identical groups and tend to react with T cells, which are carrier-specific, in preference to B cells. The binding of serum protein monomers to T cell receptors either damages the cells so severely that they do not survive or suppresses production of the signal or substance necessary to trigger the usual B cell immune response. It is often necessary to repeat the small doses of soluble antigen at intervals to maintain tolerance; otherwise, cells with surface receptors capable of reacting with the antigen carrier are recruited or arise by somatic mutation, or the damaged cells recover, and an immune response is ultimately obtained.

The native protein does not contain enough of the polymeric form to incite an immune response until the dose is increased to a moderate level. This apparently calls into play the B cell population. With a high dose of protein, immunologic paralysis occurs due to overwhelming of both T and B cells, and persistence of the antigen destroys other cells that arise.

Nossal diagrammatically represented the reaction of varying numbers of antigenic determinants or epitopes with lymphocyte receptors, as shown in Figure 4–16. Haptens alone can combine with appropriate B cell receptors, but they cause insufficient change in the membranes to induce an immunologic response. Two determinants on a carrier also do not cause a response if they are so situated that only one can combine with a receptor. Union of two or three carrier epitopes with receptor sites disturbs the membrane in such a way that an immune response results, but union of two carriers possessing three epitopes each or one carrier possessing many epitopes with immunoglobulin receptors in a given region produces tolerance. The disturbance caused by such an extensive reaction presumably severely damages and even kills the lymphocyte.

Diener et al. proposed that cellular immunologic tolerance is caused by interlinking of receptor sites. In vitro experiments with mouse spleen cell suspensions suggested that, below a certain critical level of interlinking, there is an immune

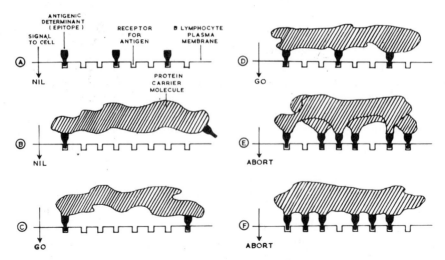

Figure 4–16. Effect of antigen epitope density on the B cell response. Epitopes alone (e.g., haptens) or widely spaced cause insufficient change in the cell membrane to incite an immunologic response (*A* and *B*). Too great an epitope density damages the B cell and prevents an immunologic response (*E* and *F*). Two or three moderately spaced epitopes cause the proper membrane perturbation for a response (*C* and *D*). (From Nossal *In* Amos, B. (Ed.): Progress in Immunology, 1971. New York, Academic Press, Inc.)

response, but above this level tolerance is produced. In the case of polymeric antigens, linear repetition of the determinant facilitates interlinking and induction of the tolerant state. With monomeric antigens, it is more difficult to achieve interlinking of receptor sites, and greater concentrations of antigen are necessary to induce tolerance.

This finding is contrary to the results obtained in vivo and led to the suggestion that a humoral factor such as antibody plays a role in the induction of tolerance against poorly immunogenic substances. This was demonstrated in vitro with mouse spleen cells that were preincubated with a poorly antigenic fraction of flagellin and antibody against polymerized flagellin. The cells became tolerant to polymerized flagellin when the ratio of antigen to antibody fell within a critical small range of values. It was then found that low zone tolerance could be induced in vitro by monomeric flagellin in subimmunizing concentrations in the presence of appropriate concentrations of antibody. It can be concluded that high zone tolerance occurs when lymphoid cell receptor sites are interlinked by polymeric antigens, whereas low zone tolerance is induced when antibody is present to mediate interlinking by lattice formation with monomeric antigen. The source of the antibody is a question. While it is generally believed that T cell surface membranes possess few immunoglobulin receptors, the recently reported 7S IgM that has been called IgT may turn out to be the antibody that participates in low zone tolerance.

MECHANISM OF T-B CELL COLLABORATION

The antigen-focusing hypothesis postulates that T cells "present" antigen to B cells in an arrangement that can incite an immune response. The carrier portions of the molecules of an antigen like serum albumin first react with T cell immunoglobulin receptor sites and bind in a pattern that permits their haptenic groups to react with B cell receptor sites. When this occurs, the B cells are stimulated to proliferate and differentiate into antibody-forming cells.

A further elaboration of the antigen-focusing hypothesis includes participation of macrophages. It is postulated that T cells are activated when the carrier protein unites with their 7S IgM (IgT) receptor sites, whereupon IgT-antigen complexes are released. The Fc portion of IgT is strongly cytophilic and can bind to macrophages. The antigen attached to the Fab sites of IgT is thus arrayed in a configuration that induces any B cells encountered to undergo a typical immune response. Feldmann and Nossal also proposed that, if the soluble IgT-antigen complexes fail to react with macrophage combining sites and reach B cells directly, the latter become tolerant.

Bretscher and Cohn (1968, 1970) postulated that B cell activity is triggered by a sequence of two signals. The B cell receives the first signal from its own receptor molecules upon contact with the antigen haptenic site, and it receives the second signal from a T cell receptor that has reacted with the carrier determinant site of the same antigen. Receipt of both signals induces a humoral response. In the absence of signal two from the T cell, the B cell is tolerized by the signal from its own receptors.

According to Kelman, Dutton, et al. (1971), signal two is a diffusible chemical mediator, not antigen-specific, released by a stimulated T cell. It can signal any B cell within reach, and there is no mandatory requirement for linked recognition; that is, the carrier antigen may be separate from the haptenic portion. Nossal, Miller, and others at the Walter and Eliza Hall Institute also postulated that signal two is short-range and nonspecific and that it may be (a) a factor that attracts macrophages and enables them to dispose of excess antigen in the vicinity of B cells, thus preventing a state of immunologic paralysis due to persisting antigen; (b) a protein (lymphokine) released by macrophages; (c) a B cell mitogen; or (d) an enzyme from activated T cells that cleaves complement. There is evidence that union of the active complement component, $\overline{C3}$, with the C3 receptor site on B cells stimulates the latter to produce IgM or IgG.

MECHANISM OF ANTIBODY FORMATION

Early Hypotheses

The specificity of antibodies strongly impressed early investigators. Buchner (1893) postulated that antibodies might be formed by the union of body proteins with part of the antigen. Doubt was cast upon this hypothesis by repeated failure to detect distinctive components of artificial antigens in homologous antibodies. Animals inoculated with a colored azo-egg albumin antigen produced antibody that contained no colored traces of the antigen. Similarly, antibodies against antigens with determinant sites containing arsenic or iodine possessed no more arsenic or iodine than normal globulin or antibodies against antigens devoid of these elements. Moreover, each milligram of an antigen may call forth the production of as much as 100,000 mg. of antibody, and since only a few atoms of arsenic or iodine may be present in such an antigen it is obviously impossible for each antibody molecule to receive the respective element from the antigen.

Ehrlich (1897) postulated that body cells possess "side chains" or "receptors" consisting of atom groups or substances having an affinity for toxins and other antigens. Chemically different receptors were presumed to combine with different antigens (Figure 4–17). Such reactions occurring upon body cells rendered the receptors useless for their normal functions. The cells therefore produced more receptors, some of which were cast off into the bloodstream. Circulating receptors protected body cells by reacting with antigen in the blood. Ehrlich's hypothesis placed the specificity of antibodies upon a chemical basis and foreshadowed the conclusions reached by Landsteiner and others. This hypothesis encountered opposition when later investigators produced antibodies against synthetic antigens that did not occur in nature and for which cell receptors were presumed not to exist.

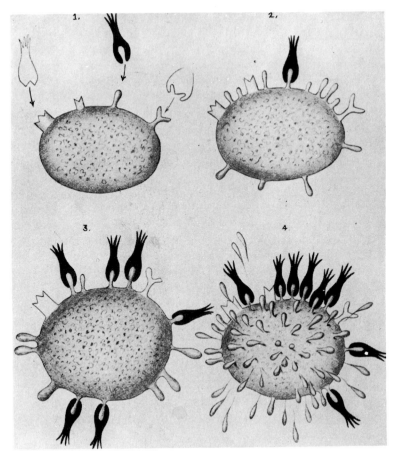

Figure 4-17. Natural chemical receptors on body cells, as pictured diagrammatically by Ehrlich, 1900. Proc. R. Soc. London, Series B, 66:424.

The Template Hypotheses

About 1930 the first of the template hypotheses appeared. According to these hypotheses, antibodies consist of globulin having a reverse structural image of the determinant group of the antigen, much as a series of identical coins represent mirror images of the die from which they are struck. This concept is reminiscent of Emil Fischer's lock-and-key idea of enzyme and substrate. Globulin synthesized in cells containing the antigen bears the imprint of the latter. For example, positively and negatively charged radicals, such as amino and carboxyl, might be arranged in a complementary pattern on the molecules of antigen and antibody.

The template hypotheses were called the "instructive" hypotheses by Lederberg, because they proposed that the antigen introduces new information to globulin-producing cells and instructs the cells to copy it in complementary form.

Breinl and Haurowitz (1930) and Mudd (1932) suggested mechanisms by which the presence of antigen provided an orienting environment that directed antibody formation. Pauling (1940) offered a more elaborate hypothesis (Figures 4-18 and 4-19). Assuming that an antibody molecule contains two specifically reactive sites capable of combining with antigen and that these sites are situated at the ends of a polypeptide chain, he postulated that the ends fold into a stable configuration in contact with determinant sites of antigen. Dissociation of one end and then the other from the

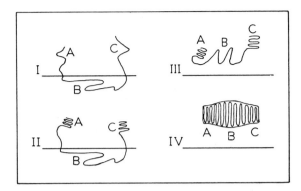

Figure 4–18. Pauling's postulated steps in the folding of a normal globulin chain into its final stable configuration. (Redrawn and reprinted with permission from Pauling, 1940. J. Am. Chem. Soc., 62:2643. Copyright 1940 by the American Chemical Society.)

antigen sets the antibody molecule free to enter the circulating blood and releases the antigen to serve as a template again.

Selective Hypotheses

For nearly 20 years, these and other investigators attempted to secure experimental evidence supporting a template mechanism. However, it gradually became apparent that this hypothesis was untenable. Sensitive techniques for determining the cellular localization of antigens using radioactive tracers were developed, and these methods showed that antibody-producing cells contained few, if any, antigen molecules. Moreover, as methods for determining protein structure improved, it appeared that the tertiary structure of a protein is determined by its amino acid sequence, and it was found that the specificity of an antibody combining site also depends upon its amino acid sequence. Inasmuch as the sequence of amino acids in a protein is dictated by the nucleotide sequence in mRNA, which in turn is transcribed from cellular DNA, it seemed evident that the structure of an antibody is under genetic control. It was even suggested that antigen specifically alters the DNA of a cell, or at least the RNA, so that the cell would synthesize an altered globulin with antibody properties. Since mutational events are known to be random, antigen must function as a selective agent rather than as a mutagenic agent, and this concept led to the selective hypotheses of antibody formation.

Figure 4–19. Pauling's postulated steps in the formation of an antibody globulin, showing how a configuration complementary to the antigen may be produced. (Redrawn and reprinted with permission from Pauling, 1940. J. Am. Chem. Soc., 62:2643. Copyright 1940 by the American Chemical Society.)

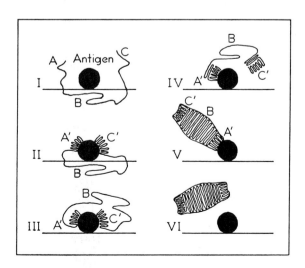

The first selective hypothesis was that of Ehrlich, previously described (see page 111). It dominated immunologic thought, albeit not uncontested, for about 30 years, or until it was eclipsed by the template hypotheses. About 1955, however, several investigators again favored some form of selective hypothesis reminiscent of that of Ehrlich.

Jerne postulated that the γ-globulin of the blood comprises a heterogeneous population of molecules, including some with reactive sites capable of combining with each antigenic determinant to which the individual can produce antibody. An antigen introduced into the body reacts in the bloodstream with one of these natural antibodies having the proper physical and chemical structure and is then removed from the circulation by a phagocytic cell that is capable of producing the antibody. The antigen therefore serves as a carrier of natural antibody to cells that thereupon produce and liberate replicas of the antibody. Antigen injected a second time quickly combines with this antibody and is taken into additional cells, so the process of antibody formation accelerates.

Talmage (1959) accepted Jerne's idea that antigen reacts with circulating natural antibody, but he proposed that production of antibody is regulated by a negative feedback mechanism. Therefore, when the concentration of a particular natural antibody is reduced by reaction with homologous antigen, the appropriate cells automatically respond by producing more of the same antibody.

Lederberg, in 1959, postulated that antibody determinant sites are characterized by unique sequences of amino acids dictated by corresponding unique nucleotide sequences in the DNA of cells where antibodies are formed. Each cell and its descendants produce only one or very few antibodies, and the large number of kinds of antibodies that an individual animal may form during its lifetime requires that its cells mutate at a high rate as they proliferate. A cell beginning to mature spontaneously produces a small amount of antibody corresponding to its own genotype. The cell is then marked specifically by the antibody and is thereby conditioned to react with a given antigen. An immature antibody-forming cell is hypersensitive to the antigen and will be suppressed by it, but a mature cell is stimulated to produce protein and develop into an active antibody-producing plasma cell. Such a cell is genetically stable and generates a cell line or *clone* preadapted to produce the homologous antibody. Even after disappearance of the antigen, the clone persists and retains the capacity to react promptly upon further contact with the antigen.

Burnet's *clonal selection hypothesis*, also formulated in 1959, is the basis for most presently accepted hypotheses of the mechanism of antibody formation. Burnet postulated that antibody-producing cells are members of a population of mobile, mesenchymal (embryonic connective tissue) cells that are constantly changing physiologically and undergoing somatic mutation. A mutant cell migrates to a suitable site, such as the spleen, a lymph node, or an inflammatory depot, settles down and proliferates, and its progeny constitute a new clone. The cells of an immunologically competent clone possess on their surfaces reactive sites analogous to antibody patterns, which can react with corresponding antigens. When stimulated by antigen, these cells produce antibody or proliferate and give rise to antibody-forming cells. A wide range of clones (10,000 or more) arises during prenatal life, owing to the assumed hypermutability of embryonic cells, but clones that encounter homologous antigenic determinants (including those of the same individual animal) are immediately destroyed. The postnatal response to contact with homologous antigen may be one of the following: (1) inhibition or destruction of the cell, (2) liberation of pharmacologically active agents from the cell, (3) proliferation, or (4) transformation to an antibody-producing plasma cell. The exact response depends upon the physiologic state of the animal, the concentration of antigen (and perhaps the timing of antigenic contact), and the site available for development of the stimulated cells.

Immunoglobulin Synthesis

When an antigen is encountered by a B cell or a T cell bearing on its surface an immunoglobulin receptor [Fab or F(ab')$_2$] with the corresponding specificity, a physical or chemical signal stimulates the cell to replicate and initiate a clone of cells capable of synthesizing the same immunoglobulin receptor. The clone becomes established first in the lymphoid tissue (e.g., lymph node, spleen) where the antigen was encountered. Upon further proliferation, cells of the same specificity may colonize other lymphoid areas. Continuation or repetition of antigenic stimulation causes B cells or their plasma cell progeny to secrete immunoglobulin, with or without the cooperation of T cells, according to the nature of the antigen and the attendant circumstances. IgM is formed first, and, according to one hypothesis, the cells that produce it shut down and switch to IgG synthesis. According to another, the IgG-producing cells are turned on more slowly than the IgM-producing cells, and accumulation of IgG exerts feedback inhibition on the latter cells.

Recent studies indicate that immunoglobulin production occurs at a fairly definite stage in the life cycle of lymphoid cells. It has become increasingly apparent in the last 20 years that eukaryotic cellular activities are performed in cyclic fashion; synthesis, growth, and division recur according to a definite pattern and time sequence unless the cell retires from the cycle to a resting phase (Figure 4–20). Starting with the G_1 phase, enzymes for DNA replication are synthesized, along with other proteins. This is followed by the S phase, in which DNA and its associated proteins are produced. Next is the G_2 phase, when proteins needed by the mitotic apparatus are synthesized, and finally mitosis occurs. Cells may enter a "resting" or G_0 state at some time during the G_1 phase.

Immunoglobulin synthesis occurs principally during the late G_1 and early S phases of lymphoid cells. These cells are normally in a resting state, but it is thought that contact with antigen stimulates them to enter an active G_1 phase and begin to proliferate. However, proliferation alone appears inadequate to account for the observed rate of immunoglobulin synthesis, so it is also postulated that cells may enter a condition in which immunoglobulin synthesis begins earlier in the G_1 phase and/or persists longer in the S phase. Alternatively, the cells may be arrested in the late G_1 state and remain actively synthesizing immunoglobulin. There is also indication that, as cells progress through the G_1 phase, the rate of immunoglobulin synthesis increases as much as

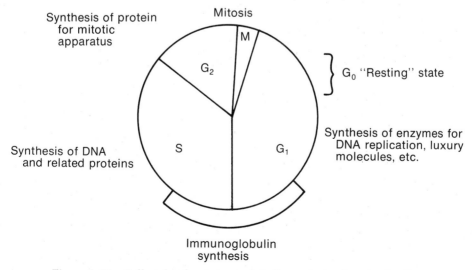

Figure 4–20. Cell cycle of an immunoglobulin-producing lymphoid cell.

fivefold without DNA synthesis or cell division. In any case, the cell is presumed to possess the proper genes and hence the capability for producing a specific immunoglobulin, but expression of the genes is repressed until a signal provided by contact with antigen permits resumption of the cycle.

The mechanism of synthesis is that considered usual for synthesis of any protein. Receipt of the proper signal triggers transcription of mRNA from the appropriate region of DNA, and this is then translated into polypeptide chains on polysomes attached to the rough endoplasmic reticulum.

It is generally accepted that the variable (V) regions and the constant (C) regions of the chains are coded by separate genes. There must be many V genes, one for each different V region, because each of these has a distinctive amino acid sequence. The amino acid sequences of C regions of chains of the same class are identical, so a single C gene suffices. The two genes appear to fuse in such a way that the V region is synthesized first, beginning at the N terminal end, and the C region is synthesized and added to the V chain without interruption.

There is question concerning assembly of the four-chain immunoglobulin from the constituent light (L) and heavy (H) chains. In some cases, two H chains appear to join via $-S=S-$ bonds first, and then one or both L chains attach to the H_2 assembly; in other cases, single H and L chains attach to one another and two HL subunits then join to form the complete H_2L_2 molecule (see Figure 4–21).

Partial assembly occurs on the polysomes, and further assembly takes place in the cisternae of the rough endoplasmic reticulum. Some of the carbohydrate is added to the polypeptide chains at or shortly after synthesis, and the remainder is added stepwise as the assembled immunoglobulin is transported via the smooth endoplasmic reticulum and the Golgi apparatus to the surface membrane, from which it is secreted (Figure 4–21). Studies with radioactively labeled amino acids indicate that 20 to 30 minutes may elapse between initiation of synthesis and secretion of the completed immunoglobulin. The level of intracellular immunoglobulin remains constant, so that the rate of synthesis equals the rate of secretion. Immunoglobulin synthesis (in lymphoid cell cultures) has been estimated to occur at 100 to 1000 molecules per cell per second. Most of the 20 to 30 minutes is therefore taken by the processes of transport from the site of synthesis and secretion from the cell.

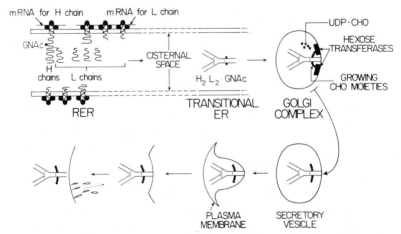

Figure 4–21. Model of the synthesis, assembly, intracellular transport, and secretion of immunoglobulin proposed by Uhr et al. (From Sherr, Schenkein, and Uhr, 1971. Ann. N. Y. Acad. Sci., 190:250.)

SUMMARY

It is presently believed that the immune response is triggered by contact of the antigenic determinant site with its corresponding lymphoid cell surface immuno-globulin receptor. For every antigen to which the animal can respond, there is at least one lymphoid cell bearing the homologous receptor site. Union of the antigen with the immunoglobulin receptor changes the surface configuration of the cell membrane. This, in turn, by an allosteric mechanism, causes the cell to proliferate and differentiate, producing a clone of cells bearing the same immunoglobulin receptor and hence able to react with the same antigen. If they are thymus-derived or T cells, they can react with the antigen directly or through the mediation of low molecular weight proteins (lymphokines), and either destroy the antigen or produce some other significant event characteristic of cell-mediated immunity or delayed-type hypersensitivity. Thymus-independent lymphoid cells develop into clones with highly active protein synthesizing and secreting machinery (rough and smooth endoplasmic reticulum, Golgi apparatus, etc.), and they respond to continued antigenic stimulation by producing immunoglobulins bearing the specific pattern of the surface receptor by which the antigenic determinant was recognized. Antigen-sensitive small lymphocytes synthesize immunoglobulins, which are then deposited in the outer membrane as receptor molecules, whereas the more highly differentiated plasma cells synthesize, transport, and finally secrete immunoglobulins into the surrounding fluid: serum, lymph, saliva, tears, gastrointestinal contents, and so forth.

Five major classes of immunoglobulin are produced—IgM, IgG, IgA, IgD, IgE—each by a different clone of cells. IgM is usually formed first, or at least it is recognized earliest because it is more readily detected by techniques involving agglutination or complement reactions. IgG is detected next. According to some investigators, the cells that produce IgG develop their synthetic capacity more slowly than those that produce IgM, and, when a sufficient concentration of IgG is attained, IgM manufacture is turned off by feedback inhibition. Other investigators maintain that the same cells first produce IgM and then switch to IgG production.

It is presumed that synthesis of immunoglobulin occurs repeatedly at a particular stage in the life cycle of the lymphoid cell, and that the only stimulus required is that necessary to call the cell from its resting state. Synthesis of the polypeptide chains is followed by assembly into the four-chain structure, with the addition of carbohydrate and any other components essential to the particular class of immunoglobulin during the secretion process.

Additional Sources of Information

Abdou, N.I., and M. Richter: The role of bone marrow in the immune response. *In* Dixon, F. J., and H. G. Kunkel (Eds.): Advances in Immunology, vol. 12, pp. 202–270, 1970. New York, Academic Press, Inc.

Abramoff, P., and M. LaVia: Biology of the Immune Response. 1970. New York, McGraw-Hill Book Company.

Amos, B. (Ed.): Progress in Immunology. 1971. New York, Academic Press.

Cinader, B. (Ed.): Regulation of the Antibody Response, 2nd ed. 1971. Springfield, Ill., Charles C Thomas, Publisher.

Cohen, S., G. Cudkowicz, and R. T. McCluskey (Eds.): Cellular Interactions in the Immune Response. 1971. Basel, S. Karger.

Friedman, H. (Ed.): Immunological tolerance to microbial antigens. *In* Annals of the New York Academy of Sciences, vol. 181, 1971.

Janković, B. D., and K. Isaković (Eds.): Microenvironmental Aspects of Immunity. 1973. New York, Plenum Press.

Katz, D. H., and B. Benacerraf: The regulatory influence of activated T cells on B cell responses to antigen. *In* Dixon, F. J., and H. G. Kunkel (Eds.): Advances in Immunology, vol. 15, pp. 1–94, 1972. New York, Academic Press.

Kochwa, S., and H. G. Kunkel (Eds): Immunoglobulins. *In* Annals of the New York Academy of Sciences, vol. 190, 1971.

Mäkelä, O., A. Cross, and T. U. Kosunen (Eds.): Cell Interactions and Receptor Antibodies in Immune Responses. 1971. New York, Academic Press, Inc.

Möller, G. (Ed.): Antigen Sensitive Cells. (Transplantation Reviews Series, vol. 1, pp. 3–149, 1969.) Copenhagen, Munksgaard.

Möller, G. (Ed.): Antigen-binding Lymphocyte Receptors. (Transplantation Reviews Series, vol. 5, pp. 3–166, 1970.) Copenhagen, Munksgaard.

Möller, G. (Ed.): Interaction between Humoral Antibodies and Cell-mediated Immunity. (Transplantation Reviews Series, vol. 13, pp. 3–141, 1972.) Copenhagen, Munksgaard.

Möller, G. (Ed.): Lymphocyte Immunoglobulin: Synthesis and Surface Representation. (Transplantation Reviews Series, vol. 14, pp. 3–210, 1973.) Copenhagen, Munksgaard.

Nelson, D. S.: Macrophages and Immunity. 1969. Amsterdam, North-Holland Publishing Company.

Nossal, G. J. V., and G. L. Ada: Antigens, Lymphoid Cells, and the Immune Response. 1971. New York, Academic Press, Inc.

Porter, R. R. (Ed.): Defence and Recognition. 1973. London, Butterworth and Company, Ltd.

Sercarz, E. E., A. R. Williamson, and C. F. Fox (Eds.): The Immune System: Genes, Receptors, Signals. 1974. New York, Academic Press, Inc.

Speigelberg, H. L.: Biological activities of immunoglobulins of different classes and subclasses. *In* Dixon, F. J., and H. G. Kunkel (Eds.): Advances in Immunology, vol. 19, pp. 259–294, 1974. New York, Academic Press, Inc.

Talmage, D. W., J. Radovich, and H. Hemmingsen: Cell interaction in antibody synthesis. *In* Dixon, F. J., and H. G. Kunkel (Eds.): Advances in Immunology, vol. 12, pp. 271–282, 1970. New York, Academic Press, Inc.

Unanue, E. R.: The regulatory role of macrophages in antigenic stimulation. *In* Dixon, F. J., and H. G. Kunkel (Eds.): Advances in Immunology, vol. 15, pp. 95–165, 1972. New York, Academic Press, Inc.

Warner, N. L.: Membrane immunoglobulins and antigen receptors on B and T lymphocytes. *In* Dixon, F. J., and H. G. Kunkel (Eds.): Advances in Immunology, vol. 19, pp. 67–216, 1974. New York, Academic Press, Inc.

Weigle, W. O.: Immunological unresponsiveness. *In* Dixon, F. J., and H. G. Kunkel (Eds.): Advances in Immunology, vol. 16, pp. 61–122, 1973. New York, Academic Press, Inc.

CHAPTER FIVE

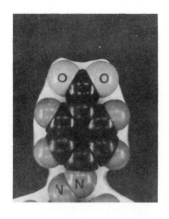

IMMUNOGENICITY AND IMMUNOLOGIC SPECIFICITY

The ability of an agent to incite an immunologic response and the specificity or selectivity of that response are interrelated because the nature of the animal often determines whether or not a response will be detected. A substance may be capable of inciting a response in one animal but not in another. Moreover, the nature of the response varies according to the nature and dosage of the inciting agent. It may consist of cell-mediated immunity, humoral immunity, or immunologic tolerance.

The specificity of immunologic reactions is a structural matter, just as a key conforms to the configuration of the lock it opens. The selective parts of the lock and the key correspond respectively to the determinant site of the immunologic agent and the receptor in the Fab portion of the immunoglobulin, whether the latter is circulating antibody or is part of a lymphoid cell surface membrane.

A cellular or macromolecular agent displaying an appropriate array of determinants incites an immune response when administered to an animal. Such an agent has traditionally been called an antigen, with the added qualification that it will react specifically in some observable way with the antibodies or sensitized cells induced.

A dual definition of this kind suffers the fault that exceptions may be found that conform to one part of the definition but not the other. It was early discovered, for example, that some microbial components do not elicit antibody formation but react observably with antibodies against the intact organism. There is therefore a growing tendency to designate as *immunogens* those agents that elicit an immune response, restricting the term *antigen* to substances that react observably with a lymphoid cell or cell product specifically engendered by an immunogen. In this sense, the word antigen overlaps partially with the word *hapten*, which Landsteiner applied in 1921 to substances that are serologically active in the test tube but do not cause formation of antibodies when injected into laboratory animals.

Topley and Wilson later defined two categories of haptens. *Complex haptens* combine specifically with homologous antibody and yield a visible reaction product but do not stimulate antibody formation. *Simple haptens* do not stimulate antibody formation nor react visibly with homologous antibody but combine with such antibody and prevent subsequent precipitation of the corresponding complete antigen or complex hapten. These relationships are particularly well illustrated by pneumococcal capsular polysaccharides. Antibodies prepared by injecting rabbits with smooth (i.e., encapsulated) pneumococci will agglutinate the intact organisms. The polysaccharide capsular material that can be removed from the organisms precipitates when mixed with the antibacterial serum. Partial hydrolysis of the polysaccharide yields a product that does not precipitate with the antiserum but still possesses specific properties. The hydrolysate combines with the antibody, and this aggregate blocks precipitation of the polysaccharide or agglutination of the intact organisms. This is the *inhibition test*.

The unit determining specificity of an immunologic reaction is small, of the order of Topley and Wilson's simple hapten or the determinant site. It seems to comprise only a few amino acid or monosaccharide residues or their equivalent—four to six residues with a molecular weight of 500 to 1000 (see Table 5–1).

FACTORS DETERMINING IMMUNOGENICITY

It will be recalled that one current hypothesis of the mechanism that triggers an immunologic response is that the inciting agent disturbs or distorts the surface membranes of a lymphoid cell. The immunologic agent reacts with immunoglobulin receptor sites on the lymphoid cell membrane. The activated receptors then migrate toward one pole of the cell, where a "cap" is formed, and the consequent perturbation or distortion constitutes the signal that induces the immunologic response. Present indications are that an appropriate degree of cross-linking must occur in order to produce a response. This necessitates a suitable number and arrangement of immunologic determinants and receptors. It has also been postulated that excessively rigid cross-linkages lead to immunologic tolerance; in this case a cap does not form, but the receptors are "frozen" and temporarily or permanently inactive.

Size of Immunogen

The requirement for an appropriate number and distribution of antigenic determinants properly presented to the lymphoid cell receptor sites suggests that immunogenic agents must be of considerable size. In general, their molecular weights are 10,000 or greater. Egg albumin, with a molecular weight slightly over 40,000, is a good immunogen, as are most blood proteins having molecular weights upward of 60,000. Very large substances, such as hemocyanins (M.W. about 6,700,000) and tobacco mosaic virus (M.W. about 17,000,000), are excellent immunogens. Among small molecules, ribonuclease (M.W. approximately 15,000) has been used to produce precipitins, as has a phenyl isocyanate of clupeine (M.W. about 5,000). Antibodies have been produced in guinea pigs against angiotensin, a decapeptide hormone with a molecular weight of 1,031, and in both guinea pigs and rabbits against the still smaller synthetic compound *p*-azobenzene-arsonate-trityrosine (M.W. 750).

Table 5–1   *Sizes of Some Antigenic Determinant Groups*

Immunogen	Determinant	Dimensions (Å)
Dextran	Isomaltohexaose	$34 \times 12 \times 7$
Poly-L-alanine-BSA	Pentaalanine	$25 \times 11 \times 6.5$
Poly-L-lysine + phosphorylated BSA	Pentalysine	$27 \times 17 \times 6.5$
Poly-γ-D-glutamic acid + methylated BSA	Hexaglutamic acid	$36 \times 10 \times 6$
Sperm whale myoglobin	C-terminal hepta-peptide	$15 \times 11 \times 9$

Structural Rigidity of Immunogens

Immunogens usually possess a large particle or molecular surface. The role of surface area is indicated by the observation that some nonantigenic low molecular weight substances become immunogenic when adsorbed onto inert particles like charcoal, quartz, aluminum hydroxide, or collodion. The important factor seems to be not the surface area per se but the opportunity to display significant determinant groups on the particle surface. A rigid structure is advantageous in formation of cross-linkages on the membrane that contribute to cap formation. The relationship between molecular size and immunogenicity has been demonstrated with Salmonella flagellin, which is isolated in a monomeric form with a molecular weight of 40,000 but can be polymerized readily into a much larger molecule. As described earlier, polymerized flagellin is strongly immunogenic in rats and induces a high titer of humoral antibody. Monomeric flagellin induces less humoral antibody and some degree of cell-mediated immunity. A partially digested flagellin, fragment A, with molecular weight of 18,000, induces little if any antibody but is markedly tolerogenic. These observations can be explained on the basis of the molecular requirement for T cell–B cell cooperation. The polymer activates both T and B cells, with the result that antibody is produced. The monomer interacts with T cells better than with B cells and hence induces less antibody and a stronger cell-mediated immune response. One explanation for the tolerogenic effect of fragment A is that it binds to T cells more readily than to B cells; therefore, little antibody is produced, and that which is formed assists in rigidly cross-linking T cell receptors and inducing tolerance.

Molecular Complexity

Studies with synthetic polypeptides indicate that immunogenicity is directly related to molecular complexity. For example, polypeptides consisting of three or four different amino acids are more highly immunogenic than those consisting of only one or two different amino acids. Among natural products, it has been observed that starch and other simple, repetitive polysaccharides are poorly immunogenic, whereas more complex polysaccharide-protein-phospholipid complexes like bacterial somatic antigens are highly immunogenic. It has long been known that gelatin is a poor immunogen, but it becomes immunogenic after attachment of a few molecules of tyrosine or tryptophan; this was formerly interpreted to indicate the necessity of aromatic rings, but it is now believed that these amino acids increase the rigidity of the molecule.

Number of Immunogen Determinant Groups

Inasmuch as the immunogenic function is accomplished as soon as immunogen determinants react with lymphoid cell receptors, it appears that only surface areas of the immunogen are effective. As indicated in Table 5–1, the size of an immunogenic determinant is reasonably small—the equivalent of four to six amino acid residues. Experience indicates that only a fraction of the surface is sufficiently distinctive to be immunogenically active, and in some cases a single amino acid or monosaccharide may be immunodominant; often this is the terminal unit in a chain. In general, there appears to be one determinant site per 5,000 molecular weight; that is, a molecule of egg albumin (M.W. 40,500) can be expected to have about eight determinant sites. This accords reasonably well with observations based on reactions with anti-egg albumin antibodies, which indicate a combining "valence" of 5 (see page 160). It can be expected that steric hindrance might interfere with expression of all eight determinant sites in formation of a precipitate; moreover, portions of the eight sites might overlap.

Foreignness

Immunologists have long been impressed by the fact that antibodies are not ordinarily produced against the body's own components. Burnet and Fenner in 1949 called particular attention to this phenomenon with their discussion of self-recognition—the ability of the antibody-producing mechanism to distinguish "self" from "not self." From what has already been said of the consequences of antigen-antibody union occurring on body cells (Chapter 2), it is obvious that formation of a high concentration of antibodies capable of reacting with body components may be disastrous. A substance is generally immunogenic only in an animal to which it is foreign. This means that the immunogenicity of a given material must be stated with reference to a particular animal; for example, rabbit serum albumin induces antibody formation in the chicken but not in the rabbit.

In exceptional cases cells or substances are immunogenic in the animal from which they are derived. The antibodies produced are known as *autoantibodies*, and the immunizing process is called autoimmunization. Gonadal tissues and proteins from the crystalline lens of the eye may induce antibodies in other members of the same species or, under special conditions, in the same individual. Guinea pigs injected with guinea pig sperm produce "spermocidin," an antibody that immobilizes homologous sperm in vitro. Moreover, guinea pigs can be sensitized with lens protein from one eye and anaphylactically shocked by injection of lens protein from the other eye. Ecker and Pillemer found considerable antigenic similarity between the ocular lens proteins of sheep, swine, and chickens (Table 5–2). Chicken lens protein even reacted with antiserum against fish lens. Antigens producing autoantibodies are normally confined to certain cells or tissues and do not gain access to antibody-producing cells. Moreover, special conditions, such as the use of a Freund's complete adjuvant suspension of the antigen, are often necessary to induce antibody formation. Rabbits subjected to local freezing (with liquid nitrogen) of various accessory sexual tissues develop IgM and IgG autoantibodies. It is significant that autoantigenic substances are serologically similar or identical in many phylogenetically unrelated species.

The erythrocytes of one individual (human or otherwise) may contain antigens that cause the production of antibodies in another individual of the same species. This process, called *isoimmunization*, will be discussed more fully in Chapter 7.

Table 5–2   Precipitation of Ocular Lens Proteins by Homologous and Heterologous Rabbit Antisera*

Antisera Against	Antigens (1:4000)			
	SHEEP LENS	SWINE LENS	CHICKEN LENS	FISH LENS
Sheep lens	+++	+++	+	−
Swine lens	+++	++++	+	−
Chicken lens	+±	++	++++	−
Fish lens	−	−	++	++++

*From Ecker and Pillemer, 1940. J. Exp. Med., 71:585.

Parenteral Immunization

An immunogen must ordinarily be introduced parenterally (i.e., beyond the epithelial tissues and hence not subject to immediate enzymatic digestion) in order to stimulate antibody formation. Intravenous and intraperitoneal injections are employed almost exclusively for antibody production in experimental animals. Each route gives excellent antisera. Intravenous inoculations are often preferred because the technique is simple and the results are comparable in the speed of antibody production and the final titers attained. The dosage of toxic substances is more critical by the intravenous method than by the intraperitoneal route. Furthermore, anaphylactic reactions are more likely to follow second or subsequent intravenous inoculations than intraperitoneal injections. Intramuscular injections yield fair titers. Subcutaneous inoculations induce slow antibody formation, and many injections must be given to obtain potent antisera. The intracutaneous route is rarely used with laboratory animals and usually yields low titers. Primary immunization of man is almost exclusively by the intramuscular route. For reimmunizing previously inoculated individuals a common practice is to inject intracutaneously. Vaccines containing "adjuvants" such as mineral oil are often employed to increase the effectiveness of subcutaneous injections. These preparations provide reservoirs of antigen from which the active material is slowly but continuously released, making fewer injections necessary.

SPECIFICITY

The feature of serologic reactions that most impressed early investigators was their specificity. It was noted, for example, that anti-typhoid serum agglutinated typhoid bacteria but not cholera bacteria, and vice versa. By the end of the nineteenth century it was known that antisera could be prepared that sharply distinguished proteins of different species by precipitation tests. Sometimes, however, more than one test antigen reacted with an antiserum, and the question arose whether the antibodies were nonspecific or of low specificity, or whether there was more than one antibody, each of a high degree of specificity. This problem was partially solved when it was demonstrated that some of the antibodies could be removed from antiserum by adsorption to the homologous antigen, leaving heterologous antibodies in the serum. This showed that each antibody is a separate entity with a single specificity.

Specificity of Bacterial Antigens

The specificity of antigenic complexes like those in bacterial cells or body fluids is governed by the same principles that control the specificity of relatively pure isolated proteins and artificially modified antigens. The fundamental structurally and immunologically significant unit is the small determinant site. The situation is complicated by the multiplicity of separate antigenic substances of which the cell or fluid is composed and the fact that each may contain several distinctive determinant sites. Before exploring the intimate chemical details of the specificity of natural and modified antigens, it seems appropriate to describe application of the cross-agglutination and reciprocal adsorption procedures to the study of bacterial specificity.

The heterogeneous collection of materials comprising the antigens of a bacterium includes principally proteins, together with polysaccharides and polysaccharide-phospholipid complexes. Some of these are associated with the flagella, others with the cell bodies, and still others with the capsules and "envelopes." Each antigenic component induces formation of homologous antibody. The whole cell, when mixed with its antiserum, reacts with all the antibodies. Any other cell possessing one or more of the same antigens will also react with that antiserum to the same or a lesser degree.

Three bacteria, 1, 2, and 3, possessing respectively antigens A and B, B and C, C and D, cause the formation of separate antibodies a and b, b and c, c and d (Figure 5–1). If Bacterium 1 is mixed with Antiserum 1, antibody a combines with antigen A and antibody b combines with antigen B, and agglutination occurs under appropriate conditions. When the same organism is mixed with Antiserum 2, agglutination occurs by action of antibody b. Bacterium 1 does not agglutinate with Antiserum 3 because this antiserum contains neither antibody a nor antibody b.

Antigen B may constitute a minor component of Bacterium *1* and cause the formation of antibody b in low titer. Antiserum *1* will therefore agglutinate Bacterium 2 in only a low dilution, regardless of the amount of B present.

Bacteria mixed with homologous antiserum combine with (adsorb) the antibody molecules in the antiserum, each antibody reacting with its corresponding antigen. A heterologous organism combines with only those antibodies for which it possesses antigens, and any other antibodies remain uncombined. If the concentration of homologous or heterologous antigen is sufficiently great or the dilution of antiserum is sufficiently high, all antibodies will be adsorbed onto the cells. The cells may be removed by centrifugation, and the supernatant fluid can be shown to contain no more antibodies by agglutination tests with the various antigens. The *adsorption* test constitutes a most important means of determining the relationships between different bacteria containing one or more common antigenic components.

The principle of adsorption is illustrated in Figure 5–2. Adsorption of Antiserum *1* with Bacterium *1* removes both antibodies, a and b, which combine with the bacterial cells. Adsorption of Antiserum 2 with Bacterium 1 results in union of antibody b with antigen B, leaving antibody c in the supernatant fluid following centrifugation. Antigen C is a common component of organisms 2 and 3 (see Figure 5–1), so antibody c can be used to distinguish them from organism 1. In this example antigen A is a distinctive component of Bacterium *1* and antigen D of Bacterium 3.

Agglutination tests in which one organism is mixed with antiserum against another organism are known as *cross-agglutination* tests. The results of a cross-agglutination experiment with three strains of *Shigella dispar* are illustrated in Table 5–3. The three organisms were isolated from the feces of patients with mild dysentery and possessed indistinguishable morphologic, cultural, and biochemical characteristics. Each organism agglutinated strongly in its homologous antiserum. Heterologous titers (strain 171 tested in antisera 167 and 205, etc.) were generally, but not always, lower. The various common antigenic components may therefore exist in different concentrations in cells of the three strains.

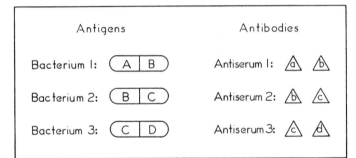

Figure 5–1. Diagrammatic comparison of the antigenic components of three bacteria and the antibodies contained in homologous antisera.

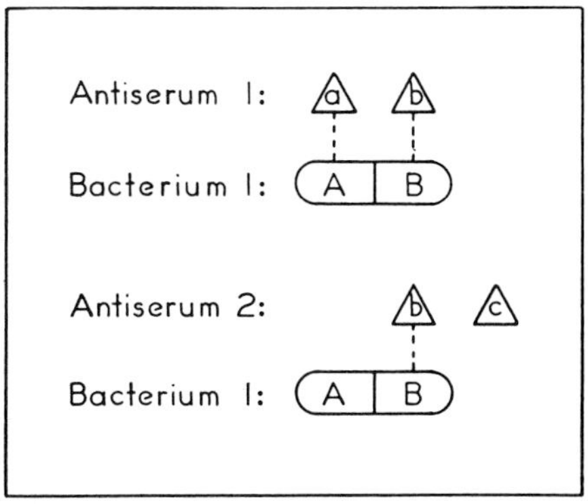

Figure 5–2. Adsorption of antibodies from homologous (antiserum 1) and heterologous (antiserum 2) antisera (diagrammatic).

Table 5–3 indicates that all three cultures possessed one or more antigens in common. Strain 171, which cross-agglutinated to titers of only 640 and 320 in antisera against 167 and 205, was obviously not identical with these organisms. A similar situation was found when antigens 167 and 205 were tested in antiserum 171. However, organisms 167 and 205 both agglutinated to high titer (10,240 or 20,480) in antisera 167 and 205, so adsorption, as previously described (see Figure 5–2), was necessary to determine whether these strains were identical. The results showed that strain 167 possessed all the antigens of 205 and one additional component of its own.

Immunogenicity and Specificity of Native Proteins

Proteins are difficult to isolate in pure form, and even when isolated there is no assurance that the chemical and physical manipulations of purification yield products identical with the original substances in their natural state. The structure of a protein is determined basically by the sequence of amino acids in its polypeptide chain, and for each sequence there is a folded state that is most stable and will be assumed under normal conditions. Moreover, under the stress of chemical or physical isolation procedures, the configuration may change. This can be expected to alter the immunogenicity and the specificity of the protein by exposing new determinant sites.

A few proteins do not stimulate antibody formation in any animal so far tested. Histones and protamines, which are relatively low in molecular weight and are among the simplest proteins, possess little or no antigenicity. Gelatin, a derived protein resulting from the hydrolysis of collagen, is not immunogenic. This may be due to the presence of very little tyrosine or histidine and no tryptophan or cystine, all of which contribute to formation of a stable configuration. It may also be suggested that most if not all animals are immunologically tolerant to this substance. As a hydrolytic deriva-

Table 5–3 *Cross-agglutination Titers of Three Strains of* Shigella dispar

Bacterial Antigens	Agglutination by Antisera		
	171	167	205
171	5,120	640	320
167	640	20,480	10,240
205	1,280	20,480	10,240

tive of collagen, found throughout the animal kingdom in skin, bone, cartilage, and other connective tissues, it may be chemically similar to portions of collagen molecules in all animal species.

The immunogenicity of animal proteins usually varies inversely with the degree of biologic relationship between the protein source and the animal immunized. For example, duck proteins induce little antibody formation in chickens but high titers in rabbits; conversely, rodent proteins are relatively poor immunogens in rabbits.

The ability of antibodies to distinguish fine differences between animal proteins (that is, their specificity for distinctive determinant configurations) is a direct function of the biologic similarity of the protein source and the animal inoculated. Rabbits and hares, as members of the family Leporidae, are closely related physiologically and morphologically. Few persons can distinguish between adults of these animals. However, rabbits are born naked and are blind for a time after birth, whereas the young of the hare possess fur and open their eyes immediately. Antiserum produced in fowls by injecting rabbit or hare serum reacts strongly with both antigens. Injection of hare serum into rabbits yields antibodies that precipitate only hare serum, thus permitting clear-cut distinction between proteins of these related species.

McGibbon utilized the same principle in immunogenetic studies of muscovy and mallard ducks and their F_1 hybrid. Rabbit antisera against red cells of the three birds agglutinated the homologous and heterologous erythrocytes in high titer. However, antisera produced by injecting the muscovy or mallard parents with hybrid red cells sharply differentiated erythrocytes of the parent species. Antibody titers developed in the ducks were only about 10 per cent of those produced in rabbits, which confirms the inverse correlation between zoologic relationship and immunogenicity.

The effect of phylogenetic relationships upon serologic cross-reactions is further illustrated by the precipitation of ovalbumins from a variety of domestic fowl by rabbit antisera against hen ovalbumin (Table 5–4). The homologous antigen reacted most strongly with the antisera; albumins from the related fowls, turkey and guinea hen, gave intermediate reactions; those from the duck and goose yielded the smallest precipitates. Reading horizontally, these results parallel the general systematic relationships between the birds and presumably reflect slight chemical differences among the various albumins. The vertical columns, except for the homologous reactions, show variation in antibody titers produced by animals A, B, and C. Individual differences in antibody-producing capacity may be observed when several animals of the same species are inoculated with identical antigens. Even siblings occasionally produce antisera of markedly different titers. Furthermore, certain breeds or "families" of animals are exceptionally potent producers of particular antibodies.

Table 5–4   *Effect of the Source of Ovalbumin on the Intensity of Precipitation with Antisera for Hen Ovalbumin**

Rabbit Anti-Hen Ovalbumin Serum	Sources of Ovalbumin Antigens				
	GALLIFORMES			ANSERIFORMES	
	Hen	Turkey	Guinea hen	Duck	Goose
	Relative volumes of precipitates				
A	100%	35%	26%	9%	9%
B	100	67	57	42	31
C	100	61	51	30	18

*From Landsteiner and van der Scheer, 1940. J. Exp. Med., 71:445.

Species and Organ Specificity

Species specificity is the immunologic property characteristic of the serum and cellular antigens of each species. It is usually attributable to proteins that are widely distributed throughout the animal body and that are not present in unrelated species. For example, Witebsky found that antiserum against hog thyroid extract reacted serologically with hog kidney, liver, heart, spleen, and other organ extracts.

It may be presumed that the serologic differences upon which species specificity are based arose as a result of evolutionary processes. Morphologic and functional evolution are the results of modifications that confer a selective advantage upon the organisms within which they occur. Both morphology and function depend upon chemical structure, so it should be possible to demonstrate correlation between the serologic properties and phylogenetic relationships of various groups of organisms.

As early as 1899, Bordet reported that the serum of a rabbit injected with fowl serum precipitated both fowl and pigeon sera, and in 1900 Myers found that antibodies against sheep globulin or beef globulin precipitated both globulins, but in each case the homologous reaction was stronger. The next year Nuttall found that antisera prepared by injecting human sera into rabbits reacted strongly with the sera of Old World monkeys but only slightly with the sera of South American monkeys.

Nuttall published a monograph in 1904 in which he tabulated and summarized the results of 16,000 precipitin tests. He employed the blood sera of man and various animals as antigens and 30 rabbit antisera against serum proteins of the various groups of animals. Results obtained in mixtures of primate sera and antihuman serum are presented in Table 5–5. Sera of orangutan, chimpanzee, gorilla, and Old World monkeys were more closely related serologically to human serum than were those of New World monkeys and marmosets. Lemurs appeared to be quite unrelated to man. These results closely follow conclusions drawn from morphologic evidence. Precipitin tests by a semiquantitative method based on precipitate volumes gave similar results (Table 5–6). The relationships were confirmed by tests with antisera against chimpanzee, orangutan, and monkey sera.

Weigle in 1961 reported a quantitative study by modern methods of the serologic relations between BSA and serum albumins of a variety of animals. He found that the

Table 5–5 Precipitation of Primate Sera by Antihuman Rabbit Serum*

Primate Sera	Number Tested	Per Cent Positive Tests
Anthropoidea		
Man	34	100
Simiidae	8	100
(orangutan, chimpanzee, gorilla)		
Cercopithecidae	36	92
(Old World monkeys, 26 species)		
Cebidae	13	77
(New World monkeys, 9 species)		
Hapalidae	4	50
(Marmosets, 3 species)		
Lemuroidea		
Lemuridae	2	0
(Lemurs, 2 species)		

*From Nuttall, 1904. Blood Immunity and Blood Relationship. Cambridge, Cambridge University Press.

Table 5–6   *Relative Amounts of Precipitate Obtained with Anti-human Rabbit Serum and Equal Amounts of Serum of Various Anthropoids and Monkeys* *

Serum	Precipitate
Human	100%
Chimpanzee	130%†
Gorilla	64%
Orangutan	42%
Cynocephalus mormon	42%
Cynocephalus sphinx	29%
Ateles (spider monkey)	29%

*From Nuttall, 1904. Blood Immunity and Blood Relationship. Cambridge, Cambridge University Press.

†Loose precipitate.

closer two species are in the phylogenetic tree, the more closely related are their antigenic constituents. This is illustrated in Table 5–7, which presents precipitation reactions of various serum albumins with a rabbit antiserum against bovine serum albumin (BSA). From the results of quantitative tests the percentage of BSA antibody precipitated by each heterologous albumin was calculated. Sheep serum albumin, for example, precipitated 74 per cent as much antibody as did the homologous antigen, beef serum albumin. Beef and sheep are closely related animal species, so this result is not surprising. The pig is less closely related to beef, and its albumin precipitated only 31 per cent of the BSA antibody. The vallaroo, at the lower end of the list, is a marsupial and quite unrelated to any of the other animals.

Table 5–7 also lists the BSA determinants present in the various albumins as indicated by the formation of lines of precipitate in Ouchterlony agar gel diffusion plates. It seems evident that the serologic behavior of the albumins shown by the quantitative precipitation tests can be attributed in part to the number of determinant sites shared.

Organ specificity is the antigenic property of an organ that distinguishes it from other organs. It is sometimes difficult to demonstrate, because species-specific antigens are often so widely distributed and so prominent in a given animal that special methods are required. Witebsky proposed two types of organ specificity: (1) *first order*

Table 5–7   *Serologic Reactions between Rabbit-anti-BSA (Bovine Serum Albumin) and Heterologous Albumins* *

Serum Albumin Antigen	Antibody Nitrogen Precipitated		BSA Determinants			
	MICROGRAMS	PER CENT	a	b	c	d
Beef	2,295	100	+	+	+	+
Sheep	1,674	74	+	+	+	+
Pig	633	31	+	+	+	−
Cat	453	25				
Human	323	14	+	+	−	−
Hamster	308	13	+	+	−	−
Rat	299	13	+	+	−	−
Dog	292	13	+	+	−	−
Horse	290	13				
Mouse	231	10	+	+	−	−
Vallaroo	144	6				
Guinea pig	124	5	+	−	−	−

*Modified from Weigle, 1961. J. Immunol., 87:599.

Table 5–8 *Cross-reactions of Thyroid Antisera with Crude Thyroid Extracts of Various Species**

Thyroid Extract	Rabbit Antiserum against Thyroid of		
	HOG	BEEF	DOG
Hog	+	+	+
Beef	+	+	+
Dog	+	+	+
Horse	+	+	+
Sheep	−	+	+
Human	−	−	+
Cat	−	−	−
Guinea pig	−	−	−
Rabbit	−	−	−

*Modified from Rose and Witebsky, 1955. J. Immunol., 75:282.

or *tissue specificity* is attributed to the presence of an antigen characteristic of a particular organ in a single species; (2) *second order* organ specificity is attributed to an antigen characteristic of the same organ in many, even unrelated, species.

First order specificity is illustrated by certain antigens found only in the red blood cells of a single animal species. There are several examples of second order organ specificity. The first to be discovered (by Uhlenhuth, in 1903) was a protein in the lens of the eye that is present in the lenses of nearly all mammals (see Table 5–2). Later, specific antigens were found in the brain, testicles, kidneys, placenta, and other organs. Witebsky and his colleagues reported that antisera against thyroid extracts reacted serologically with thyroid extracts of a variety of animals (Table 5–8), but no cross-reactions occurred with other organs of the heterologous species. They found by chemical fractionation that thyroglobulin was the principal organ-specific antigen of the thyroid but that there were also first order antigens in the gland, as well as species-specific components in the thyralbumin fraction.

An organ-specific antigen found in the adrenal of beef and sheep was absent from any other bovine organ and was also absent from the adrenals of man, rabbit, guinea pig, rat, and pig. This was considered a *species-restricted* organ-specific antigen. Insulin may also be included in this category. Crystalline insulins from a number of animal species are identical in amino acid composition and arrangement with the exception of the amino acids in positions 8 to 10 in one of the chains (see Table 5–9).

Heart antigens also exhibit organ specificity of the second order. Gery and Davies found that antisera against rabbit, guinea pig, and rat hearts reacted with heterologous and homologous heart extracts, and anti-rabbit heart sera reacted with extracts of dog, rat, guinea pig, beef, human, and chicken hearts.

Table 5–9 *Species Differences in Amino Acid Composition of Insulin**

Species	Amino Acid Number		
	8	9	10
Beef	alanine	serine	valine
Sheep	alanine	glycine	valine
Horse	threonine	glycine	isoleucine
Pork	threonine	serine	isoleucine

*From Harris et al., 1956. Arch. Biochem., 65:427.

Immunogenicity and Specificity of Modified Proteins

DENATURED PROTEINS

Denaturation is an incompletely understood process peculiar to proteins, characterized by partial or complete loss of solubility (according to the degree of denaturation) at the isoelectric point in water or dilute electrolyte. Denaturation is accomplished by numerous agents including heat, vigorous agitation, adsorption onto surfaces, strong alkalies, heavy metal salts, alcohol, ether and urea. The changes were first thought to be purely physical and irreversible, but reversibility has been indicated in some instances. Chemical changes have been reported, particularly liberation of sulfhydryl and other reducing groups. Denaturation has been attributed to the breaking of relatively unstable bonds that normally maintain the spatial configuration of a peptide chain, followed by formation of new bonds in an irregular rearrangement.

Heated proteins do not react, or react only weakly, with antisera against the native proteins. The antigenicity of heated proteins may be diminished or completely destroyed. When antibodies are formed they do not always react strongly with the native proteins but often react with other heated proteins. Cross-reactions of heated serum proteins are illustrated in Table 5–10. Antiserum against heated beef serum precipitated both heated and unheated sheep serum. Heat altered the chemical composition or structure of the antigenic constituents of horse, human, rabbit, and guinea pig sera as shown by their precipitation with antibodies against heated beef proteins. Precipitation of heated rabbit serum is especially noteworthy because the antiserum employed was obtained from rabbits. Denaturation evidently diminished the specificity of a variety of otherwise easily differentiated proteins, presumably by randomizing their configurations.

It is interesting that rabbits also can be immunized with rabbit serum that has been heated to 120° C. (i.e., autoclaved) for 30 minutes and that the antiserum produced precipitates autoclaved serum proteins of this and a number of other mammalian species.

CHEMICALLY MODIFIED PROTEINS

Obermayer and Pick in 1906 investigated specificity by joining extra elements and radicals to proteins. Nitric acid, nitrous acid, or iodine deprived proteins of their original specificity to an extent that depended upon the intensity of the treatment, and a new specificity determined by the nature of the modifying agent was introduced. Rabbits were immunized with iodoprotein prepared by treating a protein with iodine. The resulting anti-iodoprotein serum precipitated iodoproteins prepared from com-

Table 5–10 Precipitation of Native and Heated Sera by Antiserum for Heated (100° C.) Beef Serum*

	Test Antigens	Beef Serum	Sheep Serum	Horse Serum	Human Serum	Rabbit Serum	Guinea Pig Serum
Rabbit antiserum for heated (100° C.) beef serum	Native (unheated)	+++	++	−	−	−	−
	Heated (100° C.)	+++	+++	++	++	+	±

*From Furth, 1925. J. Immunol., 10:777.

pletely unrelated proteins. Anti-iodoprotein serum might or might not react with the homologous, untreated protein. Even rabbit serum proteins, similarly modified, were capable of stimulating antibody formation in the rabbit and therefore behaved as foreign proteins. More recent experiments showed that nitrate, nitrite, and halogen radicals reacted with tyrosine, histidine, and probably other aromatic amino acids of proteins. These modified amino acids rather than the introduced groups alone determined the altered specificity of treated proteins. The tyrosine of a protein may combine with iodine to form a disubstituted molecule (see Figure 5–3). That modification occurs within a protein molecule is indicated by the observation that 3,5-diiodotyrosine uncoupled to protein prevents precipitation of the homologous iodoprotein by anti-iodoprotein serum. Other substances containing the 3,5-diiodo-4-hydroxy group,

$$I \bigcup I$$
$$OH$$

such as thyroxine, also inhibit precipitation of iodoproteins.

Further evidence that substitution occurs in the tyrosine of proteins was provided when it was found that the amount of iodine necessary to iodinate a protein completely can be calculated from the tyrosine content of the protein. Complete iodination of serum globulin deprived it of the ability to react with antiserum for native globulin.

Azoprotein Antigens. In 1917 Landsteiner and his co-workers began extensive investigations of serologic specificity by joining organic radicals to proteins. A chemical to be tested as a determinant of specificity was attached to an aromatic amine, such as aniline, which was then diazotized and coupled to a protein. The resulting product was called a *conjugated antigen* or *azoprotein.*

The added radicals presumably combined with aromatic amino acids of the protein, as in nitration and halogenation. The method may be illustrated by the coupling of *p*-aminobenzene arsonic acid (atoxyl) to a protein (Figure 5–4).

Azoproteins react only weakly with antisera against the original proteins. Ordinarily, a foreign source of protein is employed, such as horse or chicken serum or egg albumin, but even rabbit serum azoproteins stimulate the formation of antibodies in rabbits. A conjugated azoprotein contains the distinctive added radical as well as normal determinant sites; each of them may engender antibodies bearing the reverse imprint of its own characteristic structure. Antibodies may therefore be formed that are capable of reacting with (1) the uncombined azo components, (2) azoproteins made from the same or other proteins, or (3) the homologous natural protein. The relative

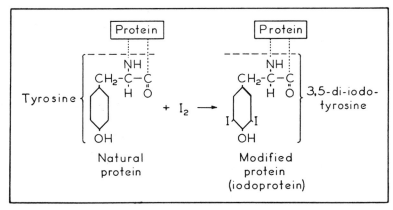

Figure 5–3. Formation of a modified protein by iodination of the tyrosine of a natural protein.

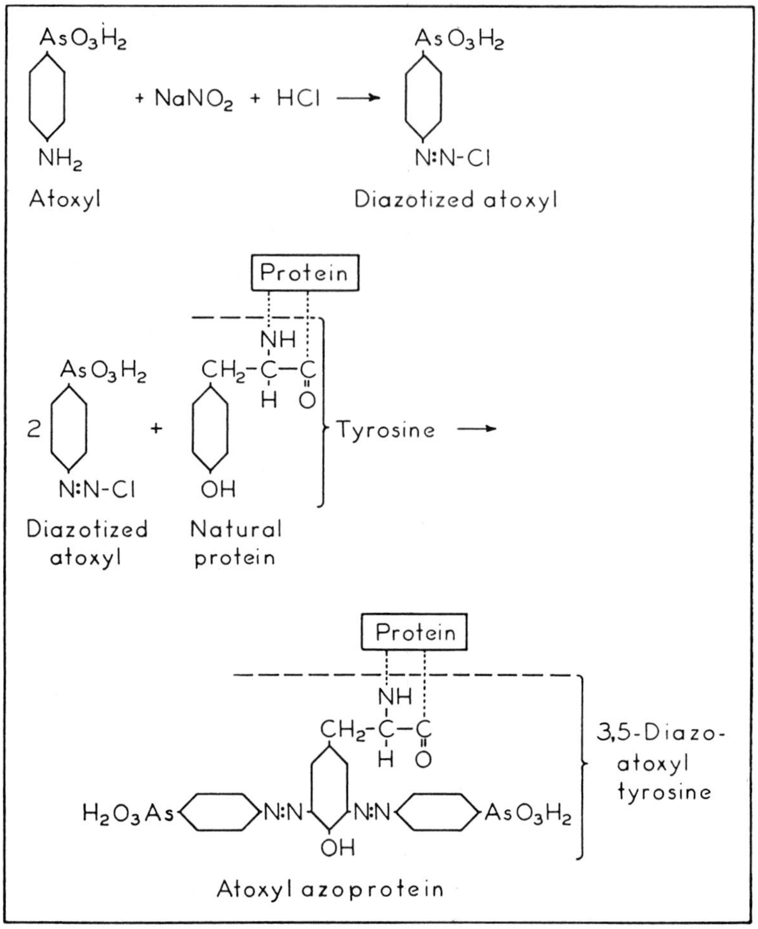

Figure 5–4. Coupling of atoxyl to the tyrosine of a protein.

amounts of the various antibodies in a given antiserum depend upon the extent of chemical modification of the immunizing antigen and often upon the inoculation dosage and number of injections. Prolonged immunization sometimes yields antisera with a broader range of reactivity than short immunization. This does not mean that the specificity of each antibody molecule is less but that a succession of antibody molecules is formed against qualitatively and quantitatively different antigenic components. Various antigenic components require different periods of time for antibody formation, with little regard for the quantity injected.

Antibodies reacting with the protein constituent may mask the effect of an added radical; therefore, tests of specificity must be performed in such a manner as to detect only antibodies capable of reacting with uncombined azo radical or determinant groups. Rabbit antiserum against an azoprotein will precipitate conjugated proteins containing the same azo group combined with a completely unrelated protein. For example, atoxyl azo-horse serum antibodies precipitate a test antigen made by coupling atoxyl to chicken serum proteins. Horse and chicken proteins are so different serologically that any reaction is associated with the atoxyl component, probably combined with the tyrosine or histidine residues of these proteins. A low molecular weight substance containing the azo component, or even the azo component itself, may be used as a simple hapten to prevent precipitation of the usual test antigen. The anaphylactic reaction can also be used to test the effect of an added radical upon specificity; a guinea pig is sensitized with one azoprotein and shocked with an unrelated protein containing the same radical.

Landsteiner immunized rabbits with proteins to which had been coupled aniline, p-aminobenzoic acid, p-aminobenzene sulfonic acid, and p-aminophenyl arsonic acid, respectively (Table 5–11). These determinants differ only in the nature of the acid radicals substituted in the *para* position on the benzene ring attached to protein by the $-N:N-$ linkage. Cross-precipitation tests employing the four antigens with all four antisera demonstrated complete specificity: aniline azoprotein antiserum reacted only with the aniline azoprotein; p-aminobenzoic acid azoprotein antiserum precipitated only its homologous antigen, and so forth. In these experiments strong acid radicals exerted a striking effect on the specificity of antigens.

Methyl and halogen radicals were not as effective determinants of specificity as acid radicals. Compounds differing only in the presence of methyl, chlorine, or bromine in the 4 position of 3-aminobenzoic acid showed considerable overlapping in precipitation tests (Table 5–12). Antiserum against 3-amino-4-chlorobenzoic acid azoprotein reacted strongly with the other test antigens. Aniline substituted by addition of chloro, methyl, or nitro groups exerted very little effect upon the specificity of azoprotein (Table 5–13).

The spatial arrangement of coupled acid radicals is an important factor in the specificity of azoproteins (Table 5–14). Antigens conjugated with aniline derivatives containing carboxyl or sulfonic radicals in the *ortho, meta,* and *para* positions were highly specific. There were only four cross-reactions. Spatial configuration dominated the effect of the acid substituent in one of these: the o-aminobenzene sulfonic acid antigen was precipitated by the o-aminobenzoic acid antiserum. The other three cross-reactions involved determinants that differed in the position of the sulfonic radical by only one carbon atom: o- and m-aminobenzene sulfonic acid antigens and antisera cross-reacted strongly, and antibody against the p-aminobenzene sulfonic compound precipitated the *meta* antigen weakly. In no case did *ortho* and *para* reagents cross-react. Cross-reactions between heterologous azoproteins and antisera

Table 5–11 *Effect of Strong Acid Radicals on the Specificity of Azoproteins**

Antisera for Azoproteins Containing:	Test Antigens: Azoproteins Containing			
	Aniline	p-Amino-benzoic acid	p-Amino-benzene sul-fonic acid	p-Amino-phenyl arson-ic acid
	NH_2	NH_2 COOH	NH_2 SO_3H	NH_2 AsO_3H_2
Aniline	+++	−	−	−
p-Amino-benzoic acid	−	+++±	−	−
p-Aminoben-zene sulfonic acid	−	−	+++±	−
p-Aminophenyl arsonic acid	−	−	−	++++

*Reprinted by permission from Landsteiner, 1945. The Specificity of Serological Reactions. Revised ed. Cambridge, Harvard University Press.

Table 5–12   *Effect of Halogen and Methyl Radicals on the Specificity of Azoproteins**

Antisera for Azoproteins Containing:	Test Antigens: Azoproteins Containing			
	3-Amino-benzoic acid COOH / NH$_2$	3-Amino-4-methyl benzoic acid COOH / NH$_2$ / CH$_3$	3-Amino-4-chlorobenzoic acid COOH / NH$_2$ / Cl	3-Amino-4-bromobenzoic acid COOH / NH$_2$ / Br
3-Aminobenzoic acid	++++	−	−	−
3-Amino-4-methyl benzoic acid	−	++	+±	±
3-Amino-4-chlorobenzoic acid	+++	+++	++++	++++
3-Amino-4-bromobenzoic acid	−	±	++±	++

*Reprinted by permission from Landsteiner, 1945. The Specificity of Serological Reactions. Revised ed. Cambridge, Harvard University Press.

therefore occurred when the determinant configurations were identical or not very dissimilar.

The effect of introducing substituents at various positions in a hapten is shown by photographs of molecular models in Figure 5–5. Large atoms or radicals can be expected to modify a determinant so that it is no longer able to react with its homologous antibody receptor site.

Experiments with levo-, meso- and dextro-tartaric acids emphasized the significance of spatial arrangement (Table 5–15). The acids were converted into aminotar-

Table 5–13   *Effect of Chloro, Methyl, and Nitro Groups on the Specificity of Azoproteins**

Antisera for Azoproteins Containing:	Test Antigens: Azoproteins Containing				
	Aniline NH$_2$	o-Chloro-aniline NH$_2$ / Cl	p-Chloro-aniline NH$_2$ / Cl	p-Toluidine NH$_2$ / CH$_3$	p-Nitro-aniline NH$_2$ / NO$_2$
Aniline	++±	+±	++±	+±	+
o-Chloroaniline	++	++±	+	+	tr.†
p-Chloroaniline	+	tr.	++	++	++
p-Toluidine	+±	+	++	++	+±
p-Nitroaniline	+	±	++±	+	++

*Reprinted by permission from Landsteiner, 1945. The Specificity of Serological Reactions. Revised ed. Cambridge, Harvard University Press.
†tr. = trace

Table 5–14 *Effect of Spatial Distribution of Acid Radicals on the Specificity of Azoproteins**

Antisera for Azoproteins Containing:	Test Antigens: Azoproteins Containing						
	Aniline	Aminobenzoic acids			Aminobenzene sulfonic acids		
		ortho-	meta-	para-	ortho-	meta-	para-
	NH_2	NH_2 COOH	NH_2 COOH	NH_2 COOH	NH_2 SO_3H	NH_2 SO_3H	NH_2 SO_3H
Aniline	+++	–	–	–	–	–	–
Aminobenzoic acids ortho-	–	+++	–	–	+++	–	–
Aminobenzoic acids meta-	–	–	++++	–	–	–	–
Aminobenzoic acids para-	–	–	–	+++±	–	–	–
Aminobenzene sulfonic acids ortho-	–	–	–	–	++++	++±	–
Aminobenzene sulfonic acids meta-	–	–	–	–	+++	++++	–
Aminobenzene sulfonic acids para-	–	–	–	–	–	+	+++±

*Reprinted by permission from Landsteiner, 1945. The Specificity of Serological Reactions. Revised ed. Cambridge, Harvard University Press.

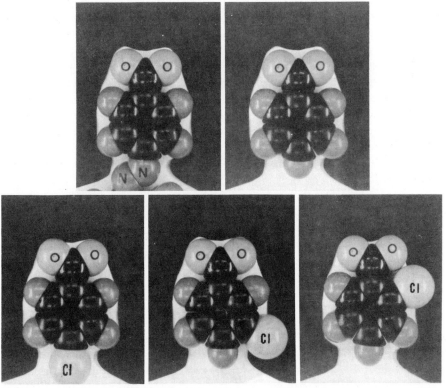

Figure 5–5. Models showing the fit of homologous and heterologous antigenic determinants into the combining region of anti-*p*-azobenzoate antibody. *Top,* Azobenzoate and benzoate are accommodated. *Bottom left, p*-Chlorobenzoate is also accommodated. The meta and ortho chlorobenzoates do not fit, owing to steric hindrance. (From Pressman and Grossberg *In* Rose et al. (Eds.): *Principles of Immunology,* 1973, p. 143. New York, Macmillan Publishing Company, Inc.)

Table 5–15   *Effect of Stereoisomerism of Determinant Radicals on the Specificity*
*of Azoproteins**

Antisera for Azoproteins Containing:	Test Antigens: Azoproteins Containing		
	Tartaric Acid		
	levo-	meso-	dextro-
	COOH | HOCH | HCOH | COOH	COOH | HCOH | HCOH | COOH	COOH | HCOH | HOCH | COOH
l-tartaric acid	++±	tr.†	−
m-tartaric acid	tr.	+++	−
d-tartaric acid	−	tr.	++±

*Reprinted by permission from Landsteiner, 1945. The Specificity of Serological Reactions. Revised ed. Cambridge, Harvard University Press.
†tr. = trace

tranilic acids before diazotization and coupling to proteins. Specificity was indicated by the strong homologous reactions. Three of the six heterologous combinations gave trace reactions and three were negative. The three trace reactions involved either the m-tartaric acid antigen or antiserum. Meso-tartaric acid differs from the levo- and dextro- forms in the arrangement of hydrogen and hydroxyl about a single asymmetric carbon atom, whereas the levo- and dextro- compounds differ from each other in the arrangement of hydrogen and hydroxyl about both asymmetric carbon atoms.

Landsteiner also demonstrated the influence of the length of aliphatic chains coupled to protein (Table 5–16). Antisera against short chain acids (oxanilic and succinanilic) were highly specific, but antisera for the longer acids reacted not only with the homologous antigens but also with those of somewhat greater or lesser chain length. A difference of one or two carbon atoms completely changed the specificity of the shorter chains, but such a difference had relatively little effect on the specificity of the longer chains.

The importance of terminal amino acids in the specificity of proteins was shown. Glycyl-leucine, for example,

$$CH_2(NH_2)-CO-NH-\underset{\underset{COOH}{|}}{\overset{\overset{H}{|}}{C}}-CH_2-CH\underset{CH_3}{\overset{CH_3}{<}}$$

Glycyl-leucine

was prepared by combining the carboxyl group of glycine with the amino group of leucine and was attached to protein. Serologic cross-reactions occurred only (but not always) when the immunizing and test antigens contained identical terminal amino acids (Table 5–17). Further experiments with tri-, tetra- and penta-peptides gave the same general results.

Stahmann and his colleagues studied the effect of added polypeptides on the immunogenicity and specificity of proteins. They developed a mild method of cou-

Table 5–16 *Effect of Chain Length on the Specificity of Azoproteins Containing Aliphatic Acids**

Test Antigens: Azoproteins Containing

Antisera for Azoproteins Containing:	p-Amino-oxanilic acid NH_2–C$_6$H$_4$–NH–CO–$COOH$	p-Amino malonanilic acid NH_2–C$_6$H$_4$–NH–CO–CH_2–$COOH$	p-Amino succinanilic acid NH_2–C$_6$H$_4$–NH–CO–$(CH_2)_2$–$COOH$	p-Amino glutaranilic acid NH_2–C$_6$H$_4$–NH–CO–$(CH_2)_3$–$COOH$	p-Amino adipanilic acid NH_2–C$_6$H$_4$–NH–CO–$(CH_2)_4$–$COOH$	p-Amino pimelanilic acid NH_2–C$_6$H$_4$–NH–CO–$(CH_2)_5$–$COOH$	p-Aminosuberanilic acid NH_2–C$_6$H$_4$–NH–CO–$(CH_2)_6$–$COOH$
p-Aminooxanilic acid	++	–	–	–	–	–	–
p-Aminosuccinanilic acid	–	–	+++	+	+++	±	–
p-Aminoadipanilic acid	–	–	+	+	++±	++±	+±
p-Aminosuberamilic acid	–	–	±	±	+±	+++	+++

*Reprinted by permission from Landsteiner, 1945. The Specificity of Serological Reactions. Revised ed. Cambridge, Harvard University Press.

Table 5–17　Effect of Amino Acid Arrangement on the Specificity of Peptide Azoproteins*

Antisera for Azoproteins Containing:	Test Antigens: Azoproteins Containing			
	Glycyl-glycine	Glycyl-leucine	Leucyl-glycine	Leucyl-leucine
Glycyl-glycine	++±	–	–	–
Glycyl-leucine	–	++±	–	tr.†
Leucyl-glycine	+	–	+++	–
Leucyl-leucine	–	+	–	++

*Reprinted by permission from Landsteiner, 1945. The Specificity of Serological Reactions. Revised ed. Cambridge, Harvard University Press.
†tr. = trace

pling peptides to proteins that produced little if any denaturation or other undesired change. The protein was allowed to react with an N-carboxyamino acid anhydride in buffered aqueous solution at pH 7.4 and 4° C. Under these conditions the reaction indicated in Figure 5–6 occurred. Coupling probably involved the free ε-amino group of lysine and free α-amino groups. Eleven to 20 polypeptide chains, each consisting of two to seven amino acid residues, were joined to proteins. Both bovine serum albumin and rabbit serum albumin, when modified by the addition of glutamic acid, lysine, phenylalanine, or leucine, were immunogenic in the rabbit. Three kinds of antibodies were formed: (1) some reacted with the unmodified protein, (2) some were specific for the polypeptide modification, and (3) some required not only the polypeptide, but also a part of the protein molecule to which it was attached.

Immunogenicity and Specificity of Synthetic Polypeptides

From the modification of proteins by addition of peptide chains, it was a logical step to the synthesis of polypeptides in an attempt to produce a complete immunogen of known size, structure, and configuration. Maurer et al. obtained a weak response in rabbits injected with a copolymer of L-glutamic acid and L-lysine in a molar ratio of 6:4 and having a molecular weight of 38,000. Gill and Doty also produced precipitating antibodies in rabbits by immunization with complete Freund emulsions of synthetic polypeptides containing various combinations of L-glutamic acid, L-tyrosine, L-lysine, and L-phenylalanine. The molecular weights were between 50,000 and 100,000. The

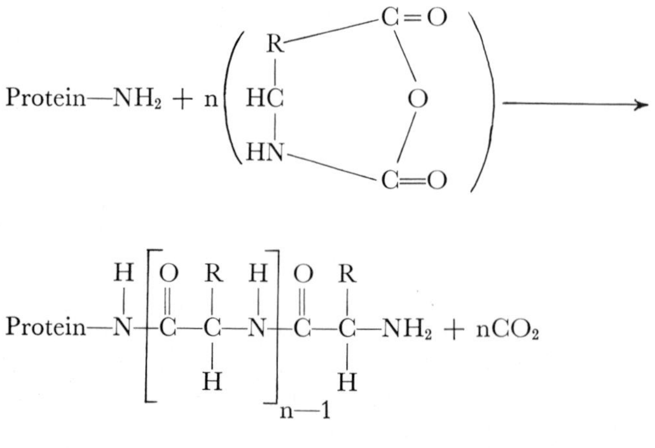

Figure 5–6. Addition of a polypeptide chain to a protein by reaction with an N-carboxyamino acid anhydride. (Modified from Becker and Stahmann, 1953. J. Biol. Chem., 204: 745.)

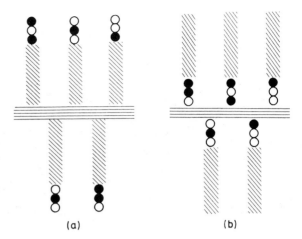

Figure 5–7. Antigenicity of the components of a synthetic polypeptide. (a) Antibodies reactive with tyrosine (●) and glutamic acid (○) were produced when their tripeptides were attached via poly-alanine side chains (diagonal hatching) to a poly-lysine core (horizontal hatching), but not when (b) the tyrosine-glutamic peptides were attached directly to the poly-lysine backbone and covered by poly-alanine. (From Sela, 1969. Science, 166:1367. Copyright 1969 by the American Association for the Advancement of Science.)

minimum requirement for antigenicity seemed to be the presence of glutamic acid and lysine in the molar ratio of 6:4. Antigenicity was improved by the addition of the aromatic acids, tyrosine or phenylalanine, although they were not essential.

Sela showed the importance of an exposed location of determinant groups by use of synthetic polypeptides consisting of a polylysine backbone with side branches of polyalanine plus tyrosine or glutamic acid (see Figure 5–7). When tyrosine or glutamic acid occupied the terminal position on the polyalanine side chain, specifically reacting antibodies were produced, but when the tyrosine or glutamic acid was attached directly to the polylysine backbone and covered by the polyalanine side chain, no antibodies were produced until the side chains had been separated some distance apart.

Specificity of Native Globular Proteins

The specificities of a number of native globular proteins, such as myoglobin, hemoglobin, lysozyme, cytochrome c, and β-galactosidase, have been studied to ascertain the antigenic determinants responsible for their serologic specificity. Most of these studies indicate that the structures of the determinants depend upon the overall conformation of the entire molecule. Therefore, the molecular basis of their antigenic structures can be understood for only those proteins whose three-dimensional architecture is known.

A two-dimensional representation of the configuration of a molecule of whale myoglobin is shown in Figure 5–8. Immunologically active peptides that react with antibody against the entire molecule are marked. There appear to be five or six regions that possess reactivity. Some of these consist of 10 to 15 amino acid residues. Inasmuch as an antibody combining site is no larger than six residues, it appears that some of these determinant areas are larger than the actual combining site and that different antisera may react with different portions of the determinant. This conclusion has also been reached by study of other globular proteins. Another conclusion from these studies is that determinants are limited to the protein surface and preferably to the more exposed areas like "loop" regions and "corners" of folded chains.

It has already been mentioned that the density of determinants appears to be about one per 5,000 molecular weight. Frequently, however, a single amino acid residue can

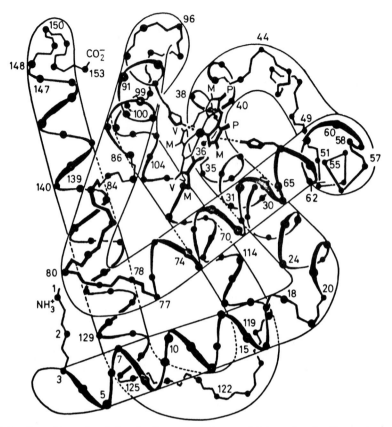

Figure 5–8. Two-dimensional sketch of sperm-whale myoglobin molecule. The amino acid residues, numbered from the N terminus, are arranged in alternating helical and nonhelical segments, folded into a globular structure. Immunologically active peptides occupy exposed positions encompassing residues 15–29, 56–69, 70–76, 77–89, 139–149, and 147–153. (From Crumpton *In* Porter, R. R. (ed.): Defence and Recognition, 1973, p. 152. Butterworth & Co., Ltd., London, England. University Park Press, Baltimore, Maryland.)

make a significant contribution to the specificity of an entire molecule, particularly when it is in a terminal or otherwise exposed position.

It has also been noted that determinants are usually found in regions of a polypeptide chain that are phylogenetically not conserved. This observation is consistent with the "self–not self" principle, according to which an animal does not produce antibody against its own components or closely related components.

In addition to the determinant sites, a globular protein contains portions that can be considered as the carrier region. The internal peptides and the comparatively nondistinctive surface peptides serve this function. It will be recalled that T cells react particularly with the carrier portion of an antigenic protein and B cells with determinant or haptenic portions.

Polysaccharides

Polysaccharides are serologically important components of most cells. Many are not immunogenic but dominate the serologic specificity of proteins with which they are combined.

Starches, dextrans, glycogens, and similar substances have generally been reported nonimmunogenic under ordinary conditions. Glycogen adsorbed onto a colloidal carrier, such as aluminum hydroxide, has been said to stimulate weak formation of antibody.

The serologically active polysaccharides are chiefly substances isolated from microorganisms. Bacterial polysaccharides were discovered by Zinsser and others and were called *residue antigens*. Goebel, and Heidelberger and Avery found that the specificity of the pneumococcus types was dependent upon their capsular polysaccharides. These substances were precipitated by antisera for the respective whole bacteria. Certain polysaccharide-protein complexes, either with or without lipids, are also important bacterial constituents because of their toxicity.

A typical polysaccharide is composed of a number of monosaccharide molecules joined by the $\equiv$C—O—C$\equiv$ linkage. The monosaccharides most frequently found in serologically important polysaccharides are pentoses and hexoses. Each monosaccharide may be substituted at one or more positions (e.g., by methyl, amino, acetyl, or other groups), one carbon (often the number 6 carbon of a hexose) may be oxidized to —COOH, one or more carbons may be reduced to —CH$_2$—, and the sugars may be joined by either α or β linkages. In all, a considerable variety of structures and configurations is possible. However, the same structures are found widely distributed among a surprising diversity of microbes, plants, and animals.

The immunogenic pneumococcus 3 polysaccharide is composed of cellobiuronic acid molecules joined by glucoside linkages:

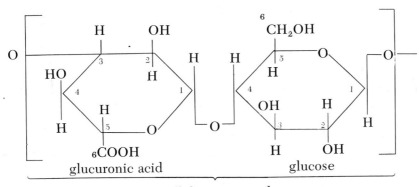

cellobiuronic acid

The minimum molecular weight of the polysaccharide is about 62,000, equivalent to approximately 180 cellobiuronic acid residues. Cellobiuronic acid is also present in type 8 pneumococci and *Rhizobium radicicolum* and is responsible for serologic cross-reactions among these organisms. It is of interest that partially oxidized cotton contains cellobiuronic acid and reacts with antisera against types 3 and 8 pneumococci.

Polysaccharides used in early work were considerably altered in the process of purification. Type 1 pneumococcal polysaccharide, for example, lost acetyl groups as a result of drastic methods of isolation. Procedures that avoided heat and strong acids or alkalies permitted separation of type 1 pneumococcal polysaccharide from cells or culture filtrates in a form that proved to be immunogenic for mice, man, horses, and a few other animals, but not for rabbits. This polysaccharide, artificially combined with protein, is a better immunizing agent than the pure substance. The polysaccharide-protein complex, unlike the polysaccharide itself, immunizes rabbits against challenge with capsulated pneumococci, and the animals produce antibody demonstrable by passive protection in other rabbits, by agglutination of homologous pneumococci, and by precipitation of the polysaccharide hapten. Small amounts of protein may suffice to render a polysaccharide immunogenic in the animal body. This fact was not appreciated at first, and conflicting reports of the immunogenicity of polysaccharides are common.

Cellular extracts containing "Vi antigen" in various degrees of purity have been obtained from *Salmonella typhosa*, *Paracolobactrum ballerup*, *Escherichia coli*, and other organisms. This substance appears to consist principally of polymerized O-acetyl and N-acetyl aminohexuronic acids. It is now known to be highly stable to heat and chemicals, is very soluble in distilled water and saline, and is readily extracted in active form by boiling suspensions of Vi containing bacteria for an hour. The supernatant fluid from boiled cultures is capable of inducing formation of Vi antibody. Previous reports that heated Vi cultures failed to agglutinate in Vi antisera can be explained on the basis of the loss of antigen from the cell surfaces.

The type-specific substances by which the human blood groups are recognized contain serologically active polysaccharides (see page 213). The terminal monosaccharides, to which Springer et al. attribute a large part of their specificity, appear to be as follows: A substance, N-acetyl-D-galactosamine; B substance, D-galactose; H(O) substance, L-fucose. These polysaccharides, which are found in the erythrocytes, are also present in various tissues and secretions of man, numerous other animals, plants, and many bacteria, and serologic cross-reactions can be demonstrated between the same substances from different sources.

There are many other serologic cross-reactions among materials of animal, plant, and bacterial origin in which polysaccharides are concerned; therefore, it seems likely that only a limited variety of polysaccharides is widely distributed in nature.

Lipids

Lipids are poorly defined substances. They are esters of organic acids with various alcohols, plus other radicals such as phosphate and sulfate, nitrogenous bases, etc. It has been assumed in immunologic literature that substances extracted by solvents like alcohol, benzene, ether, and chloroform are restricted to lipids, but it is now known that an amount of protein sufficient to cause antibody formation may be found in these extracts.

There are relatively few lipids and, in general, they are widely distributed in nature. They possess little if any immunogenicity. Presumably, they are first formed during embryonic or neonatal life, and animals become immunologically tolerant to their own and, hence, to other identical lipids from any source. Therefore, they should lack the ability to stimulate antibody production and, with few exceptions, this is true.

Some lipids function as haptens, altering the specificity of proteins to which they are attached. Sachs and Klopstock reported that cholesterol or lecithin in combination with swine serum induced in rabbits formation of antibodies that fixed complement and flocculated with the respective lipids. Other authors maintained that these results, although capable of duplication, were caused by traces of impurities in the lipid preparations. On the other hand, antibody formation has been obtained against a synthetic distearyl-lecithin and against several times recrystallized cholesterol.

Alcoholic extracts of animal organs that alone do not cause antibody formation may be capable of stimulating antibody production when mixed with foreign protein such as swine serum. This procedure has repeatedly been followed with successful results and is called "combination immunization." Landsteiner thought the lipid might form a loose union with serum proteins. Sachs, Klopstock, and Weil suggested that the protein merely served as an "envelope" that permitted entry of the nonprotein matter into the cells and referred to the protein as a "schlepper" or "conveyer." It may be suggested that the protein, as a "carrier," activates T cells to perform their helper function in association with B cells activated by the lipid. Combination immunization has been employed with extracts of brain, testicle, and other organs, and antibodies have been induced in an animal against its own tissues. Lewis produced antibodies in rabbits by injecting alcoholic extracts of rabbit brain mixed with normal horse serum. These antibodies completely fixed complement when reacting with as little as 0.02 milligram of the lipoid (alcohol-soluble) material from rabbit brain.

THE FORSSMAN ANTIGEN

The Forssman antigen is an example of a heterophile antigen; that is, a substance isolated from a living form that stimulates production of antibodies capable of reacting with tissues of other organisms—animal, plant, or microbial.

Forssman discovered in 1911 that emulsions of guinea pig liver, kidney, adrenals, testicles, and brain produced in rabbits high concentrations of antibodies capable of lysing sheep red blood cells in the presence of complement. Guinea pig erythrocytes and serum did not cause production of these antibodies. The active substance was later called the Forssman antigen, and the hemolysin was designated the Forssman antibody. Forssman antigen free from protein can be extracted by alcohol from tissues of certain animals. This material combines with Forssman antibody but when properly extracted has no immunizing power unless artificially combined with a protein such as swine serum.

Forssman antigens can be boiled or autoclaved for several hours without being completely destroyed. At the present time the composition of the Forssman antigen is not definitely known, but it seems to contain nitrogen and upon hydrolysis liberates a reducing sugar that may be glucosamine. There is also evidence of fatty acids and other components, but apparently no sulfur or phosphorus.

The Forssman antigen has been found in the horse, dog, cat, mouse, fowl, tortoise, and many other animals. It is present either in the organs or in the erythrocytes but usually not in both. It is found in erythrocytes of sheep and man (blood groups A and AB) but is absent from both organs and erythrocytes of the rabbit, cow, pig, and rat. Hawes and Coombs reported its presence in nearly all guinea pig tissues examined in addition to those mentioned above: spleen, lung; epithelium of the bronchi and trachea, bladder, urethra, gallbladder, esophagus, and duodenum; vascular endothelium, pericardium, peritoneum; and skeletal and cardiac muscle; it was not found in smooth muscles or the epithelium of the jejunum. The Forssman antigen is also present in certain strains of Salmonella and Pasteurella, *Sh. dysenteriae, Diplococcus pneumoniae,* and *B. anthracis.*

Forssman antibody can be produced by injecting rabbits with sheep erythrocytes, saline suspensions of guinea pig kidney, and other tissues containing Forssman antigen. Rabbits injected with sheep cells produce, in addition, antibodies against the species-specific substances of the cells. These are called *isophile* antibodies. The heterophile titers are invariably much greater than the isophile titers. Anti-sheep cell sera having titers of 20,480 possess isophile titers of only 320 to 640, as shown by adsorption with boiled sheep erythrocytes.

The incompatibility between Forssman antigen and antibody can be demonstrated dramatically in vivo by intravenously injecting a guinea pig, whose tissues contain the antigen, with normal or immune serum containing sufficient of the antibody. The animal immediately dies with symptoms resembling acute anaphylactic shock.

There are many heterophile systems, of which the Forssman antigen is only one. Unfortunately the terms *Forssman antigen* and *heterophile antigen* have frequently been used synonymously. The designation *Forssman antigen* should be limited to the antigen discovered by Forssman in guinea pig tissues, and *heterophile antigen* should be used to denote a broad group of antigens present in various plants and animals and possessing characteristics similar to those of the Forssman antigen.

The heterophile systems that involve sheep hemolysins or hemagglutinins constitute a confusing example of serologic complexity. The sera of many normal humans contain sheep hemagglutinins in titers as high as 320. These normal antibodies are completely or almost completely removed by adsorption with guinea pig kidney but not by beef red blood cells and are, therefore, for the most part Forssman antibodies. Forssman sera prepared by immunizing rabbits with saline emulsions of guinea pig kidney contain high titers of sheep hemolysin. Adsorption of these antisera with guinea pig kidney removes all sheep cell antibodies, but adsorption with beef erythrocytes does not affect the sheep cell titers.

Human sera in infectious mononucleosis contain moderate amounts of both sheep hemolysins and hemagglutinins. They also agglutinate beef erythrocytes. The sheep agglutinins are reduced slightly if at all by adsorption with guinea pig kidney but are almost completely removed by beef red blood cells. These heterophile antibodies therefore appear to be non-Forssman in nature.

Sera from patients with serum sickness (produced by horse serum injection) contain moderate titers of sheep hemagglutinins that are partially removed by adsorption with guinea pig kidney and completely removed by beef red cells. Rabbit erythrocytes, which lack Forssman antigen, also adsorb sheep agglutinins from some sera. These observations indicate that horse serum probably contains more than one heterophile antigen capable of inducing increased sheep hemagglutinin titers, only one of which is the Forssman antigen.

The picture is further complicated by the observation that human blood cells of groups A and AB possess the Forssman antigen. However, sheep hemagglutinins and hemolysins in infectious mononucleosis and serum sickness do not produce apparent reactions in vivo with such blood cells, which indicates that the heterophile antigen in human A and AB cells is not identical with that of infectious mononucleosis or serum sickness.

SEROLOGIC ROLE OF LIPIDS

Lipids take definite part in certain serologic reactions. The test antigen used in the Wassermann test for syphilis is an alcoholic extract of beef heart; the purified hapten isolated in 1941 by Pangborn is known as cardiolipin. These reagents are made more sensitive by addition of pure lipids, such as cholesterol or lecithin, which may function by increasing the dispersion of the specific active substance or by converting a monovalent (hapten) molecule into a polyvalent aggregate, which can then react with antibody to form an immune complex.

Hartley reported that if a protein antigen such as horse serum and homologous immune serum were extracted with ether, they did not flocculate when mixed, although antigen and antibody apparently combined and the mixture became opalescent. Horsfall and Goodner removed the agglutinating and precipitating activity from anti-pneumococcal horse serum by extraction with alcohol and ethyl ether; activity was restored by addition of a small amount of purified lecithin. Removal of lipids did not seem to affect the combining power of the antiserum with homologous pneumococcal antigen. Similarly, Hartley found that diphtheria antitoxin, extracted with alcohol and ether, retained its ability to neutralize toxin, as indicated by skin tests in guinea pigs, but no longer flocculated toxin in vitro.

Boivin Antigens, Somatic Antigens, Endotoxins

The search for toxic bacterial components led to discovery of complex substances that were termed *Boivin antigens* after one of their discoverers. Boivin and his co-workers, Raistrick and Topley, Morgan and Partridge, and others, extracted bacterial cells with trichloracetic acid or diethylene glycol or digested them with trypsin. Toxic antigenic substances were secured from smooth gram-negative bacteria, particularly Salmonella and Shigella species. These substances represented 5 to 20 per cent of the weight of the dried organisms. Boivin's trichloracetic acid extract of *S. typhosa* was lethal for mice in doses of 0.05 to 0.1 milligram intraperitoneally or intravenously. The minimal lethal dose for mice of similar material from *Sh. dysenteriae* was also about 0.1 milligram. These toxic agents were believed to be endotoxins. They consist of a *loose* complex of polysaccharide, phospholipid, and often protein.

The term *endotoxin* applied to the bacterial component under discussion is, in a sense, an historical misnomer dating from 1893, when Pfeiffer observed that bacteriolysis of *Vibrio cholerae* in experimental animals apparently released a toxin from within the cells, thus producing the disturbances that led to death. It was later shown that endotoxin is actually situated at the bacterial surface, in the cell wall, but it apparently is not normally released to the surrounding medium (in vivo or in vitro) until cell lysis takes place.

The pathologic effects of endotoxins from all species are similar. Injection of a lethal dose into an experimental animal initiates a sequence of events leading to irreversible shock and death, often within 24 hours. For an hour or two after injection the animal appears normal but then becomes lethargic, refuses food and water, and has profuse diarrhea; if it survives beyond 1 or 2 days its weight decreases markedly. Other physiologic changes preceding death include increased and later decreased blood sugar, initial leukopenia and subsequent leukocytosis, and either hyperthermia or hypothermia according to the dose and other circumstances. Autopsy reveals intestinal hemorrhage with swelling and necrosis of Peyer's patches and the underlying mucosa; degeneration occurs in the liver, spleen, kidney, and heart. Many of the above physiologic changes also occur in humans infected with the intestinal pathogens.

Sublethal doses of the polysaccharide-phospholipid-protein complex incite the formation of agglutinating antibody. The sera of animals immunized against Boivin endotoxins neutralize only a few minimal lethal doses of the endotoxins.

Extraction of gram-negative bacteria such as Salmonella with trichloracetic acid yields a lipopolysaccharide-protein complex that induces antibody formation and has potent endotoxic activity. When the bacteria are extracted with 45 per cent phenol, the lipopolysaccharide (LPS) is obtained free from protein. It is only weakly immunogenic but retains its endotoxicity. It is also antigenic in the sense that it reacts specifically with antisera against the whole bacteria or the LPS-protein complex. Mild acid treatment of the bacteria or LPS yields two fractions, the polysaccharide and lipid A. In Salmonella, the latter is a disaccharide composed of two glucosamine molecules heavily substituted by β-hydroxymyristic acid and other long chain fatty acids. Its molecular weight is 2,000 to 3,000; in pure form it is insoluble in water, but in association with the polysaccharide or with a protein it is soluble and is highly toxic. Lipid A therefore appears to be the toxic component of LPS.

The polysaccharide is responsible for the serologic specificity of the so-called O (somatic) antigens of gram-negative bacteria—those nonflagellar antigens which, in the Salmonella and Escherichia groups, are used in diagnostic schemata. Rosen reported that anti-endotoxin can combine with the isolated polysaccharide; moreover, the antibody is specific for the bacterial source of endotoxin. It may be mentioned parenthetically that each kind of bacterium contains many proteins and other substances that could be called somatic antigens in a general sense. Some incite antibody formation and are readily detected; others on occasion fail to induce antibody production: the animal host may be immunologically tolerant to them, or they may be digested before they reach antibody-forming cells.

The chemical basis for the specificity of the O antigens of the enteric bacteria has been found in the nature and arrangement of the simple sugars in the polysaccharide chains. Staub and Kauffmann and their respective collaborators determined the significant sugars in the O antigens from strains of Salmonella and Escherichia of known antigenic types by means of inhibition tests. Table 5–18 and Figure 5–9 indicate the terminal or immunodominant sugars in several antigens. S. paratyphi, for example, has long been known to contain antigens 1, 2, and 12. Glucose is the terminal sugar in the antigen 1 molecule and paratose in antigen 2; antigen 12 is a complex and possesses two chains, one ending with rhamnose, the other with glucose. Certain sugars, such as some of the dideoxyhexoses, were first discovered in bacterial O antigens (see Figure 5–10).

The O antigen determinants of gram-negative bacteria appear to be principally trisaccharides that occur as repeating units on the surface of a bacterial cell (see Table 5–18). Often, but not always, the terminal sugar residue is immunodominant. The specific O antigen polymers may be repeated 25 to 30 times in a linear array (see Table 5–19). They are attached to the cell membrane via an oligosaccharide composed of glucose, galactose, and N-acetylglucosamine, comprising the "outer core" of the LPS, and an "inner core" of a heptose and KDO (2-keto-3-deoxyoctonate) plus pyrophosphoryl-ethanolamine (see Figure 5–11). KDO attaches to lipid A, which is embedded in the outer cell membrane. The overall structure has been described as an array of specific O antigen "whiskers" on the outside of the cell.

Most smooth strains possess the complete LPS. Rough forms lack the O antigen polymer repeating units, and may lack part or all of the outer core oligosaccharide. Mutants designated as "extremely rough" also lack the heptose; the "backbone" of KDO and lipid A represents the minimum necessary for continued viability.

Study of the endotoxins and somatic antigens of bacteria is not entirely academic. The practical aspect of these investigations lies in the attempt to prepare potent but nontoxic agents for human immunization. Typhoid and other bacterins may produce considerable inflammation at the site of inoculation, general malaise, fever, nausea, and other unpleasant reactions. It was hoped that chemical extraction would yield antigens producing better protective antibodies with no undesirable side reactions, but at present typhoid immunization is still performed with killed whole bacteria.

Table 5–18 *Partial Structures of the Determinants of Certain Salmonella Somatic Antigens*

Antigen	Partial Structure
1	Glucose-galactose-
2	Paratose-
3	Mannose-rhamnose-galactose-
4	Abequose-galactose-mannose-
9	Tyvelose-mannose-
12	Glucose-galactose-mannose-rhamnose- Rhamnose-
15	Galactose-mannose-
35	Colitose-

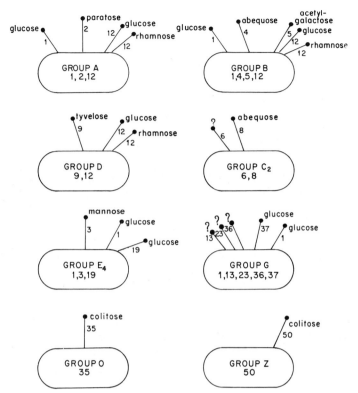

Figure 5–9. Terminal or immunodominant sugars in some Salmonella O antigens, as indicated by serologic inhibition. (From Lüderitz, Staub, and Westphal, 1966. Bacteriol. Rev., 30:192.)

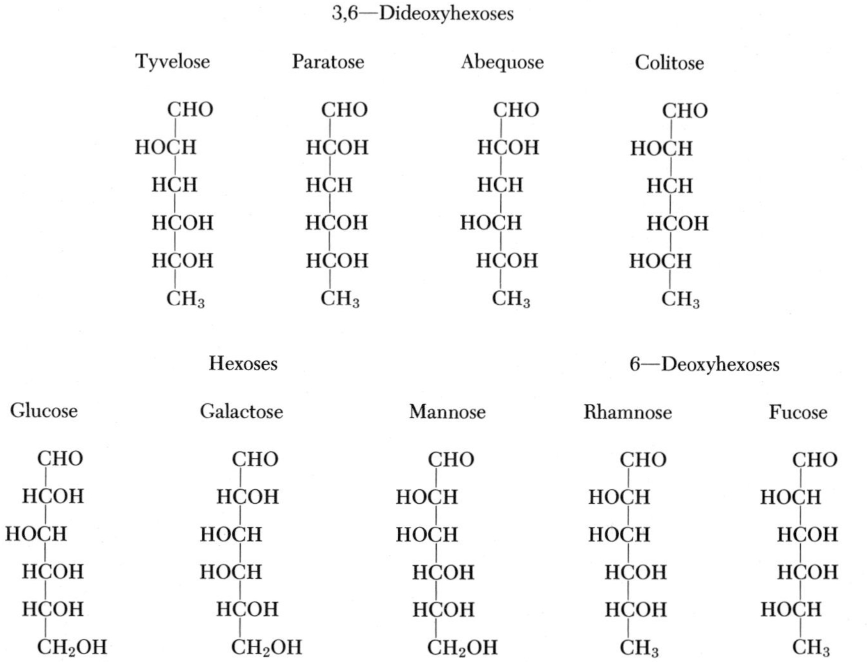

3,6—Dideoxyhexoses

Tyvelose | Paratose | Abequose | Colitose

$$\begin{array}{cccc}
\text{Tyvelose} & \text{Paratose} & \text{Abequose} & \text{Colitose} \\
\text{CHO} & \text{CHO} & \text{CHO} & \text{CHO} \\
\text{HOCH} & \text{HCOH} & \text{HCOH} & \text{HOCH} \\
\text{HCH} & \text{HCH} & \text{HCH} & \text{HCH} \\
\text{HCOH} & \text{HCOH} & \text{HOCH} & \text{HCOH} \\
\text{HCOH} & \text{HCOH} & \text{HCOH} & \text{HOCH} \\
\text{CH}_3 & \text{CH}_3 & \text{CH}_3 & \text{CH}_3
\end{array}$$

Hexoses | 6—Deoxyhexoses

$$\begin{array}{ccccc}
\text{Glucose} & \text{Galactose} & \text{Mannose} & \text{Rhamnose} & \text{Fucose} \\
\text{CHO} & \text{CHO} & \text{CHO} & \text{CHO} & \text{CHO} \\
\text{HCOH} & \text{HCOH} & \text{HOCH} & \text{HOCH} & \text{HOCH} \\
\text{HOCH} & \text{HOCH} & \text{HOCH} & \text{HOCH} & \text{HCOH} \\
\text{HCOH} & \text{HOCH} & \text{HCOH} & \text{HCOH} & \text{HCOH} \\
\text{HCOH} & \text{HCOH} & \text{HCOH} & \text{HCOH} & \text{HOCH} \\
\text{CH}_2\text{OH} & \text{CH}_2\text{OH} & \text{CH}_2\text{OH} & \text{CH}_3 & \text{CH}_3
\end{array}$$

Figure 5–10. Structures of monosaccharides important in Salmonella and Escherichia somatic antigen determinant groups.

Table 5–19   *Examples of Salmonella O Antigen Polymers*

Subgroup	O Factors	O Antigen Repeating Unit
B	1,4,12	Abe $\xrightarrow{\alpha\text{-}1,3}$ → Man $\xrightarrow{\beta\text{-}1,4}$ Rha $\xrightarrow{1,3}$ Gal (Glc $\xrightarrow{\alpha\text{-}1,6}$) $\xrightarrow{\alpha\text{-}1,2}$
B	1,4,5,12	2-Ac-Abe $\xrightarrow{\alpha\text{-}1,3}$ → Man $\xrightarrow{\beta\text{-}1,4}$ Rha $\xrightarrow{1,3}$ Gal (Glc $\xrightarrow{\alpha\text{-}1,6}$) $\xrightarrow{\alpha\text{-}1,2}$
D_1	9,12	Tyv $\xrightarrow{\alpha\text{-}1,3}$ → Man $\xrightarrow{1,4}$ Rha $\xrightarrow{\alpha\text{-}1,3}$ Gal (2-Ac-Glc $\xrightarrow{\alpha\text{-}1,4}$) $\xrightarrow{\alpha\text{-}1,2}$
E_1	3,10	→ Man $\xrightarrow{\alpha\text{-}1,4}$ Rha $\xrightarrow{1,3}$ Gal (Ac ↓) $\xrightarrow{\alpha\text{-}1,6}$
E_2	3,15	→ Man $\xrightarrow{\alpha\text{-}1,4}$ Rha $\xrightarrow{1,3}$ Gal $\xrightarrow{\beta\text{-}1,6}$

Abbreviations:

Abe	Abequose
Ac	Acetyl
Gal	Galactose
Glc	Glucose
Man	Mannose
Rha	Rhamnose
Tyv	Tyvelose

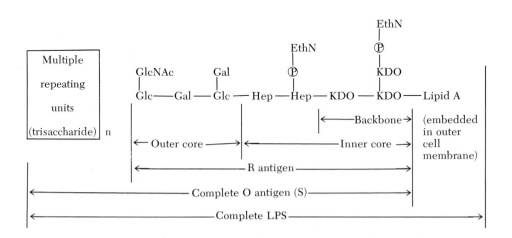

GlcNAc	N-acetylglucosamine
Glc	Glucose
Gal	Galactose
Hep	Heptose
EthN	Ethanolamine
Ⓟ	Phosphate
KDO	2-Keto-3-deoxyoctonate

Figure 5–11.   Structure of lipopolysaccharide of Salmonella.

THE SHWARTZMAN PHENOMENON

The Shwartzman phenomenon is a severe local or general reaction demonstrable in rabbits injected twice under specified conditions with bacterial cultures or endotoxic filtrates. Originally described in 1924 by Sanarelli, it was rediscovered in 1928 by Shwartzman. Because of its apparently nonimmunologic basis, despite its gross similarity to a form of hypersensitivity and other toxic reactions, it has been of considerable interest to immunologists.

A rabbit is prepared for the local Shwartzman reaction by injecting intracutaneously 0.25 ml. of the filtrate of a culture of *S. typhosa* or certain other bacteria. After 24 hours (not less than 2 nor more than 48 hours) an intravenous injection of 0.01 ml. of the same material provokes violent hemorrhagic necrosis at the cutaneous site, appearing within 2 or 3 hours and reaching its maximum by 5 hours. A generalized Shwartzman reaction is elicited by use of the intravenous route for both injections; this is essentially the phenomenon discovered by Sanarelli, in which death occurred either immediately after the second injection or within a few hours. Shwartzman's initial observations were made on meningitis patients with severe purpuric skin lesions. In the Waterhouse-Friderichsen syndrome the adrenals are severely damaged, and it has been postulated that they become hypersensitive to the meningococcal endotoxin.

Additional Sources of Information

Chase, M. W., and W. J. Kuhns (Eds.): Specificity of Serological Reactions: Landsteiner Centennial. *In* Annals of the New York Academy of Sciences, vol. 169, pp. 1–293, 1970.

Davis, B. D., and L. Warren (Eds.): The Specificity of Cell Surfaces. 1967. Englewood Cliffs, N.J., Prentice-Hall, Inc.

Inman, F. P. (Ed.): Contemporary Topics in Immunochemistry, vol. 1. 1972. New York, Plenum Press.

Nowotny, A.: Cellular Antigens. 1972. New York, Springer-Verlag.

Plescia, O. J., and W. Braun (Eds.): Nucleic Acids in Immunology. 1968. New York, Springer-Verlag.

Pressman, D., and A. L. Grossberg: The Structural Basis of Antibody Specificity. 1968. New York, W. A. Benjamin, Inc.

CHAPTER SIX

ANTIGEN-ANTIBODY INTERACTIONS

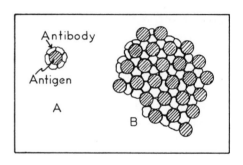

The basic immunologic reaction is union of an antigenic determinant or hapten (simple hapten in Topley and Wilson's terminology) with an antibody receptor—that is, the Fab portion of an immunoglobulin. The result of union is not ordinarily observed directly; the fact that it takes place is inferred from subsequent tests of the activity of one or the other reagent, utilizing a macromolecular or particulate system that can be assayed visually or in some other quantifiable way. The general term *ligand* is applied to an antigenic determinant with reference to its property of reacting with an antibody site, whether the determinant is free as a simple hapten or part of a more complex antigen or immunogen.

REACTIONS OF ANTIBODY WITH HAPTEN

Methods of Study

Theoretic studies of hapten-antibody reactions are best performed with reagents that are as pure as possible in order to decrease confusing extraneous reactions. Antibodies against simple haptens can be prepared by immunizing animals with conjugated antigens containing the haptenic radical, as was done by Landsteiner in his study of azoproteins (see page 131). For example, antibodies against 2,4-dinitrophenol are formed in rabbits injected with an immunogen consisting of a protein, such as BGG or BSA, to which dinitrofluorobenzene or dinitrobenzene sulfonate has been coupled. The antibody is removed from the antiserum by precipitation or adsorption, with the hapten coupled to a carrier unrelated to the protein of the immunogen (e.g., cellulose, polystyrene, or agarose). A high concentration of the hapten may then be added to displace the adsorbent competitively, yielding soluble complexes of antibody and hapten. Various procedures such as dialysis, chromatography, and gel filtration are available for separating the antibody from the hapten and for purifying it.

Antibodies against types 3 and 8 pneumococcal polysaccharide are purified by elution from specific antigen-antibody precipitates with 10 to 15 per cent NaCl. Preparations have been obtained from which 80 to 100 per cent of the protein nitrogen was precipitated by homologous antigen.

When a solution containing a small univalent ligand (possessing only a single determinant site per molecule) is mixed with antibody, ligand molecules unite reversibly with antibody molecules in proportions that depend on their relative concentrations; the number of antibody combining sites occupied increases as the amount of ligand increases up to a maximum, when all the accessible combining sites have reacted. This represents the immunologic "valence" of the antibody: 2 in the case of

IgG, 10 in the case of IgM. The reaction between a ligand and an antibody combining site can be represented as follows:

$$L + A \underset{k_d}{\overset{k_a}{\rightleftharpoons}} LA$$

in which L denotes a molecule of ligand and A an antibody combining site. If k_a and k_d are the association and dissociation rate constants, respectively, the *intrinsic association constant*,

$$K = \frac{k_a}{k_d}$$

represents the intrinsic affinity of the antibody combining site for the ligand. It can be evaluated from the relationship:

$$K = \frac{k_a}{k_d} = \frac{[LA]}{[L][A]}$$

in which the bracketed expressions refer to the concentrations at equilibrium of bound antibody sites $[LA]$, unbound antibody sites $[A]$, and unbound ligand molecules $[L]$. From the total concentration of antibody binding sites $([A] + [LA])$ and ligand molecules $([L] + [LA])$ and quantitative determination at equilibrium of either $[LA]$, $[A]$, or $[L]$, the association constant, K, can be calculated. Free ligand $[L]$ is often determined, and there are several methods by which it can be distinguished from bound ligand $[LA]$.

EQUILIBRIUM DIALYSIS

One of the most useful methods is equilibrium dialysis. A low molecular weight hapten is placed on one side of a membrane that is permeable to small molecules (e.g., M.W. less than 1,000), and the antibody, which is too large to pass through the membrane, is placed on the other side. For example, a dialysis sac containing antibody in known concentration is immersed in a solution of hapten. At intervals, samples from the sac and the surrounding liquid are analyzed for free haptens (colored or radioactively labeled haptens are easily determined). Within a few hours an equilibrium is reached (see Figure 6-1). If no antibody is present in the sac, at equilibrium the concentrations of ligand inside and outside the sac will become equal. However, if antibody is present, it will react with some ligand entering the sac, so additional ligand will enter until the concentration of *free* ligand in the sac equals that outside. The difference in total concentration of ligand inside and outside the sac represents the amount bound by antibody. From this figure and the known concentrations of ligand and antibody originally employed, it is possible to calculate the intrinsic association constant of the antibody. Actual values vary greatly among antigen-antibody systems and even within the same system from one antiserum to another or from time to time during immunization; the range is usually between 10^3 and 10^{10} liters per mole.

The effect of a structural change in a hapten on its binding affinity for an antibody site can be expressed by its relative combining constant, K_{rel}:

$$K_{rel} = \frac{K}{K_{ref\ hapten}}$$

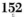

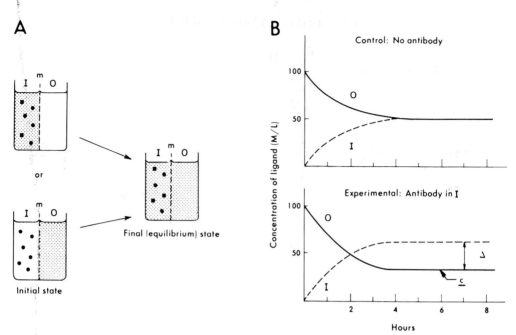

Figure 6-1. Equilibrium dialysis. *A, bottom,* Antibody in compartment I (inside) is initially separated from a hapten by a membrane (m) permeable to the hapten but not to the antibody. *B, bottom,* Periodic assay of free hapten in the outer compartment (solid line) and the inner compartment (dashed line) indicates that equilibrium is attained by 4 hours; $\underline{c}$ is the concentration of unbound hapten at equilibrium, and Δ is the concentration of hapten bound to antibody in compartment I at equilibrium. In the absence of antibody (*B, top*), the concentration of hapten becomes the same inside and outside the membrane. Since the reaction is reversible, the same final equilibrium is attained, whether antibody and hapten are initially in different compartments or in the same compartment (*A, top*). (From Davis et al., 1973. Microbiology, 2nd ed., p. 361. Hagerstown, Md., Harper and Row, Publishers, Inc.)

in which its association constant is compared with that of a reference hapten. Table 6-1 illustrates the type of data obtainable and shows, with reference to the 2,4-dinitrophenyl system, that both nitro groups are necessary for good combination with the antibody site (K_{rel} = 3.7 and 2.2 vs. 0.012 and 0.01 with *p*- and *o*-nitroaniline). The high K_{rel} obtained with the DNP-lysine suggests that attachment of dinitrophenyl to protein in the immunogen may occur via ϵ-amino groups.

FLUORESCENCE QUENCHING

Another method of determining the equilibrium constant that is very rapid but less generally applicable than equilibrium dialysis is based upon the fact that tryptophan residues of protein fluoresce when exposed to ultraviolet light and that the fluorescence of antibody protein is quenched when particular antigens or haptens are bound by the antibody. The degree of quenching is proportional to the number of antibody sites combined, so this provides a method of evaluating the concentration of hapten-antibody complexes and hence determining the association constant, K. Titrations are made by measuring the fluorescence of the antibody solution after adding each of a series of small increments of hapten. The data permit calculation of the concentration of binding sites and the value of K. The method requires only 10 to 20 minutes and a small amount of antibody (20 to 200 μg.), but it is limited to purified antibody preparations and to yellow-colored haptens.

HAPTEN INHIBITION OF PRECIPITATION

A very common method of determining K_{rel} is by inhibition of precipitation. When a univalent hapten combines with an antibody site, it prevents subsequent union of that site with bivalent antigen and hence decreases precipitation. Two series of analyses are needed: one with various amounts of test hapten and the other with various amounts of reference hapten. Each is added to the antiserum and followed later

Table 6–1 Binding of Haptens to Antibody Against

2,4-Dinitrophenyl

Hapten		K_{rel}
m-Dinitrobenzene (reference hapten)		1.00
2,4-Dinitroaniline		3.7
2,4-Dinitrotoluene		2.2
p-Nitroaniline		0.012
o-Nitroaniline		0.01
ε-DNP-L-lysine		38

by the antigen. An end point is chosen, such as 50 per cent inhibition of precipitation, and K_{rel} is given by the equation:

$$K_{rel} = \frac{\text{(total conc. ref. hapten added to give 50\% inhibition)}}{\text{(total conc. hapten added to give 50\% inhibition)}}$$

Effects of Temperature, pH, and Ionic Strength on Rate of Hapten-Antibody Reaction

Antibodies are relatively stable proteins, so they are active over a wide range of conditions. Temperature variations within a range from 4° to 40° C. have no effect on some systems; that is, they do not change the association constant, K. Heidelberger reported that egg albumin and its antibody combined in less than 20 seconds, even at 0° C., and that union between pneumococcal polysaccharides and antibodies was 90 per cent complete in less than 3 seconds at 0° C. With other systems the value of K decreases as the temperature increases; in other words, binding is exothermic. Boyd detected evolution of heat by microcalorimetry immediately upon mixing hemocyanin and its antibody; the reaction was complete in about 3 minutes, with evolution of approximately 40,000 gram calories per mole of antibody. No antibody-ligand system has been found in which there is increasing affinity with increasing temperature.

The effect of temperature on serologic reactions is probably limited chiefly to the secondary or visible result of hapten-antibody union, which is usually slower than the primary reaction. Figures such as those in Table 6–2, obtained by observation of secondary reactions, still indicate a wide range of reactivity, from 0° to 60° C. Reaction was so nearly complete, even at 0° C., that increased temperature had little if any stimulating effect.

Inhibition above 55°C. can be attributed in part to increased dissociation and in part to denaturation of the reagents. Dissociation of some antigen-antibody complexes occurs when the temperatue is raised. "Cold hemagglutinins" (see page 203) react with erythrocytes at low temperatures but dissociate from them upon incubation at 25 to 37° C. Agglutinins may be separated from certain bacteria by a similar procedure. Stuart and Carpenter observed flagellar agglutination of normal and intermediate Escherichia and paracolon strains after 2 hours at 37° C., but agglutination of approximately 65 per cent of the strains was partially or completely reversed when the tests were placed at 55° C. overnight. Reincubation at 37° C. of tests in which dispersion had occurred at 55° C. resulted in complete reagglutination.

Table 6–2   *Effect of Temperature on Union of Sheep Hemolysin with Homologous Erythrocytes**

Temperature (°C.)	Per Cent Adsorption of Hemolysin
0	90
15	94
25	94
37	90
40	88
45	82
50	78
55	60
60	38

*From Cromwell, 1922. J. Immunol., 7:461.

Binding of ionic ligands is affected by changes in pH and ionic strength, whereas nonionic ligands are relatively unaffected. The reaction of p-aminobenzoate with its antibody decreases as the pH falls from 7 to 4 and as the NaCl concentration increases from 0.1 M to 1.0 M, in contrast to the reaction of 2,4-dinitroaniline with its antibody. Apparently binding of the former ligand involves interaction between the —COO⁻ radical and a positively charged group in the antibody site, but ionic interactions are less significant in the case of the neutral dinitrobenzene ligand.

Practical utilization of the effect of high ionic strength was made by Heidelberger in the purification of anti-pneumococcal antibodies. The polysaccharide ligands contain ionizable groups (e.g., —COOH), which dissociate from antibody when the NaCl concentration is raised from the normal 0.15 M to 2.5 M. Agglutinated bacteria or precipitated polysaccharide are therefore treated with additional salt, whereupon pure antibody can be recovered (see page 63).

The rate of reaction between antibody and ligand is extremely rapid. The binding of small haptens is one of the fastest biochemical reactions known. The rate constant, k, is only about ten times less than that of diffusion-limited reactions; that is, a theoretic limit of 10^9 liters per mole per second. The fact that the activation energy of the forward reaction is low (as indicated by the comparatively slight effect of temperature on K) suggests that the antibody combining site is rigid and requires little conformational adjustment to accommodate the hapten. This is in contrast to the case with enzymatic reactions, which often include complicated sequences of conformational modification.

REACTIONS OF ANTIBODY WITH SOLUBLE MACROMOLECULAR ANTIGENS

Whereas the reaction between antibodies and haptens cannot be visualized directly, reactions with macromolecular antigens like proteins and polysaccharides may lead to a visible result such as precipitation. It must be borne in mind, however, that the primary reaction is the same, whether the ligand is a soluble, univalent hapten or one of many determinant sites on the surface of a large carrier molecule or, as will be seen, on an erythrocyte or bacterial cell.

Two-stage Nature of Serologic Reactions

Serologic reactions involving macromolecular or particulate antigens are two-stage processes. The first step consists of the reaction just described—union of antibody combining site with antigenic determinant. The nature of the second step is determined by the physical state of the antigen and by accompanying conditions. Precipitation and agglutination have been most used in studies of the theoretic aspects of visible antigen-antibody reactions.

In the absence of a proper concentration of electrolyte a potent antityphoid serum does not agglutinate typhoid bacteria that have been adequately freed from electrolyte by washing with distilled water. However, addition of sodium chloride or various other electrolytes is promptly followed by agglutination. Specific agglutination by antiserum obviously requires the presence of three reagents: antiserum, antigen, and electrolyte. The same requirement can also be demonstrated in precipitation. Antigen and antibody separately do not flocculate in the presence of electrolyte, so it appears that agglutination and precipitation are two-stage reactions. The first stage is the union of antigen and antibody, and the second stage is the visible effect caused by electrolyte.

In bacteriolysis, hemolysis, and bactericidal action, the second stage is mediated by complement, the nature and activity of which will be described more fully in

Chapter 8. Opsonic action is visualized only through the activity of phagocytic cells. Anaphylaxis and other examples of immediate-type hypersensitivity are demonstrable with tissues sensitive to histamine, serotonin, and the other chemicals liberated in the primary antigen-antibody reaction.

PRECIPITATION REACTIONS IN SOLUTION

The Zone Phenomenon. A peculiarity of many serologic reactions is the zone phenomenon, illustrated in the case of precipitation by the results shown in Table 6–3. Five-tenths of a milligram of egg albumin yielded the maximum amount of precipitate when mixed with 1 ml. of undiluted antiserum. All the antigen combined with all the antibody in the mixture, as shown by examination of the supernatant liquid after removal of the precipitate. Decreased precipitation with larger amounts of antigen is called the "inhibition" or prozone phenomenon. Within the antigen excess inhibition zone there was insufficient antibody to precipitate all the antigen, although part of the antigen combined with the antibody. Some of the antigen-antibody complexes were evidently of such small size (low molecular weight) that they did not precipitate. The reaction mixture also contained uncombined antigen, which was detected by addition of antiserum to the supernatant liquid. Lesser amounts of antigen also yielded smaller precipitates than that obtained with 0.5 mg. of egg albumin. All the available antigen was combined, so the decreased amounts of precipitate can be attributed to insufficient antigen to combine with the antibody present. Excess (uncombined) antibody was present in the supernatant fluid. Many antigen-antibody systems are not particularly sensitive to slight excesses of antigen, so there is often a range of antigen concentrations within which neither antigen nor antibody is present in the supernates. This is known as the "equivalence zone." Maximal precipitation occurs either within this zone or in mixtures containing a small excess of antigen.

Precipitates formed in the equivalence zone may disappear when more antigen is added. A point usually not made clear is that "dissolution" of the precipitate is merely conversion of a large aggregate into small, invisible complexes, owing to dissociation and reassociation into aggregates containing a higher concentration of antigen. An antigen-antibody precipitate is usually pictured as a chain or network of alternating antigen (G) and antibody (A) molecules:

$$
\begin{array}{ccc}
| & | & | \\
A & A & A \\
| & | & | \\
-G-A-G-A-G- \\
| & | & | \\
A & A & A \\
| & | & |
\end{array}
$$

Table 6–3   The Zone Phenomenon in Precipitation

Egg albumin (mg. in 1 ml.)	2.0	1.0	0.5	0.25	0.125	0.0625
Rabbit anti-egg albumin serum (undiluted)	1 ml.	1 ml.	1 ml.	1 ml.	1 ml.	1 ml.
Precipitation	±	+++	++++	+++	++	+
Tests of supernates:						
*with antiserum	+	+	−	−	−	−
**with egg albumin	−	−	−	+	+	+

*+ in this row indicates excess antigen
**+ in this row indicates excess antibody

A large network yields a visible precipitate, but when the reaction mixture possesses a high antigen:antibody ratio or when further antigen is added to a precipitate, small complexes are formed, such as

$$G—A—G$$

These are invisible and of such low molecular weight that they are referred to as "soluble complexes."

Early work suffered from ignorance of the zone phenomenon or lack of appreciation of its significance. Visible reaction sometimes does not occur if only one or a few dilutions of antigen are tested, depending upon the position of the dilutions in relation to the equivalence zone. Adequate study of a precipitating system requires tests with several dilutions of first one reagent and then the other.

Simple mixtures of antigen and antiserum, observed macroscopically for relative turbidity or amount of precipitate, yield only limited information. Precipitates are sometimes measured roughly by centrifugation in graduated tubes. Photoelectric devices have been adapted to determine the cloudiness or turbidity of precipitating mixtures. Tests of this sort are usually read after a specified time interval because the amount of precipitate increases to some extent with continued incubation. Dean and Webb employed the reaction times of simple mixtures to determine the end point of a titration procedure that bears their names. Antigen dilutions were mixed with a constant amount of antiserum and closely observed. The mixture in the series that flocculated most rapidly was noted. A typical set of results, cited by Wilson and Miles, is shown in Table 6–4. The first visible reaction occurred at a particular ratio of antiserum to antigen (40:1). Dean and Webb found that the "optimal ratio" was constant for a given lot of antiserum. If the antiserum illustrated in Table 6–4 were used in a dilution of 1:5, it would flocculate most rapidly with antigen diluted 1:200, and so forth. Such a relationship makes it possible (1) to determine the amount of an antigen in an unknown solution by use of a standardized antiserum, and (2) to determine the relative amounts of antibody in two or more antisera.

The result obtained by the Dean and Webb method is called the constant antibody optimal ratio. When antigen is kept constant and antibody is varied, a mixture is often found that reacts most rapidly in a series of antiserum dilutions. This method is used in the Ramon flocculation test of diphtheria antitoxic sera (see Chap. 8). Both titration procedures employed with the same antigen and antibody yield results like those in Table 6–5. Each horizontal row represents a constant antibody titration in which antigen concentration is varied and contains a mixture flocculating more rapidly than any other mixture in the same row. For example, 1:20 antibody reacted most rapidly with 1:800 antigen, and 1:40 antibody reacted most rapidly with 1:1600 antigen. The

Table 6–4 *Effect of Antigen Dilution on the Flocculation Time of Antigen and Antibody (1:10 Rabbit Antihorse Serum)**

Antigen (Horse Serum) Dilution	Flocculation Time (min.)
1:50	14.5
1:100	12.0
1:200	8.0
1:400	6.0
1:800	8.5
1:1,600	13.0
1:3,200	28.0

*From Wilson and Miles, 1946. Topley and Wilson's Principles of Bacteriology and Immunity, 3rd ed. London, Edward Arnold and Company, Ltd.

Table 6–5   *Constant Antibody versus Constant Antigen Precipitation Reactions**

Antibody Dilutions	Antigen (Horse Serum) Dilutions						
	1:50	1:100	1:200	1:400	1:800	1:1,600	1:3,200
	Flocculation time (minutes)						
1:2.5	2.75	2.25†	2.50	3.25	6.00	17.00	60.00
1:5	4.00	3.50	2.75	3.75	7.00	14.00	40.00
1:10	14.50	12.00	8.00	*6.00*	8.50	**13.00‡**	**28.00**
1:20	134.00	39.00	30.00	19.00	*13.50*	18.50	**28.00**
1:40	–	–	83.00	65.00	50.00	*38.00*	45.00

*From Wilson and Miles, 1946. Topley and Wilson's Principles of Bacteriology and Immunity, 3rd ed. London, Edward Arnold and Company, Ltd.

†Italicized figures are minimal flocculation times in constant antibody titrations (horizontal rows).

‡Bold face figures are minimal flocculation times in constant antigen titrations (vertical columns).

constant antibody optimal ratio was 40:1. Each column of the table represents a constant antigen titration, antibody being varied. Minimum flocculation times in the last two vertical columns indicate that the constant antigen optimal ratio was approximately 160:1.

Flocculation time is determined by several factors, including the antigen:antibody ratio and the chemical compositions and molecular weights of the antigen and antibody. These factors and differences in solubility of various antibodies and antigen-antibody complexes probably account for the observation that constant antibody and constant antigen optimal ratios rarely, if ever, coincide.

Application of quantitative chemical procedures to the analysis of precipitates formed in mixtures of antigens and antibodies furnished a method of determining the amounts of the reaction substances that appear in precipitates. These procedures, developed by Heidelberger and his associates, made it possible to describe antigen-antibody reactions precisely and provided an objective basis for an hypothesis of the mechanism of reaction between antigen and antibody.

The quantitative method is based upon the fact that antibody is protein and hence contains nitrogen, which can be determined with high accuracy by the micro-Kjeldahl or various other methods. Mixtures containing known amounts of antiserum and antigen are incubated under conditions of temperature and time favorable for maximal precipitation (1 to 7 days at 0° C.). The precipitates are washed and quantitatively analyzed for total nitrogen. The nitrogen content of the antigen alone is also determined. Subtraction of the amount of nitrogen in the antigen from the total in the precipitate yields the antibody nitrogen in the precipitate, when a test of the supernatant fluid indicates that all the antigen was precipitated. Excess (uncombined) antigen in the supernate can be determined quantitatively by a second precipitation with additional antiserum. Certain antigens possess distinctive chemical characteristics by which their concentration in a precipitate can be ascertained. For example, hemocyanin contains copper, and synthetic azoprotein antigens often contain readily determinable elements, such as arsenic, iodine, or radioisotopes. Moreover, some polysaccharide antigens contain no nitrogen, so all the nitrogen in their specific precipitates represents antibody.

The variation in composition of an antigen-antibody precipitate is illustrated by quantitative data obtained with egg albumin and a rabbit anti-egg albumin serum (Table 6–6 and Figure 6–2). Addition of increasing amounts of egg albumin to a constant amount of anti-egg albumin yielded precipitates which increased to a maximum (0.830 mg. N), and throughout this range all the antigen was precipitated.

*Table 6–6 Analyses of Precipitates Formed by Adding Various Amounts
of Egg Albumin to 1.0 ml. Rabbit Anti-egg Albumin Serum**

Egg Albumin N Added	Total N Precipitated	Egg Albumin N Precipitated	Antibody Nitrogen by Difference	Ratio in Precipitate: Antibody N / Egg Albumin N	Tests of Supernatant Liquid
mg.	mg.	mg.	mg.		
0.0091	0.156	Total	0.147	16.2	Excess Ab†
0.0155	0.236	Total	0.220	14.2	Excess Ab
0.050	0.632	Total	0.582	11.6	Excess Ab
0.065	0.740	Total	0.675	10.4	Excess Ab, tr. Ea‡
0.074	0.794	Total	0.720	9.7	No Ab or Ea
0.082	0.830	Total	0.748	9.1	No Ab, < 0.001 Ea N
0.090	0.826	0.087	0.739	8.5	Excess Ea
0.124	0.730	0.087	0.643	7.4	Excess Ea
0.195	0.414	(0.048)	(0.366)	(7.6)	Excess Ea
0.307	0.106	(0.004)			Excess Ea

(Values in parentheses uncertain.)
*From Heidelberger and Kendall, 1935. J. Exp. Med., 62:697.
†Ab = antibody.
‡Ea = egg albumin (antigen).

The first four supernates contained excess antibody. Beyond the maximum, decreasing amounts of egg albumin precipitated, the excess remaining in the supernates, and the total quantity of precipitate diminished. The relative amounts of antibody and antigen in the precipitates varied markedly throughout the range of the experiment. The ratio of antibody nitrogen to antigen nitrogen was about 16 to 1 in the region where considerable antibody remained uncombined, whereas in the region of antigen excess the antibody:antigen nitrogen ratio was approximately 7.5 to 1. The ratio in the zone of equivalence was about 9 to 1. Assuming that the molecular weights of egg albumin and of rabbit antibody are 42,000 and 165,000, respectively, the molecular antibody:antigen ratio at equivalence was approximately 2.5 to 1. These and similar data with other

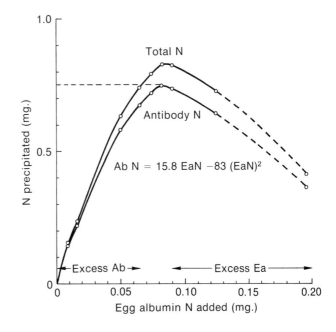

Figure 6–2. Total and antibody nitrogen precipitated from 1.0-ml. aliquots of a rabbit anti-egg albumin serum by various amounts of egg albumin. The graphic method of estimating the antibody content of an antiserum is illustrated. (Plotted from the data of Table 6–6.)

systems permit calculation of the molecular compositions of precipitates or complexes formed when antigen and antibody in various proportions are allowed to react (Table 6–7).

Mathematical Relations in Antigen-Antibody Reactions.   The antibody:antigen ratio (r) in some precipitates formed in the antibody excess zone can be represented by an equation of the following type:

(1) $r = a - bG$

in which G = mg. antigen nitrogen (Ag N) precipitated and a and b are constants whose values can be calculated from the data. With excess antibody, all or nearly all the antigen is precipitated, as shown in Table 6–6, so G is essentially equal to the amount of antigen nitrogen added. If both sides of equation (1) are multiplied by G, it becomes:

(2) Ab N precipitated $= aG - bG^2$

When the data of Table 6–6 are plotted to show the relationship of r, the antibody:antigen ratio in the precipitate, to the amount of antigen added to a constant amount of antibody, the straight line shown in Figure 6–3 is obtained. The equation for this line can readily be calculated as follows:

r = 15.8 – 83 Ea N

It is evident from the linear relationship between r and the amount of antigen precipitated in the region of antibody excess that the composition of the precipitate changes uniformly throughout most of this zone, decreasing from a maximum value of approximately 16. A ratio of 9 is attained in the equivalence zone, and thereafter the linear relationship does not hold.

The equation for the curve in Figure 6–2 becomes:

Ab N precipitated $= 15.8$ Ea N $- 83$ (Ea N)^2

where the values 15.8 and 83 are substituted for a and b in equation (2).

Heidelberger and Kendall derived an equation based on the mass law of chemical reactions:

(3) Ab N precipitated $= 2\,RG - \dfrac{R^2}{A}G^2$

Table 6–7   *Molecular Composition of Precipitates with Rabbit Antisera**

Antigen	Inhibition Zone (prozone)		Equivalence Zone		Extreme Antibody Excess in Supernate
	Soluble Compounds	Antigen Excess	Slight Antigen Excess	Slight Antibody Excess	
Egg albumin (E)	(EA†)	EA$_2$	E$_2$A$_5$	EA$_3$	EA$_5$
Pneumococcus 3 specific polysaccharide (S)	(S$_5$A)	S$_4$A	S$_2$A	S$_3$A$_2$	SA
Hemocyanin (H)		HA$_{36}$	HA$_{83}$	HA$_{120}$	
Diphtheria toxin (T)		T$_2$A	T$_2$A$_3$	TA$_4$	TA$_8$

*Reprinted by permission from Landsteiner, 1945. The Specificity of Serological Reactions, revised ed. Cambridge, Harvard University Press.
†A = antibody.
Composition of compounds in parentheses is uncertain.

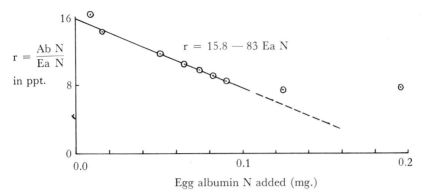

Figure 6–3. Straight line illustrating the linear relationship between the antibody:antigen ratios in precipitates and the amount of antigen added in the antibody excess and equivalence zones. Plotted from the data of Table 6–6.

in which A = mg. antibody N precipitated at the equivalence point and $R = \dfrac{A}{G}$ at the equivalence point. From this it is apparent that the constants a and b in equations (1) and (2) are $2R$ and $\dfrac{R^2}{A}$, respectively.

The data of some systems do not fit a curve of the form described by equation (2) but agree better with the following:

(4) Ab N precipitated $= cG - dG^{\frac{3}{2}}$

in which c and d are constants.

Several factors adversely affect the agreement between the observed results of a quantitative precipitation experiment and those calculated by one of the above equations. Kabat listed several as follows:

1. The system may contain more than one antigen capable of reacting with the antiserum. This is discussed in more detail below (see page 163).

2. Complement in the antiserum may react with the antigen-antibody aggregate and cause a higher apparent antibody:antigen ratio than anticipated.

3. Use of only two points to draw the antibody:antigen ratio line and to calculate the values of a and b may lead to error if the points are chosen poorly or the analytical data are inaccurate; three or more points are advisable.

4. Some antigens, especially those of high molecular weight, do not yield a linear relationship with any of the above equations.

5. Certain sera contain antibodies that do not give a straight line relationship.

Quantitative Determination of Precipitin in Antiserum. The quantitative precipitin test just described permits precise determination of the amount of antibody in an antiserum. From the data presented in Table 6–6 and Figure 6–2, the amount of antibody N precipitated from the anti-egg albumin serum was calculated by subtracting the antigen nitrogen precipitated from the total nitrogen precipitated. It is apparent that the antiserum contained about 0.75 mg. of antibody nitrogen capable of reacting specifically with the homologous antigen. This figure represents the highest point of the antibody nitrogen curve.

The total antibody content of an antiserum can be calculated from the equation describing the relationship between antigen added and antibody precipitated. The general equation

(2) Antibody N precipitated $= aG - bG^2$

was found to fit the data for the egg albumin–anti-egg albumin curve, and the constants were

$$a = 15.8$$
$$\text{and } b = 83$$

The anti-egg albumin content of the serum (i.e., the amount precipitable at equivalence) is therefore obtained by the following:

$$\text{Antibody N} = (15.8 \times 0.082) - 83(0.082)^2$$
$$= 0.738 \text{ mg./ml.}$$

The value found graphically agrees very closely with this.

The quantitative technique has been widely employed in studies of the nature of antigen-antibody reactions. Certain antisera produced in the horse, for example, yield a different type of reaction curve from that illustrated in Figure 6–2, which was obtained with rabbit antiserum. The reaction between diphtheria toxin and homologous horse antitoxin is shown in Figure 6–4. Flocculation occurs only within a certain range of toxin concentrations and is completely inhibited both below and above this zone. This reaction is referred to by some authors as the "flocculation reaction" in contrast to the "precipitin reaction," typified by the behavior of rabbit antiserum against egg albumin. The precipitin reaction is characterized by a narrow equivalence zone and by gradually decreasing precipitates on either side of equivalence. The antibody content of flocculating antiserum is indicated by extrapolation of the straight portion of the curve to the vertical axis. Throughout most of the zone of flocculation all the antigen and antibody are precipitated, neither appearing in the supernatant liquid. Flocculating antibodies are observed only in antisera derived from the horse, but not all horse antisera are of this type. Flocculating antibodies have been described for diphtheria, tetanus, scarlet fever, and botulinum toxins, chicken ovalbumin and conalbumin, human and rabbit serum albumins, and hemocyanin.

The quantitative precipitin technique is useful for the assay of specifically reacting substances for which no other analytic method is available. One advantage of this

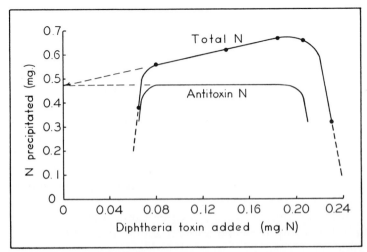

Figure 6–4. Total nitrogen and antitoxin nitrogen precipitated from 1.0 ml. of a diphtherial horse antitoxin, showing complete inhibition of flocculation outside the equivalence zone. (Plotted from data in Pappenheimer and Robinson, 1937. J. Immunol., 32:291.)

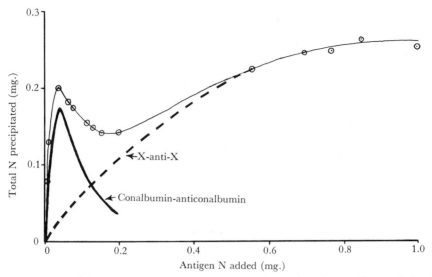

Figure 6–5. Bimodal quantitative precipitation curve obtained with partially purified egg conalbumin and its rabbit antiserum. The impurity, X, probably amounted to not more than 5 per cent of the total protein; its precipitation curve was drawn by extrapolation backward from the point corresponding to 0.55 mg. antigen-N. The conalbumin-anticonalbumin curve is the mathematical difference between the other curves. (From Cohn et al., 1949. J. Immunol., 61:283.)

procedure is that the substance does not have to be in pure form but may be mixed with other components if the antiserum contains no antibodies capable of reacting with the heterologous substances. Globulins and albumins in normal and pathologic sera, lymph, edema and ascitic fluids have been measured quantitatively by means of homologous antisera. Blood group polysaccharides in a variety of secretions have also been estimated by specific precipitation.

Reactions of Impure Antigens. Protein and other antigens are rarely pure as encountered in nature; usually they occur in mixtures with other antigenic substances, from which they cannot be separated easily. Antiserum prepared by immunizing an animal with such a mixture contains separate antibodies for each antigenic component. Minute traces of a contaminating antigen often induce the formation of a disproportionately large amount of antibody. When a precipitation reaction is performed with this antiserum and the mixed antigens, each specific antibody reacts with its antigen in a quantitative relationship that is characteristic of the antigen-antibody system and is often different from that of the other antigen-antibody system in the mixture.

The experimental result is that even at the apparent equivalence point the fluid from which a precipitate has been removed may contain both antigens and antibodies, and in no mixture will all the antigens and antibodies be precipitated. Moreover, precipitates formed with larger amounts of the mixed antigens will not decrease sharply toward zero, as would be the case with a pure antigen. Instead, small amounts of precipitate may form, even with great excess of the antigen mixture; if the impurity is very highly antigenic there may even be a second increase in the amount of precipitate formed. Figure 6–5 illustrates this situation. Rabbit antiserum was prepared against conalbumin isolated from egg white by precipitation with alcohol and purified by reprecipitation. The quantitative precipitation curve obtained with these reagents showed two peaks: one when about 0.04 mg. antigen N was added to 1 ml. of antiserum and the other with about 0.8 mg. antigen N. The first peak appeared to represent the conalbumin–anti-conalbumin reaction, whereas the second peak was attributed to a highly antigenic impurity that made up no more than 5 per cent of the isolated protein.

The bimodal curve was interpreted to be the sum of two separate antigen-antibody curves. The curve showing the reaction of the impurity with its antibody was approximated by extrapolating backward to zero from a point at approximately 0.5 mg. antigen N (curve X–anti-X). The difference between this extrapolated curve and the first peak of the bimodal curve was then plotted as the conalbumin–anti-conalbumin curve.

In the region between the two peaks of a bimodal curve, the supernates, after precipitation has ceased, contain unreacted antigen of the first system (e.g., conalbumin) and also unreacted antibody for the second antigen (e.g., X). It is obvious that the quantitative precipitation reaction is an important means of determining the serologic purity of isolated antigenic substances such as proteins.

PRECIPITATION REACTIONS IN GELS

The homogeneity and identity of antigens and antibodies are also indicated by the results of precipitation reactions in gels. Antigen and antibody diffuse toward one another through the gel, and where they meet in optimal proportions they form a visible precipitate in a disc, band, or line. Each antigen-antibody system that has a unique optimal reaction zone produces a separate precipitate.

Oudin reported in 1946 that when antiserum is gelled with agar and overlaid with a single, pure antigen, the zone of precipitate that forms migrates downward into the serum-agar, the distance of migration being inversely related to the square of the time elapsed. Two or more unrelated antigens tested in the same tube against a mixture of their homologous antibodies yielded a corresponding number of zones of precipitate, usually migrating at different rates because of differences in the concentrations and diffusion constants of the various antigens (see Figure 6–6).

The Oudin procedure depends upon *simple* or *single diffusion* in one dimension. The method permits determination of the *minimum* number of antigenic substances in a mixture such as blood plasma or cell extract and detection of antigenic impurities in protein solutions. It has been used for such purposes as determination of the number and succession of proteins during development of the frog from the egg through the embryonic stages to the adult stage.

Double diffusion in one dimension was described in 1953 by Oakley and Fulthorpe, and a modification known as the Preer technique was reported in 1956. Serum is placed in the bottom of a tube 1.7 to 2.0 mm. in inside diameter, and plain

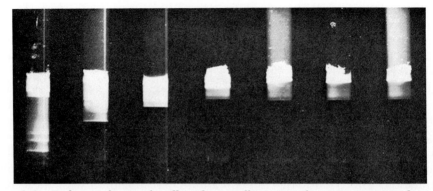

Figure 6–6. Oudin test showing the effect of recrystallization on the antigenic purity of egg albumin. Antiserum against egg white in agar was overlaid with (left to right) egg white, egg albumin crystallized once, twice, thrice, etc. The number of separately precipitating antigenic fractions decreased with repeated recrystallizations. (From Munoz *In* Cole, W. H. (Ed.): Serological Approaches to Studies of Protein Structure and Metabolism, 1954. New Brunswick, N. J., Rutgers University Press.)

agar is carefully overlaid and allowed to solidify; antigen is then added as the top layer. Planes of precipitate appear in the agar layer at points where antigen and antibody meet in serologically equivalent proportions and, in general, each antigen-antibody system produces one precipitate disc. Precipitates may be visible within a few hours or after several days. When antibody is constant and tubes are prepared with various concentrations of antigen, the distance from the antigen layer to the band is proportional to the antigen concentration. Conversely, with constant antigen, the greater the concentration of antibody, the greater is the distance from the antibody layer to the band of precipitate. If the initial ratio of antigen to antibody corresponds to serologic equivalence, the band does not move, but if either reagent is in excess the plane of precipitate moves away from the source of that reagent. The Preer test is very sensitive; as little as 0.0001 per cent egg albumin can be detected, and 0.01 ml. of reagent suffices when tubes 1.7 mm. in diameter are employed.

The technique of double diffusion in two dimensions was developed by Elek and Ouchterlony independently in 1948. It is particularly useful for the study of complicated antigen-antibody systems because of its high resolving power and the ease with which one system can be compared with another. Agar containing buffered saline and a preservative is poured on a flat glass surface (Petri dish, glass plate, microscope slide) and allowed to harden. Holes or troughs are cut and the agar is removed. The wells are filled with appropriate antiserum and antigen solutions, and the plates are kept moist for several days or weeks. Under favorable conditions lines of precipitates appear within a few hours between wells containing homologous reagents; weak reactions may not be evident for several days. The number of lines of precipitate indicates the minimum number of distinct antigenic substances present in the antigen solution. Although in general different antigens diffuse at different rates, this is not always the case, so it is possible that two precipitates will coincide. Antibody molecules are assumed to diffuse independently.

When antigen and antibody are in reservoirs of identical size and shape, the curvature of the precipitate line depends in part upon the relative molecular weights of antigen and antibody. If both are of the same molecular weight, the line is usually straight; otherwise, the line tends to be concave toward the reagent of higher molecular weight.

Ouchterlony distinguished three principal types of reaction that may be observed when related antigens in adjacent wells react with antibodies against the various antigenic determinants diffusing from a central reservoir (see Figure 6–7). Type I, the so-called *reaction of identity*, is characterized by fusion of bands of precipitate. In Type II, the *reaction of nonidentity*, the precipitate lines intersect or cross because the samples contain no antigenic determinant in common. Type III is the reaction obtained when the two antigens compared possess common determinants but also display antigenic differences; it is distinguished by spur formation. In Figure 6–7,C, anti-A diffuses toward Antigens AB and A and reacts with the A component to produce a band of precipitate showing the reaction of identity. Antibody B, however, diffuses through the A-anti-A precipitate and forms a precipitate with antigen B; most of this is in the same band as the A-anti-A precipitate, but a little extends beyond as a spur. Double spur formation (Figure 6–7,D) occurs when each of the cross-reacting antigens is somewhat different from the antigen used to produce the antiserum.

Use of the word "identity" has been criticized because the method offers only evidence that two antigen components produce a single, visible precipitate with the same antiserum. They might actually comprise different structures.

Application of the Ouchterlony technique to the study of cross-reactions of hen and duck egg albumin and products of partial enzymatic digestion of these proteins is illustrated in Figure 6–8. The antigenic preparations to be compared were arranged in

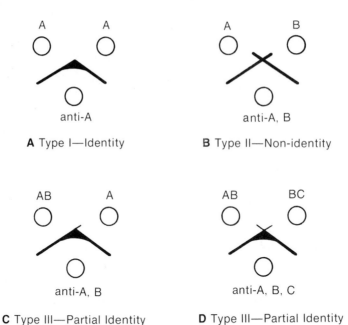

A Type I—Identity

B Type II—Non-identity

C Type III—Partial Identity

D Type III—Partial Identity

Figure 6–7. Types of reaction in Ouchterlony gel diffusion precipitation tests. A, B, and C represent determinant groups on cross-reacting antigen molecules, which are placed in neighboring wells, equidistant from a well containing antiserum (anti-A, anti-A, B, etc.).

rows, and the antisera were placed in troughs parallel with the rows of antigen reservoirs. Spur formation indicated many reactions of Type III; for example, anti-HEa reacted with both HEa and DEa, but the spur between these two bands of precipitate showed that HEa possessed a component not found in DEa. Conversely, the reactions of the same antigens with anti-DEa showed that DEa possessed a component absent from HEa.

Radial immunodiffusion is used to quantitate an antigen (e.g., an immunoglobulin or a hormone). Agar containing the appropriate antiserum is poured on glass plates or slides, and wells are cut. After a solution containing the antigen is placed in a well, a ring of precipitate forms, the diameter of which depends upon the concentration of the antigen. Known concentrations of pure antigen are used to prepare a standard curve, and the concentration of the unknown is read from the curve (see Figure 6–9).

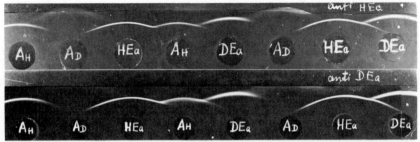

Figure 6–8. Cross-reactions of native and partially digested hen and duck egg albumins with anti-hen and anti-duck egg albumin sera. Antigens were placed in the circular wells, antisera in horizontal troughs above each row of wells. Numerous reactions of partial identity are indicated by spur formation. It is evident that hen and duck albumins share antigenic components, but each also possesses distinctive components. (HEa, hen egg albumin; DEa, duck egg albumin; AH, partially digested hen egg albumin; AD, partially digested duck egg albumin.) (From Kaminski, 1962. Immunology, 5:322.)

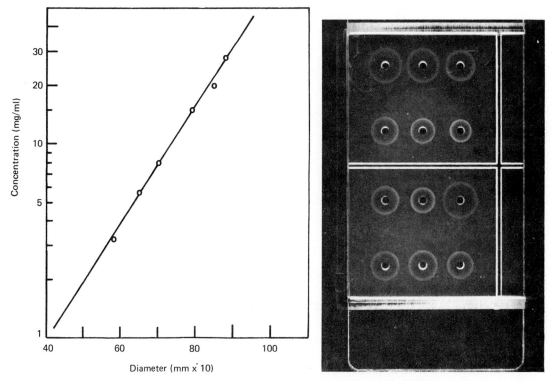

Figure 6–9. Measurement of antigen concentrations by radial immunodiffusion. Known concentrations of human IgG were placed in wells in agar containing goat anti-human IgG (*right, top*). The diameters of the circular precipitates were plotted to obtain the standard curve (*left*). Tests with six different human sera are shown at the right, bottom. (From Davis et al., 1973. Microbiology, 2nd ed., p. 390. Hagerstown, Md., Harper and Row, Publishers, Inc.)

REACTIONS OF ANTIBODIES WITH PARTICULATE ANTIGENS

The agglutination that follows union of antibody with determinants on the surface of particulate antigens, such as bacteria, erythrocytes, or inert particles (e.g., collodion, bentonite) coated with a soluble antigen, is similar in most respects to the precipitation of antigens in solution, with the important difference that much less antibody is required to produce the visible result. Since IgG antibody is bivalent, one molecule theoretically suffices to bind two antigenic cells together (if the binding force between antibody receptors and antigenic determinants is great enough). Actually, many antibody molecules probably participate in union of two antigenic particles, and moreover there is good evidence for "monogamous binding" of antibody, each molecule attaching to two determinant sites on a single antigenic particle (see Figure 6–10); this may involve many molecules of IgG per particle of antigen.

Most natural cellular antigens contain a number of different determinants distributed over their surface, and an antiserum usually contains a variety of antibodies, each of which is specific for one of these determinants. It was noted earlier, for example (Figure 5–9), that *S. paratyphi B* possesses somatic antigens 1, 4, 5, and 12, which contain glucose, abequose, acetyl galactose, and rhamnose as terminal or immunodominant sugar residues. Therefore, antibodies with receptors for any one of these sugars in the proper oligosaccharide sequence will assist in agglutinating the organism.

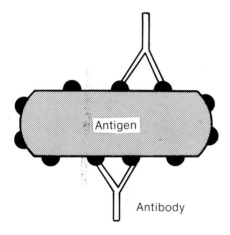

Figure 6–10. Monogamous binding of bivalent anti-body to two determinant sites on an antigenic particle.

Factors Affecting Agglutination

Electrolytes are necessary for agglutination, although they may not be required for union of antibody with determinant. Too high a concentration of salt may agglutinate bacterial suspensions in the absence of antibody ("salt agglutination"), as it may precipitate ("salt out") proteins nonspecifically.

Combination with antibody apparently protects antigenic particles against loss of cohesiveness in electrolyte solutions, so that aggregation occurs even with univalent cations when the surface potential is below 15 mv. In the absence of antibody, bacteria behave as though they are hydrophilic, whereas after union with antibody they become hydrophobic.

The visible stage of serologic reactions is usually accelerated as the temperature rises from 0 to 20 or 30° C. and in some cases to higher temperatures. The increased rate of precipitation or agglutination results in part from accelerated Brownian movement, which causes more frequent collisions between the reacting molecules or particles. Greater rates of molecular or particle contact are also obtained by incubating precipitation or agglutination tests with the water bath level at two-thirds the depth of the fluid within the test tubes. Convection currents created by the cooler top surface of the liquid promote faster visible reaction. Above 56° C. the rate of precipitation or agglutination usually decreases.

Some antigens and antibodies agglutinate only at very low temperatures. The cold isohemagglutinins or autohemagglutinins clump erythrocytes of the same species or individual from which they were obtained at 0 to 35° C. but not at normal body temperature. Moreover, certain animals such as the rabbit contain cold hemagglutinins for human erythrocytes of any or all blood groups as well as for erythrocytes of the rabbit, guinea pig, horse, and sheep. Cells agglutinated at low temperature redisperse when warmed and reagglutinate when again cooled. Antibody is eluted from the cells by warming but recombines upon cooling.

The optimum temperature for bacterial agglutination varies with the type of organism and antigen (somatic or flagellar). Within a large group of related organisms there may be a temperature gradient through which the different organisms or antigens agglutinate optimally. Flagellar agglutination varies widely with the bacterial species. For certain organisms it is best at room temperature, for others at 37° C., and for some others best results are obtained at temperatures as high as 50 to 55° C. Little if any somatic agglutination may occur after several hours at 37° C., whereas marked agglutination to high titers is obtained at 55° C.

Mechanical shaking accelerates the visible stage of antigen-antibody reactions, apparently by providing increased opportunity for contact between molecules or particles of the reagents. Agglutination, precipitation, complement fixation, and cytolysis are hastened by frequent mixing, and gentle agitation of phagocytosis tests seems to permit more efficient ingestion.

SPECIFICITY AND THE NATURE OF THE FORCES JOINING ANTIGEN AND ANTIBODY

The reaction between antigen and antibody derives much of its theoretic interest from its specificity. Antigens are chemically heterogeneous. Most proteins, some polysaccharides, and possibly a few lipids are antigenic. It is therefore impossible to postulate a single type of attractive force or chemical reaction between antigen and antibody. The alternative appears to be a specific pattern or arrangement of nonspecific forces.

Landsteiner and others demonstrated that highly polar radicals (with which strong fields of force are associated) are important determinants of the specificity of synthetic antigens. Less strongly polar but larger radicals also exert considerable influence upon specificity. It must be presumed that antibody molecules displaying specificity toward these determinant radicals contain sites having an affinity or attraction for the determinants and capable of reacting with them.

Marrack considered that specific attraction between antibody and antigen is the result of intermolecular forces whose specificity is attributable to atoms or radicals with suitable (and presumably opposite) fields of force so arranged that they can come into apposition.

Pauling postulated that the attraction of antigen for antibody consists of several short-range forces, any or all of which may be effective under appropriate conditions. One of the most obvious is Coulomb attraction between positive and negative charges, such as those associated with $-NH_3^+$ and $-COO^-$ ions. The cationic side chains of lysine, arginine, and histidine and the terminal $-NH_3^+$ of any polypeptide chain may interact with $-COO^-$ in side chains of glutamic and aspartic acids, terminal amino acids of peptide chains, and acidic polysaccharides. This force alone is too weak to yield a stable aggregate, but hydrogen bond formation may increase the strength of interaction sufficiently to provide a fairly strong union between the groups.

Hydrogen bonds may form between certain pairs of atoms, among which oxygen and nitrogen yield the strongest bonds. It is believed that protein molecules are held in stable configurations by hydrogen bonds connecting amino and carboxyl radicals:

$$-N-H \cdot \cdot \cdot \cdot O:C\big\langle$$

This linkage provides a moderately firm union.

One of the least specific intermolecular forces exerted between every pair of molecules is van der Waals attraction. This force attracts every atom in one molecule toward every atom in neighboring molecules. It is attributed chiefly to the polarization of any two atoms as they approach each other. Its magnitude is inversely related to the sixth or seventh power of the distance between atoms. The mutual attraction between molecules can be great only if they possess large configurations sufficiently complementary to allow them to approach each other closely.

Electric dipole or multipole forces may play some part in the attraction of one molecule to another but are relatively unimportant in antigen-antibody interactions.

Hydrophobic forces are probably most significant. These are the forces that cause coalescence of oil droplets suspended in water. Protein surfaces, also consisting largely of hydrophobic groups such as hydrocarbon chains and other nonpolar radicals, have a tendency to appose one another. If the "fit" between them is good enough, water molecules are squeezed out and arrange themselves in a more stable (lower free energy) state than that which obtains when they are in contact with a nonpolar surface. The hydrophobic surfaces will therefore be held more firmly together.

The various forces of attraction described are not specific by themselves. However, two molecules with suitable surface structures may be mutually attracted by strong hydrophobic and van der Waals forces as they approach each other under the influence of Brownian motion. An appropriate arrangement of hydrogen bond-forming groups and radicals of opposite electric charge strengthens the force between the two molecules. Pauling postulated that the configuration of the specific combining sites of antigen and antibody correspond to within 1 or 2 Ångstroms. A lower degree of correlation in structure and arrangement provides less tendency for interaction. According to this concept, both specificity and mutual attraction are determined by the extent to which the molecules possess complementary surface configurations.

Najjar preferred a modified lock-and-key hypothesis of the relationship between antigen and antibody on the ground that it better accounts for certain observed irregularities or contradictions, such as the occasional immunogenicity of antibody in the individual who produced it and the formation of specific antibody to one antigen in response to stimulation by another. He proposed that corresponding reactive sites of antigen and antibody are *subcomplementary* in configuration rather than complementary, that is, they fit well enough to interact but do not fit perfectly. When antibody reacts with antigen, forces of attraction (ionic, van der Waals, etc.) cause an adjustment in orientation and spatial accommodation so that the various parts fall into place and a good fit is obtained. The stress exerted on the molecules breaks bonds ordinarily concerned in the secondary and tertiary structures of the proteins and produces a change in configuration of both antibody and antigen. If this occurs in vivo, the antibody may acquire sufficiently "foreign" characteristics to become antigenic in the animal that produced it. The antigen also may acquire new or modified antigenic sites. In consequence, new antibodies may form against (1) the primary antibody, (2) the modified antigen, and (3) the antigen-antibody complex.

MECHANISM OF PRECIPITATION AND AGGLUTINATION

Early investigators dealt with what appeared to be simple systems in their studies of the reactions between antigens and antibodies. Observations were carefully made and adequate in scope and were interpreted in a straightforward manner to yield the simplest hypothesis consistent with the known facts. That some of these hypotheses seem a little naive today is readily understood when it is appreciated that little was known of the chemical and physical properties of the reacting ingredients. In recent years the characteristics of antigens and antibodies have been ascertained in considerable detail, and the proportions in which they can interact have been determined. Hypotheses of the mechanism of antigen-antibody reaction have become more sophisticated and, it is hoped, more nearly in accord with the truth.

Ehrlich's Side Chain Hypothesis

Ehrlich (1906) postulated that the reaction between antigen side chains and antibody receptors is a firm chemical union in constant proportions. This hypothesis encountered opposition when it was shown that a given quantity of antitoxin may completely neutralize varying quantities of toxin. It was then proposed that toxic bacterial filtrates contain substances with differing degrees of toxicity and/or affinity for antitoxin, and such names as toxone, prototoxoid, syntoxoid, and epitoxoid were applied to them. It is of interest that the term *toxoid* is still in widespread use to designate toxin so modified that it does not produce symptoms in an experimental animal although it can combine with antitoxin; this is the same description as that given by Ehrlich.

Ehrlich's hypothesis emphasized the now well established chemical basis of specificity and the chemical nature of antigen-antibody reaction. It gradually became cumbersome as attempts were made to fit new discoveries to the old framework, but it persisted for a number of years. Recent observations, particularly concerning the serologic properties of viruses and erythrocytes, are currently described in terms reminiscent of Ehrlich.

Arrhenius and Madsen's Mass Action Hypothesis

Arrhenius (1907) was the first physical chemist to attempt an interpretation of the reaction between antigen and antibody. He and Madsen concluded from their studies of the neutralization of toxins by antitoxins that they were dealing with a reversible reaction like that between a weak acid and a weak base. They proposed that antigen-antibody reactions follow the law of mass action and attain a state of equilibrium in which both free and combined antigen and antibody are present in concentrations that agree with the familiar mathematical relationship.

The most significant feature of this hypothesis is its emphasis upon reversibility. This was vigorously opposed by Ehrlich, to whom the reaction between toxin and antitoxin seemed to resemble that between a strong acid and a strong base. This question was never adequately investigated by either Ehrlich or Arrhenius and Madsen because of the lack of accurate technical methods at that time.

Bordet's Adsorption Hypothesis

Bordet (1920) attempted to account for the union of antigen and antibody in variable proportions and for the participation of electrolytes in agglutination and precipitation. He regarded the reaction as essentially colloidal in nature and postulated that it consists of the adsorption of antibody by the antigen. The amount of antibody adsorbed is governed by the surface area of the antigen and the concentration of antibody according to the physical laws of adsorption. Antigen with its adsorbed antibody behaves essentially as a particle of globulin and is "salted out" by electrolyte in the visible reaction of agglutination or precipitation. This "second stage" of antigen-antibody reaction was considered to be nonspecific. Eagle later proposed that combination with antigen produces a change in the structure of antibody protein similar to denaturation so that the solubility of antibody is decreased. This presumably requires considerable distortion of the antibody molecules when joined to antigen. The most serious objection to Bordet's hypothesis was its failure to account adequately for specificity.

The Lattice Hypothesis

The lattice or framework hypothesis utilizes portions of earlier hypotheses. The chemical basis of specificity, originally postulated by Ehrlich, is now universally accepted, as is union in variable proportions, as proposed by Bordet, and the participation of electrolytes in agglutination and precipitation.

The lattice hypothesis was described by Marrack (1938), and modifications were proposed by Heidelberger, Pauling, and various other workers. The basic concept is that an antigen-antibody aggregate consists of a lattice or framework of alternating antibody molecules and antigen molecules or particles.

Marrack attributed the solubility of antibody globulin to its polar radicals, and postulated that these are brought into close apposition and attract each other instead of water molecules when antibody combines with antigen (Figure 6–11,A). This complex precipitates if the remaining free polar groups are insufficient to keep it in solution and if the surface potential is below a critical level. Assuming that both antigen and antibody are multivalent, large complexes may build up through specific links provided by further antigen molecules and thus form a network or lattice (Figure 6–11,B).

Pauling supported the lattice hypothesis of Marrack, but saw no need for multivalent antibody except in certain situations involving polyhaptenic antigens. He postulated that antibody is bivalent and antigen multivalent. The reactive sites of an antigen and its antibody correspond closely in physical configuration (Figure 6–12), and the molecules join alternately to form a large aggregate (Figure 6–13). If the determinant areas do not conform in structure to within one or two Ångströms, they will not react or will react only weakly (Figure 6–14).

The agglutination of cells was represented diagrammatically as in Figure 6–15, the cells being held together at the regions of "contact" by antibody molecules. The relative sizes of antigen and antibody obviously limit the effective valence of antibody to two. Pauling likewise reasoned that the maximum possible valence of any antigen is determined by the ratio of its surface area to the area effectively occupied by one antibody molecule. It is likely that the actual valence of an antigen is never this high, because only a small proportion of its surface consists of determinant or combining sites.

Precipitation under optimal conditions was represented as in Figure 6–16, A. A network formed with a greater than optimal proportion of antibody is indicated in Figure 6–16,B, and networks or complexes with less than optimal antibody in Figure 6–16,C, D, E.

It should be pointed out that these diagrams antedate present knowledge of the physical structure of immunoglobulins. They are, however, based on the concept that antibodies are bivalent, as is known to be true of IgG and some of the other classes of immunoglobulin. Figure 6–17 is a truer representation of the structure of an aggregate composed of a bivalent hapten and its antibody, and Figure 6–18 represents a cellular antigen agglutinated by bivalent antibody.

Singer reported physical studies of soluble BSA—anti-BSA antigen-antibody aggregates that provide objective evidence that antibody molecules contain two combining sites. Since the molecular weights of BSA and rabbit IgG are about 69,000 and

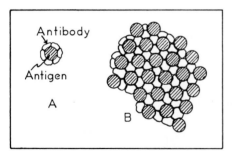

Figure 6–11. Two of Marrack's postulated arrangements of antigen and antibody molecules in the antigen-antibody complex. A, Simple unit. B, Complex structure at optimal proportions. (Redrawn from Marrack, 1938. The Chemistry of Antigens and Antibodies. London, Her Majesty's Stationery Office.)

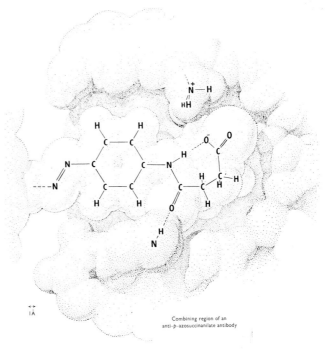

Figure 6–12. A reactive site of an azoprotein antigen and the corresponding site of its antibody. A *p*-azosuccinanilate hapten coupled to a protein (*left*) is surrounded by the combining region of antibody. (From Pauling, 1948. Endeavour, vol. 7, No. 26.)

160,000, respectively, they and small complexes containing them can be readily distinguished by ultracentrifugation. Analysis of BSA—anti-BSA mixtures in slight to great antigen excess showed the presence of three principal components or complexes (see Figure 6–19). The major component in a mixture made with great excess of antigen had a sedimentation constant corresponding to that of BSA. There was also a considerable amount of material (a) with a larger sedimentation constant, which could be attributed to a complex with the formula $(BSA)_2Ab$, and a very small amount of a

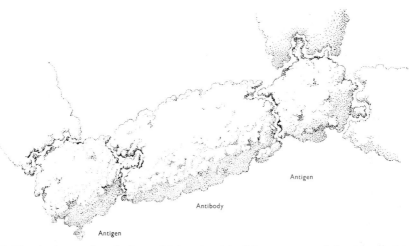

Figure 6–13. Antigen and antibody combining sites join if they correspond closely enough in physical configuration, and a complex of alternating antigen and antibody molecules forms. (From Pauling, 1948. Endeavour, vol. 7, No. 26.)

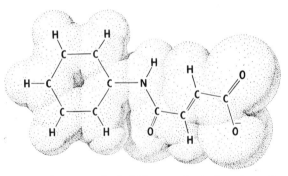

Figure 6-14. The fumaranilate ion, which differs in physical configuration from the succinanilate ion (see Figure 6-12) and hence can combine only weakly with anti-*p*-azosuccinanilate. (From Pauling, 1948. Endeavour, vol. 7, No. 26.)

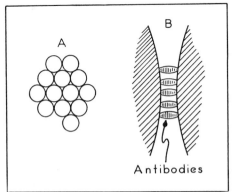

Figure 6-15. Pauling's pictorial representation of (*A*) agglutinated cells, and (*B*) the region of contact of two cells, showing the postulated structure and mode of action of agglutinin molecules. (Adapted and reprinted with permission from Pauling, 1940. J. Am. Chem. Soc., 62:2643. Copyright 1940 by the American Chemical Society.)

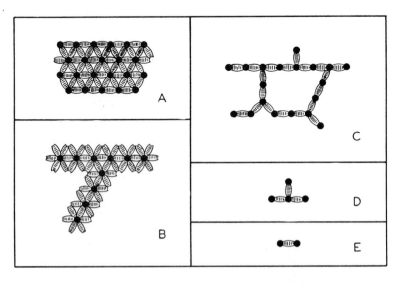

▥ Antibody   ● Antigen

Figure 6-16. Complexes formed with soluble antigen and antibody postulated by Pauling. *A,* An ideal framework. *B,* A network formed with antibody excess. *C,* A network formed with antigen excess. *D* and *E,* Soluble complexes formed with excess antigen. (Adapted and reprinted with permission from Pauling, 1940. J. Am. Chem. Soc., 62:2643. Copyright 1940 by the American Chemical Society.)

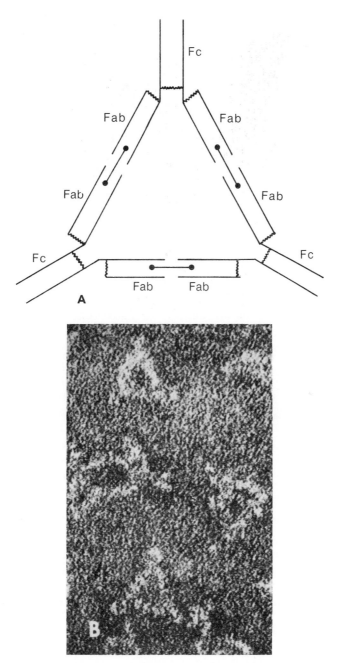

Figure 6-17. A, A triangular hapten-antibody aggregate; the hapten, dinitrophenol (●——●) binds three IgG molecules via their Fab combining sites. *B*, Electron micrograph of complexes formed when bivalent dinitrophenol (DNP) reacts with rabbit anti-DNP × 1,000,000. (*B* after Valentine and Green, 1967. J. Mol. Biol., 27:615.)

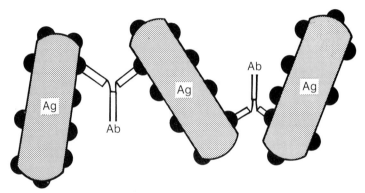

Figure 6–18. Agglutination of bacterial cells by antibody (diagrammatic). Antibody Fab combining sites react with homologous antigenic determinant sites on the bacterial surface.

still larger complex (b) whose sedimentation constant was consistent with the composition $(BSA)_3Ab_2$. In mixtures prepared with a small excess of antigen, less uncombined BSA appeared and a greater proportion of the heavier complex (b) as would be expected.

Acidification of the BSA—anti-BSA system below pH 4.5 caused reversible, progressive dissociation of the antigen-antibody complexes, as shown by the ultracentrifugal pattern, and at pH 2.4 only γ-globulin and BSA were detected. The value of the calculated hydrogen ion association constant was consistent with the assumption that a single carboxyl group (and presumably a corresponding positively charged complementary group) was critically present in each antigen-antibody bond. This accounted for about half the energy of the bond, the remainder possibly being attributed to hydrogen bonds, dipole interactions, hydrophobic attraction, and other forces.

To determine whether carboxyl radicals might react with amino radicals in the antigen-antibody linkage, free amino groups of anti-BSA were blocked by acetylation, whereupon the ability of the antibody to react with BSA was lost. Similar treatment of BSA had little effect upon its ability to combine with antibody. It therefore appeared reasonable to postulate that the combining site on the antibody molecule contains a single amino group, which reacts with a single carboxyl group on the antigen.

SUMMARY

The development of ideas regarding the mechanism of antigen-antibody reactions provides an interesting illustration of the increasing complexity that accompanies acquisition of factual knowledge. In fact, proper understanding of present hypotheses requires considerable familiarity with chemistry, physics, and mathematics. The original explanation of Ehrlich, that agglutinin and precipitin molecules possess

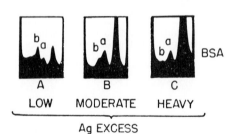

Figure 6–19. Ultracentrifuge diagrams of BSA–anti-BSA soluble complexes. The direction of sedimentation is from right to left in each pattern. The peaks labeled *a* and *b* are referred to in the text. (From Singer, 1957. J. Cell. Comp. Physiol., 50(Suppl.):51.)

"zymophore" radicals that cause the visible reactions, left much to the imagination of the student but was perfectly intelligible if he did not seek to know what zymophore radicals actually are. Its emphasis upon chemical structure accorded well with present concepts of specificity, which have only been more clearly defined by recent investigators. The later concept, that particles of multivalent antigen coated with antibody agglutinate or precipitate because of some attraction or lack of repulsion, is also fairly understandable. Inasmuch as the reaction of hapten or antigen with antibody does not involve covalent bonding but depends upon a variety of short-range, intermolecular forces, it appears that the specificity of immunologic reactions is a sine qua non of their actual occurrence—in the absence of the lock-and-key relationship, there can be no antigen-antibody interaction.

The present situation may be stated as follows:

1. Immunologic reactions consist of rapid union between antigen and antibody, followed by a visible stage that is often slower and is modified by the nature of the antigen and the antibody, temperature, electrolytes, and other factors.

2. Antibody combines with antigen through relatively small surface structures possessing complementary physical configurations and patterns of force.

3. The antigen-antibody complex consists of a network of alternate antigen and antibody molecules. This indicates bivalence or multivalence of one or both reagents, which makes possible union in variable proportions.

4. The necessity for electrolyte implies that reduction in the number or effectiveness of polar radicals, which normally attract water, plays an important part in the visible reaction. This may consist of mechanical blocking of polar radicals, mutual neutralization, or reduction of charge by electrolytes.

Additional Sources of Information

Day, E. D.: Advanced Immunochemistry. 1972. Baltimore, The Williams and Wilkins Company.

Sell, S.: Immunology, Immunopathology, and Immunity. 1972. Hagerstown, Md., Harper and Row, Publishers.

CHAPTER SEVEN

IN VITRO ANTIGEN-ANTIBODY REACTIONS: PRECIPITATION AND AGGLUTINATION

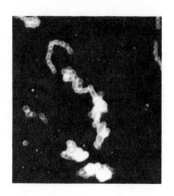

Aggregated growth of bacteria in homologous immune serum was observed in 1889, but the first systematic study of agglutination was that of Gruber and Durham, described in 1896. Even in this first report, its usefulness as a diagnostic aid was suggested, and within months Widal applied the method successfully.

The precipitin reaction was first reported by Kraus in 1897. Bacteria-free filtrates of *Vibrio cholerae* and *Salmonella typhosa* mixed with homologous antisera became cloudy after a short period of incubation; by 24 hours finely flocculent precipitates settled to the bottoms of the tubes. The specificity of the reaction was shown by failure of anticholera serum to precipitate the typhoid culture filtrate and vice versa. It was not known at that time that the same antibody might be responsible for both precipitation and agglutination, so Kraus applied the name *precipitin* to the antibody reacting in precipitation and called the antigen that elicited its formation *precipitinogen*.

Two years later Tchistovitch, studying the toxicity of eel serum, inoculated this material into rabbits, guinea pigs, dogs, and goats. Blood serum from animals surviving the toxic effects of the antigen yielded a copious precipitate when mixed with eel serum. About the same time Bordet reported that milk, injected into rabbits, stimulated the appearance of antibodies that caused flocculation when mixed with milk. Likewise Myers, in 1900, obtained precipitins for egg albumin by intraperitoneal injection into rabbits.

Agglutination and precipitation are fundamentally a single phenomenon: aggregation of antigen and antibody through formation of a framework in which antigen particles or molecules alternate with antibody molecules. Because of the difference in dimensions of the antigen units, different quantitative relations obtain in the primary reaction—union of antigen with antibody—and in its visible, secondary manifestation. Precipitation is the term applied to aggregation of a soluble (i.e., molecular) test antigen, and agglutination is the aggregation of a particulate (e.g., cellular) test antigen.

PRODUCTION AND TESTING OF ANTISERA

Precipitating Antisera

PRECIPITIN FORMATION IN MAN

Precipitating antibody is often formed in the normal course of an infection. The stimulus is provided by soluble antigenic bacterial constituents liberated by autolysis and other means of disintegration. Antibacterial precipitin tests are not often performed because suitable concentrations of antibody are difficult to obtain.

Precipitating antibodies are sometimes found in the sera of individuals who have had parenteral contact with foreign proteins. Such antibodies have been detected in the blood of patients with serum sickness. Precipitins have also been demonstrated by highly sensitive techniques in the sera of patients hypersensitive to egg, insulin, and tuberculin. The concentration of antibody is often low in such conditions, and negative results are not infrequent.

PRECIPITIN PRODUCTION IN THE LABORATORY

Precipitins may be produced against most proteins and some carbohydrates and carbohydrate-lipid complexes. Certain purified pneumococcal polysaccharides and dextrans and levans are not antigenic in the rabbit or the guinea pig but are antigenic in man and in mice. Immunization of the rabbit with whole pneumococci, however, induces formation of antibodies that will precipitate the purified polysaccharide. Some substances like ragweed pollen extract that are usually considered poorly antigenic induce precipitin formation when injected with complete Freund adjuvant (see page 91). It has also been reported that nonantigenic carbohydrates such as glycogen, adsorbed onto aluminum hydroxide particles, produce antibodies and that the antigenicity of lipids is greatly enhanced by adsorption onto kaolin or other inert particles. It appears, therefore, that the species of animal injected and the presence of contaminating or other adjuvant substances affect the formation of precipitating antibodies.

Procedures for production of precipitins in rabbits vary greatly according to the nature of the antigen and the animal species. For some purposes a single injection may suffice but, in general, higher antibody yields are obtained by administering a series of injections. Protein solutions for immunization of rabbits contain 1.5 to 10.0 mg. per ml. (0.15 to 1.0 per cent) in saline. Intravenous injections usually start at 1.0 ml. and increase to 5.0 ml.; intraperitoneal doses of 2.0 to 5.0 ml. are easily tolerated. Two to four injections are given per week for about 4 weeks, and the animal is bled 5 to 7 days later. The total amount of antigen is 10 to 100 mg.

Satisfactory precipitin titers against some substances such as egg albumin and bovine serum albumin are obtained only after prolonged immunization, although small doses of many antigens suffice to yield detectable antibodies; positive results have been obtained with 0.35 mg. of a synthetic dye-egg albumin antigen. Very small amounts of bacterial extracts induce high titers of precipitating antibody in rabbits: 0.002 to 0.005 mg. per kg. of body weight.

Precipitin formation is enhanced by the use of certain adjuvant substances or conditions. Proteins precipitated with alum often induce a stronger antibody response than saline solutions. The protein is precipitated by adding alum (potassium aluminum sulfate) and neutralizing with N/10 NaOH until maximum turbidity (caused by the developing precipitate) is produced. This suspension can be injected intravenously in the same dosages used with protein solutions. Freund adjuvant (see page 91) is also widely used in laboratory research. Antigens emulsified in paraffin oil, with or without killed mycobacteria, are injected subcutaneously or intramuscularly into one to four sites on the animal. A single injection or set of injections may suffice, or they may be repeated once or twice at weekly intervals. Final bleeding is usually a month or two after the last injection.

Precipitin formation parallels the ability of the various animal species to produce antibodies in general and is usually better in rabbits, horses, chickens, and man than in guinea pigs, dogs, and rats. Wide individual differences within any species are common.

Precipitins are titrated in sera from trial bleedings before and at intervals during the course of immunization. When the antibody concentration is sufficiently great, the animal may be bled out by cardiac puncture. Larger quantities of serum can be secured by bleeding the animal partially (e.g., 40 to 50 ml.) at 2- or 3-day intervals. After each large bleeding an equal volume of sterile saline is injected intraperitoneally to replace the lost fluid.

PRECIPITATION TESTS

General Principles.   The reagents required for precipitation tests are antigen, antibody, and saline. All solutions must be perfectly clear because traces of turbidity or cloudiness obscure the results. Filtration or centrifugation of the reagents is frequently necessary.

Precipitin tests, in contrast to agglutination tests, are usually set up with serial dilutions of antigen and a constant, high concentration of antibody (either undiluted or diluted not more than 1:5). Apart from the serodiagnosis of syphilis, precipitin tests are rarely employed in laboratory diagnosis. A single precipitin test ordinarily requires 1.0 ml. of antiserum, an amount that suffices for 40 or more agglutination tests.

The amount of precipitate and titer rapidly decrease as antiserum is diluted and antigen is added in constant amount. The necessity for more concentrated antibody in precipitation than in agglutination is related to the size of the "particles" being aggregated and the fact that theoretically a single molecule of antibody suffices to attach one antigenic unit to another. A milligram of antigen in molecular form (e.g., a protein solution) obviously comprises vastly more units than a milligram of antigen in particles the size of bacterial cells.

The temperature at which precipitation tests are incubated varies according to the nature of the test and the particular antigen-antibody system employed. The rate of precipitation usually increases as the temperature rises to 40 or 45° C., so that qualitative tests are often incubated at 37° C. or slightly higher. More complete precipitation, however, is frequently obtained at 0 to 4° C., and quantitative precipitation tests practically always include an interval of one or more days of refrigeration before chemical analysis. The optimal temperature and time of incubation must be determined for each new antigen-antibody system investigated.

Simple Mixtures.   A quick qualitative or rough test is made by placing decreasing amounts of antigen—2 drops, 1 drop, ½ drop, by Pasteur pipette (approximately 0.06, 0.03, 0.015 ml.)—into successive 6- × 50-mm. test tubes, adding 1 drop of antiserum to each and shaking the tubes very vigorously.

Semiquantitative tests are made by mixing undiluted or slightly diluted (e.g., 1:3 to 1:5) antiserum with dilutions of antigen. Sufficient dilutions are employed to ensure a positive result that might otherwise be missed because of inhibition by too concentrated antigen. It should be reemphasized that diluting the antiserum only slightly causes a disproportional reduction in the titer observed by this procedure. It is therefore important in comparing antisera that the same concentration of antiserum be employed in all tests with the same antigen. Likewise, the same concentration of a given antiserum must be employed in tests against different antigens.

Tests are observed continuously or at intervals of only a few minutes. In the rough test, a highly potent antiserum produces opalescence, turbidity, and flocculation in succession almost immediately in the first tube. In a semiquantitative test, one tube in the dilution series reacts more quickly than the others, becoming opalescent, turbid, and then flocculent. The tubes on either side (i.e., with greater and lesser concentrations of antigen) react more and more slowly, and finally some tubes become only opalescent or do not change. Heavy precipitates settle rapidly; light precipitates may require several hours or overnight. The tube in which definite flocculent particles of precipitate first appear is the indicating tube and received the optimal ratio of antibody and antigen. If antiserum diluted 1:2 were placed in each tube and the most rapid reaction occurred with antigen diluted 1:1000, the antibody:antigen optimal ratio (O.R.) is 500:1. Inasmuch as more antibody molecules are required to produce an O.R. with a higher concentration of antigen, it is apparent that another antiserum with which an O.R. of 250 is obtained contains twice as much antibody and is therefore a stronger antiserum.

Interfacial or Ring Test. The interfacial or ring test introduced by Ascoli in 1902 is a simple and yet sensitive form of the precipitin reaction. Very small test tubes or capillary tubes are employed to conserve antiserum, and the reagents are added in such a manner that mixing does not occur; antiserum usually constitutes the bottom layer and antigen the top layer. With large enough test tubes the antiserum may be allowed to run down the wall of the tube and flow under the antigen, or it may be added with a Pasteur pipette inserted to the bottom of the tube beneath the antigen. If small test tubes (e.g., 3 mm. inside diameter) are employed, the antigen may be added slowly with a Pasteur pipette as a layer above the antiserum. This method often gives sharper results but is more time consuming and tedious.

Tests are incubated either at room temperature or at 37° C. for periods up to 4 hours. Formation of a visible ring or layer of precipitate at the interface between antiserum and antigen may occur within a few minutes, depending upon the antibody content of the serum and the concentration of antigen. The end point or titer is represented by the highest antigen dilution giving a positive result. This method does not suffer greatly from inhibition by antigen excess because diffusion at the interface provides a zone of nearly optimal proportions in which precipitation occurs. A positive result may be obtained with antigens diluted one million times or more. This procedure is used to detect specific antigens but gives little information regarding the antibody content of an antiserum. It is commonly employed to identify proteins, as in the forensic determination of the origin of blood stains (see Figure 7–1).

Quantitative Test. This has already been described (see page 158).

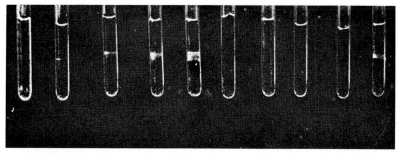

Figure 7–1. Interfacial test demonstrating the origin of a blood stain. The five tubes at the left contain antihuman serum overlaid by increasing concentrations of a blood stain extract. There is no ring of precipitate in the first tube, but there are increasingly strong zones of precipitate in the next four tubes. The remaining tubes are controls; the last, containing known human blood layered over antihuman serum, has a moderately strong precipitate. (From Boyd, 1956. Fundamentals of Immunology, 3rd ed. New York, Interscience Publishers, Inc.)

Agglutinating Antisera

IMMUNIZATION OF RABBITS

Rabbits are immunized by inoculation with living, killed, or extracted bacteria or other cells. The details of preparation of immunizing suspensions vary from one laboratory to another and depend somewhat upon the nature of the antigen. After an appropriate course of injections, the animal is bled and the serum is removed and preserved.

A bacterial antigen should consist of a single species. The culture should be genetically pure, but variations such as smooth-rough, opaque-translucent, phase 1-phase 2, motile-nonmotile, and so forth make it difficult to know the exact serologic state of the antigen at any given moment. Organisms are usually grown on a suitable agar medium, although broth cultures are sometimes preferred. Traces of agar in immunizing antigens have been reported to induce anti-agar antibodies that agglutinate completely unrelated bacteria grown on agar medium.

The bacteria, suspended in saline, may be killed by moderate heat (e.g., 56° C.) or by chemicals such as formaldehyde, phenol, or Merthiolate. The method of sterilization should be as mild as possible because drastic physical or chemical treatment sometimes alters the specificity of cell antigens. For this reason living bacterial vaccines are often preferred, although they may be more dangerous to the animal. Despite the fact that rabbits are not susceptible to infection by most of the organisms with which they are immunized for experimental purposes, even small doses sometimes kill the animals for reasons not clearly understood. Very small initial doses can usually be tolerated, however, and larger amounts are withstood as immunity develops. An alternative procedure is to administer a few injections of killed bacteria followed by a series of doses of living organisms.

The vaccine is usually standardized to contain a specified number of bacteria, such as 500,000,000 or 1,000,000,000 per ml. Suspensions are counted directly with the microscope, using a counting chamber, or by the Wright method. In the Wright procedure equal volumes of bacterial suspension and blood are mixed, smeared, and stained. Comparative numbers of erythrocytes and bacteria are determined in several fields, and the number of bacteria is calculated, assuming a normal number of red cells (5,000,000,000 per ml. of blood). Vaccines to be sterilized by heat must be standardized before sterilization because heat disrupts the cells. Vaccines are also standardized to a certain turbidity, either photoelectrically or by comparison with known suspensions. Some vaccines for commercial use are diluted to a specified nitrogen content.

Rabbits are generally used for production of agglutinating sera in the laboratory, but commercial houses employ horses or other animals for large scale manufacture. The animals selected should be healthy. The age of the animal is a matter of debate. Young adult rabbits usually produce antibody most rapidly and yield highest titers. It is not difficult to secure antisera against gram-negative bacteria that have agglutination titers of 10,000 after a relatively short series of injections requiring less than 3 weeks. Older and larger animals often produce antibody more slowly but have the advantage of yielding more blood.

Rabbits usually are given a series of injections into the marginal ear vein. Intravenous inoculation provides most rapid distribution and absorption of antigen. The intraperitoneal route gives somewhat slower distribution and absorption, and subcutaneous inoculations are even slower. The later injections in a series, particularly those following several days of rest, are often given subcutaneously because slow dissipation of antigen from the site of inoculation is less likely to produce toxic reactions.

Inoculation schedules are highly variable, but it is usually considered desirable to secure the maximum attainable titer as quickly as possible. Injection routines are often dictated more by convenience than by the requisites of efficient antibody production. Daily injections yield antisera of high titer more rapidly than weekly injections. A common schedule consists of three injections at 5- to 7-day intervals, followed by bleeding 5 to 7 days after the last injection. Some investigators administer 12 or 16 injections at the rate of three or four per week, followed by bleeding 1 week later. Excellent titers are obtained against members of the Enterobacteriaceae by a series of six daily injections followed by one more injection after 5 days and bleeding 5 to 7 days later.

The frequency, dosage, and route of injections should be judged from daily observations of the animal's condition. The usual response of an animal to injection of foreign material is similar to that of a human: fever, malaise, loss of appetite. Fever is only transient unless a living vaccine produces actual infection, the temperature ordinarily rising several degrees within 2 or 3 hours but returning to normal by the next day. Loss of appetite and activity are the simplest indications of an unfavorable reaction. If an animal reacts unfavorably it is best to change the route of injection, decrease the dosage, or omit an injection or two.

Periodic "trial" bleedings of a few milliliters during the course of immunization provide opportunity to determine the progress of antibody formation by agglutination tests and indicate when a final bleeding may be made to secure a large amount of serum. Antiserum preserved with 0.45 per cent phenol or 0.01 per cent Merthiolate keeps for years at refrigerator temperature with little loss of potency. Such sera occasionally develop a protein and/or lipid precipitate, but this does not affect the antibody titer appreciably. Perhaps the most satisfactory preservation is obtained by adding an equal volume of glycerin (highest purity), but this has the disadvantage of requiring double the storage space. Serum may be kept indefinitely in the frozen state without chemical preservative.

TITRATION OF AGGLUTININ BY THE TUBE TEST

Dilutions of serum are prepared in serologic tubes and a constant amount of the antigen suspension is added to each. The tubes are shaken thoroughly and incubated, preferably in a water bath, and the degree of agglutination in each is recorded. The titer of antibodies in the serum is expressed as the reciprocal of the highest dilution giving definite agglutination. Details of the procedure vary with individual preference. Usually the total volume of reagents is 0.5 to 1.0 ml. Serum dilutions are doubled in succeeding tubes (e.g., 1:10, 1:20, 1:40, etc.), and sufficient dilutions should be made to provide one or more tubes without agglutination. A control tube containing antigen and saline is always included and must show a negative result. Agglutination in the control indicates that the antigen was at fault (perhaps a "rough" bacterial strain) or that there was some error in technique; in this case the whole test is meaningless and must be discarded. The end point of the titration is the last tube in the serum dilution series in which definite agglutination (1+ in a 4+ scale of reading) occurs, and the titer of the antibody is expressed as the reciprocal of the dilution.

Preparation of bacterial antigen for the agglutination test varies with the organism and with the information desired. Cultures may be taken from broth or from agar slants. Broth cultures are usually centrifuged and the packed cells resuspended in saline. Agar slants are washed off with saline and diluted. It is difficult to state a rule for diluting bacterial antigens; usually they should be as dilute as possible and still give readable results. Living antigens of many organisms are used, but it is safer to kill pathogens if the nature of the experiment permits; 0.3 per cent formalin or 1:10,000 Merthiolate is sometimes added to the saline used for this purpose.

Preparation of the test suspension is also determined by the particular antigenic fraction whose antibody is to be titrated. Motile bacteria contain at least two different kinds of antigenic substances: one associated with the cell bodies and known as somatic (O) antigens, the other presumably associated with the flagella and called flagellar (H) antigens. Somatic antigens are resistant to heat, whereas flagellar antigens are destroyed by heat. Fortunately, formalin used to kill bacteria does not affect either the somatic or flagellar antigens, and therefore animals immunized with living or formalin-treated bacteria produce both somatic and flagellar antibodies. Pure somatic antibodies are obtained either by immunizing with a nonmotile variant or a boiled suspension, or by adsorbing flagellar antibodies from antiserum against a motile strain. Pure flagellar antibodies are secured by adsorbing somatic antibodies from antiserum produced with a motile organism.

Somatic test antigens are prepared by heating a suspension of the organisms. Such antigens, or suspensions of nonmotile bacteria, react with homologous antisera to form compact sediments that break up into sharply defined granules when shaken. Flagellar test antigens consist of living or formalin-treated suspensions; they produce loose, flocculent sediments with homologous antisera that break up on shaking into almost indistinguishable clumps. These characteristic types of agglutination are common, but gradients between the two extremes are encountered in which it is impossible to determine the type of agglutination by inspection.

The temperature and time of incubation of tube agglutination tests differ according to the nature of the organism and the antigen preparation. Recommendations for flagellar agglutination tests range from incubation at 37° C. for 2 hours to incubation at 50° to 55° C. for 4 hours. It is generally agreed that somatic agglutination of bacteria requires a higher incubation temperature or a longer time or both than flagellar agglutination. Recommendations vary from 15 to 24 hours at 50° to 55° C. Certain bacteria agglutinate only with difficulty. Brucella species are often incubated for 2 days at 37° to 55° C. Very light phenolized suspensions of highly mucoid bacteria require 1 or 2 days at 37°C. The optimum conditions for each organism or group of organisms must be worked out individually by trial and error.

When results are needed quickly, agglutination can be hastened by centrifuging the tubes lightly (e.g., 2000 r.p.m. for 10 to 15 minutes). All tubes *including the control* are then carefully shaken together in a rack before reading. Passage of the cells through the serum dilution provides opportunity for antigen-antibody contact and reaction, and packing speeds the process of aggregation. Final shaking redisperses cells that did not agglutinate and allows a reading to be made.

Bacteria possessing certain somatic or envelope antigens fail to agglutinate in high titer homologous O antisera. Such organisms are called O-inagglutinable. The K antigens of *E. coli* and the Vi antigen of *S. typhosa* are examples of antigens that confer O-inagglutinability.

Three kinds of K antigen are known, designated L, A, and B. (1) L antigens are thermolabile, and cultures containing them regain O-agglutinability after boiling for 1 hour. Antisera containing L antibodies may be prepared by immunizing with appropriate living organisms; the O antibodies that are also formed can be removed by adsorption. Colonies of strains containing L antigens are somewhat more opaque than those lacking them. (2) The A antigens are thermostable capsular polysaccharides. They resist boiling for 2½ hours but are destroyed in 2 hours at 120° C. Bacteria containing A antigen give a *Quellung* reaction in homologous antiserum. (3) B antigens, like L antigens, are thermolabile, being destroyed by boiling for 1 hour. They differ from L antigens in the ability of heated suspensions to adsorb homologous B antibody, although such heated suspensions do not agglutinate in B antiserum.

The Vi antigen is relatively heat stable, despite reports that seem to indicate the contrary. When strains of *S. typhosa* containing Vi antigen in addition to the usual O antigens are heated at 100° C., they lose their agglutinability by Vi antiserum within 30 minutes, although their O agglutinability is retained. Vi antigen extracted from bacteria by boiling saline suspensions of the cells 1 hour or longer induces high titers of Vi antibody in rabbits. Heat therefore easily removes the Vi antigen from cells, particularly in aqueous media, but the antigen itself retains its immunologic character.

O agglutination of a culture containing Vi antigen may be obtained in anti-O serum by use of a suspension boiled 30 minutes. Antiserum against Vi antigen is prepared by immunizing rabbits with saline extracts, as just mentioned, or with living organisms. Vi agglutination tests employ living or formalized (0.5 per cent formalin) test suspensions and are incubated at 37° C. for 2 hours followed by storage at room temperature or refrigeration overnight. Vi agglutination also occurs to full titer of the serum if tests are kept at room temperature or in the refrigerator for 20 hours without preliminary 37° C. incubation.

Other Methods of Demonstrating Precipitins and Agglutinins

In addition to the procedures just described, precipitating antibodies are demonstrated by the gel diffusion and Dean and Webb optimal ratio procedures, described on pages 157 and 164. Further methods include the following:

AGGLUTINATION OF ANTIGEN-COATED INERT PARTICLES

Agglutination of inert particles to which soluble antigen has been adsorbed provides a serum dilution method of titrating precipitin and also demonstrates the similarity between precipitation and agglutination. Collodion, bentonite, latex particles, colloidal charcoal, or cells unrelated to the antigen (e.g., bacteria or erythrocytes) are coated with the antigen and employed in constant amount in an agglutination test against serial dilutions of antiserum.

Collodion particles are prepared by adding a water-acetone mixture in a fine stream to a constantly stirred solution of collodion in acetone. The particles are freed from acetone by washing with distilled water. Particles between 1 and 5 micrometers in diameter are secured by differential centrifugation, mixed with the antigen solution to permit adsorption, and finally washed several times to remove unadsorbed material. Coated particles diluted to proper turbidity are employed as test antigen in the agglutination reaction. This procedure is very sensitive. Positive results have been obtained with sera from patients hypersensitive to egg, insulin, or tuberculin.

Bentonite, a colloidal hydrated aluminum silicate, has also been used as an inert particulate carrier to adsorb soluble antigens. The particles are treated with the antigen and with a dye (thionin) to facilitate reading flocculation. In tests performed on large microscope slides, a drop of antigen is added to 0.1 ml. of serum dilution, the slide is rocked and tilted mechanically for 15 minutes, and flocculation is read with the low power of the microscope. This test has been used to detect antibody in sera of patients with trichinosis, using a test antigen prepared from trichina extract. The flocculation reaction was as sensitive as complement fixation and apparently gave no falsely positive reactions.

Polystyrene latex particles approximately 0.8 μm. in diameter (available commercially) adsorb antigen or antibody and become a sensitive reagent useful in diagnostic serology. Antibacterial antibodies can be detected in patients' sera by adding a mixture of latex particles and intact or disintegrated bacteria in buffer at pH 8.2 to serum dilutions; after incubation 3 to 5 minutes at 56° C. and brief centrifugation at 2500 r.p.m., the tubes are shaken and read as in an agglutination test. Satisfactory results can be obtained with sera from patients with tularemia, brucellosis, typhoid fever, and other infections. It has been postulated that, unlike inert carrier particles in other tests, the latex adsorbs antibody globulin, which then reacts with the bacterial antigen and produces an agglutinated mass. The mechanism of the latex agglutination test for rheumatoid arthritis is similar. Latex particles coated with γ-globulin agglutinate when mixed with patients' sera containing rheumatoid factor, an IgM anti–γ-globulin autoantibody produced by the patient.

A colloidal suspension of charcoal (also available commercially) can be used as a carrier for viruses or bacterial endotoxins and serves as a test antigen in a macroscopic slide agglutination test. A single adsorption of the antigenic material suffices to coat the particles, and after suitable washing they are ready to be mixed with serial dilutions of antiserum for the test.

Passive Hemagglutination. Erythrocytes treated with extracts of bacterial cells, rickettsiae, pathogenic fungi, or protozoa, or with purified polysaccharides or proteins constitute a very sensitive reagent for detecting and titrating the corresponding antibodies. The *indirect* or *passive hemagglutination test* is performed with washed sheep, human group O, rabbit, or other erythrocytes, which are incubated at 37° C. with a solution of the antigenic material. The cells are then washed thoroughly and employed as test antigen in a tube or macroscopic slide agglutination procedure with antiserum or patient's serum. Controls are necessary to ensure that positive results are caused by antibodies against the adsorbed antigen rather than natural anti-erythrocyte antibodies. The latter must often be removed from sera by preliminary adsorption with unmodified erythrocytes.

Normal red blood cells adsorb polysaccharides and lipopolysaccharides and are used with various crude or purified microbial extracts. Vi antibodies, for example, have been titrated in the sera of normal and immune individuals by use of erythrocytes treated with Vi antigen from bacteria. Titers as high as 240 have been reported in humans 2 weeks after immunization with 40 mg. of Vi antigen, and a titer of 10,240 was obtained with an antiserum against *Paracolobactrum ballerup*. Erythrocytes can adsorb several antigens simultaneously, and it appears that specific receptors may exist for different antigens.

Erythrocytes pretreated with tannic acid adsorb proteins readily and can be used to titrate antibodies present in very small concentrations in experimental or diagnostic sera. (Tannic acid-treated cells also adsorb polysaccharides, but not so rapidly.) The procedure consists of mixing thrice-washed red blood cells with 1:20,000 tannic acid in saline buffered at pH 7.2 and incubating 10 minutes at 37° C. The cells are washed again and treated with the protein antigen at pH 6.4 for 15 minutes at room temperature. After washing to remove unadsorbed protein, a suspension of the "tanned" cells is added to test serum dilutions prepared with 1:100 normal rabbit serum as diluent. Normal rabbit serum added to the saline prevents spontaneous agglutination of the modified red blood cells. After suitable incubation, agglutination of the cells is read according to the pattern of settling in test tubes or in cups on a macroscopic slide (see Figure 7–2). In a strong reaction the cells form a compact, granular agglutinate; weaker reactions are characterized by a small mat with folded or ragged edges; a negative reaction consists of a small discrete red button of cells that have settled and slid to the bottom of the tube or depression without sticking to the walls.

There is considerable variation in the amounts of different proteins needed to sensitize tanned red cells optimally. The following amounts have been suggested:

Chicken serum globulin	0.025 mg. per ml. of 2.5% RBC
M. tuberculosis P.P.D.	0.15 mg. per ml. of 2.5% RBC
Streptococcus protein	0.5 mg. per ml. of 2.5% RBC

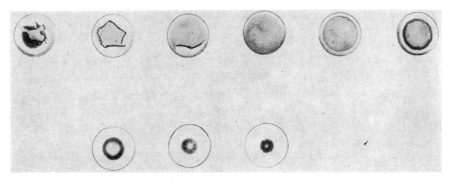

Figure 7–2. Appearance of patterns of hemagglutination. Top row, left to right: ++++, +++, +++, ++, +, ±; bottom row; ±, −, −. (From Stavitsky, 1954. J. Immunol., 72:360.)

Horse serum albumin	0.5 mg. per ml. of 2.5% RBC
Horse serum globulin	1.0 mg. per ml. of 2.5% RBC
Egg albumin	5.0 mg. per ml. of 2.5% RBC

Erythrocytes must usually be freshly prepared for use each day—a time-consuming process and one which presents the possibility of day-to-day variation. For large scale work, the cells may be treated with formalin first, then with tannic acid, and finally with the antigen. Formalinized red cells are stable for at least 5 months.

As previously noted (Table 4–2), passive hemagglutination is one of the most sensitive methods for detecting antibodies against proteins or polysaccharides. As little as 0.02 to 0.04 μg. of antibody can produce detectable agglutination. It has been calculated that this represents about fifty molecules per erythrocyte.

LABELED ANTIBODIES

Inasmuch as only a small fraction of an immunoglobulin comprises the specific antibody combining site, it is not surprising that antibodies can be labeled with various distinctive substances, which presumably attach principally to the Fc region and constant portions of the Fab regions. These antibodies can then be detected by appropriate techniques and their location determined in vivo, or their participation in antigen-antibody reactions can be ascertained and in some cases visualized.

Fluorescent Antibodies. Labeling of antibodies by coupling with fluorescent dyes to permit their detection by direct microscopic examination was suggested by Coons et al. in 1941. The chemical manipulations did not seriously impair antibody activity, and a fluorescent antibody reacted specifically with its homologous antigen. The first application of the fluorescent antibody (FA) technique in microbiology was the demonstration of soluble pneumococcal polysaccharide in tissue sections from infected mice. Polysaccharide stained with pneumococcal antibody to which fluorescein had been attached appeared greenish blue when illuminated with ultraviolet light.

A fluorescent substance is one which, when it absorbs light of one wavelength, emits light of another (longer) wavelength. In fluorescent antibody microscopy, the incident or "excitation" light is often blue-green to ultraviolet; it is provided by a high-pressure mercury arc lamp with a primary (e.g., blue-violet) filter between the lamp and the object which passes only fluorescence-exciting wavelengths. The color of the emitted light depends on the nature of the substance. Fluorescein gives off yellow-green light, and the rhodamines fluoresce in the red portion of the spectrum.

The color actually observed in the fluorescence microscope depends upon the secondary or "barrier" filter, used in the eyepiece; a yellow filter absorbs the green fluorescence of fluorescein and transmits only yellow.

Fluorescent antibody solutions are prepared from the globulin fraction of antiserum, which may be separated from whole serum in sufficient purity by precipitation with half-saturated ammonium sulfate. Labeling with fluorescein is accomplished by stirring an alkaline (pH 9) buffered solution of the protein with fluorescein isothiocyanate overnight at 0 to 2° C. Uncombined dye is then removed by prolonged dialysis against buffered saline or by adsorption on an anion-exchange resin followed by dialysis. Fluorescent antibodies used to detect microbial or other foreign antigens in animal tissues may stain the tissue nonspecifically. This is prevented by adsorbing the fluorescent antibody solution with liver (e.g., hog) powder, or by use of anion-exchange resin in preparing the antibody solution.

Direct staining of fixed tissue sections or microbial smears requires 10 to 60 minutes of exposure to the fluorescent antibody; this is followed by washing to remove excess antibody and mounting in buffered glycerol. A darkfield method of observation is commonly employed so the fluorescent cells or structures appear bright (e.g., green, yellow, red, according to the dye and the secondary filter) against a dark background. Controls are necessary to guard against confusion by innate and other nonspecific fluorescence. An unknown antigen can be identified by its fluorescence when stained with a known fluorescent antibody (see Figure 7–3).

The *inhibition* reaction is a blocking test in which an antigen is first exposed to unlabeled antibody, then to labeled antibody, and is finally washed and examined. If the unlabeled and labeled antibodies are both homologous to the antigen, there should be no fluorescence, a result that confirms the specificity of the FA technique. Antibody in an unknown serum can also be detected and identified by the inhibition test.

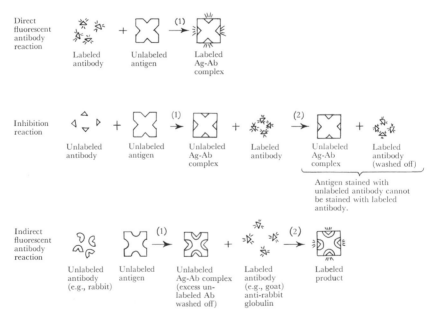

Figure 7–3. Diagrammatic representation of the direct, inhibition, and indirect fluorescent antibody reactions. (Modified and redrawn from Cherry et al., 1960. Fluorescent Antibody Techniques in the Diagnosis of Communicable Diseases. Public Health Service Publication No. 729. Washington, D. C., U. S. Government Printing Office.)

The *indirect* fluorescent antibody reaction is also a two-stage test. The antigen is treated with unlabeled homologous antibody first, and the antigen-antibody complex that forms then reacts with labeled antiglobulin corresponding to the species of unlabeled antibody used in the first step. For example, unlabeled rabbit anti-streptococcal serum is allowed to react with homologous streptococci, and the excess serum is washed off; the preparation is treated with labeled goat anti-rabbit globulin, which reacts with the rabbit anti-streptococcal antibodies joined to the bacteria and confers fluorescence upon the cells.

This procedure can be used to identify an unknown antigen by use of unlabeled antiserum in the first stage. The labeled antiglobulin employed in the second stage makes the antigen visible in the fluorescence microscope if the first antigen and antibody were homologous. The indirect FA test will also detect and titrate antibodies in an unknown serum. Dilutions of the unknown serum are added to smears of the antigen on microscope slides; after incubation, the uncombined antibody is removed by washing, and the smears are treated with labeled antiglobulin homologous to the species whose serum was the primary reagent. Tests with unlabeled positive and negative control sera must be included.

Early work with the FA technique consisted of study of the fate of foreign proteins, polysaccharides, hormones, rickettsiae, viruses, protozoa, fungi, and other substances in the animal body. Later, procedures were devised for the laboratory diagnosis of infectious disease. FA methods are particularly well suited for this purpose because they permit detection of small numbers of specific microorganisms (40 to 100 per ml.), even in the midst of large amounts of debris and of other, normal microorganisms. This great sensitivity hastens the identification of slowly multiplying organisms, such as Brucella and Pasteurella (see Figure 7–4). Rickettsiae and viruses, which are too small for ordinary microscopy, can be detected specifically by means of fluorescent antibodies.

Ferritin-conjugated Antibodies. Conjugation of antibody globulins with ferritin provides a specific reagent for determining the exact location of antigenic molecules in cells or tissues. Ferritin is a protein with a molecular weight of about 700,000. It contains approximately 23 per cent iron, largely as ferric hydroxide and phosphate, concentrated within the molecule in four particles or micelles forming a central core 55 to 60 Å in diameter. The iron micelles are electron-dense and give a characteristic appearance to electron photomicrographs of the protein.

When ferritin is coupled to antibody globulin, the antibody activity of the protein is retained. This has been demonstrated by use of ferritin-conjugated anti-vaccinia globulin to study the localization of antigenic material of the virus in infected HeLa (human tumor tissue culture) cells. Electron microscopy showed that the ferritin granules appeared at the surface of the virus particles, thus marking the site of antigen-antibody interaction (see Figure 7–5). Bacterial and mycotic antigen localization has been examined in the same manner, and *Clostridium botulinum* toxin, coupled with ferritin and injected into mice, has been found in the neuromuscular junctions, particularly at the motor end plates of the intercostal muscles.

Radioisotope-Labeled Antibodies. Antibodies can be labeled internally or externally with various radioisotopes. Internal (biosynthetic) labeling occurs when an animal that is producing antibody is administered amino acids containing ^{14}C, ^{35}S, or ^{3}H. Some of the isotope appears in the immunoglobulin molecules synthesized. External labeling of antibodies or antigens may be accomplished by diazotization and coupling of ^{35}S-sulfanilic acid. Three isotopes of iodine are also useful for specific purposes as antibody labels: ^{125}I, ^{130}I, and ^{131}I. Labeled antigens, antibodies, and antigen-antibody aggregates can be detected in vitro or in vivo by appropriate counting methods and by autoradiography, a technique in which isotopes such as ^{125}I and ^{131}I are dete ted by the spots they produce on an X-ray film. They can be used to determine the

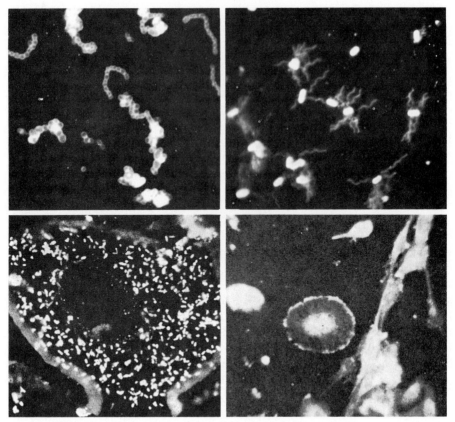

Figure 7–4. Microorganisms stained with homologous fluorescent antibodies.
Upper left, Group A hemolytic streptococci. (From Moody et al., 1958. J. Bacteriol., 75:553.)
Upper right, Salmonella typhosa, stained with labeled combined 9,12;Vi;d antibodies. (From Thomason et al., 1957. J. Bacteriol., 74:525.)
Lower left, Rickettsia rickettsii in young oocyte of infected female tick; numerous rickettsiae within the yolk, none within the cell nucleus. × 800. (From Burgdorfer, 1961. Pathol. Microbiol., 24[Suppl.]: 27.)
Lower right, Vesicular stomatitis virus in swine kidney tissue culture cells; the virus is found throughout the cytoplasm of most cells, sometimes on the periphery. × 870. (From Hopkins et al., 1962. Am. J. Vet. Res., 23:603.)

in vivo localization of reagents or to study the distribution of various labeled fractions separated by paper electrophoresis.

MICROSCOPIC SLIDE AGGLUTINATION

The Widal agglutination reaction as originally performed was a microscopic slide test used in the laboratory diagnosis of typhoid fever. Drops of the patient's blood were collected on a glass slide, aluminum foil, or glazed paper. The specimen, allowed to dry, might then be stored for considerable time if necessary. The dried blood was moistened with a small loopful of saline and gently emulsified. Sufficient of this solution to yield a delicate orange tint was mixed with a loopful of 24-hour broth culture of the typhoid organism on a cover glass, which was then inverted and sealed with petrolatum over the depression of a hollow ground slide. A control in which saline was substituted for serum was also prepared. After incubation for 30 to 60 minutes at room temperature or 37° C., both slides were observed with the high power dry objective. Positive results consisted of clumping of the organisms in the serum mixture but not in the control. The serum dilution represented by the "delicate orange tint" probably

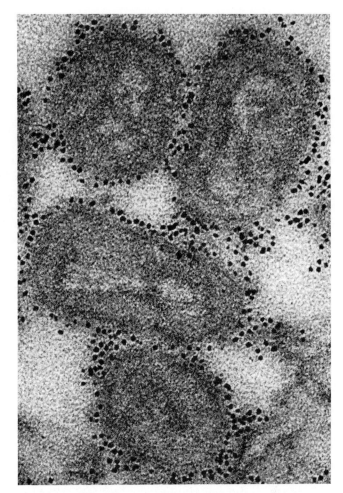

Figure 7–5. Vaccinia virus particles within a HeLa tissue culture cell tagged with ferritin-conjugated antivaccinial globulin. The black (electron-dense) ferritin granules surround each virus particle, because the labeled vaccinial antibody has reacted with its homologous antigen. (From Morgan et al., 1961. Virology, 14:292.)

corresponded to about 1:80. A typhoid antibody titer of 80 or more in a patient's serum almost always indicates active infection (see Table 7–1). The principal objection to this test was that it provided only one serum dilution, and occasionally a prozone gave a falsely negative result.

The process of agglutination may be followed continuously with the microscope in slide preparations. A hanging drop is prepared with a loopful of diluted serum and a

Table 7–1 *Interpretation of Agglutination Test in Diagnosis of Typhoid Fever**

Antibody Titer		Significance
H (FLAGELLAR)	O (SOMATIC)	
80 or higher	80 or higher	Almost always indicates active typhoid infection
80 or higher	Less than 80	Found in typhoid carriers or after previous infection or immunization; rare in active infection
Less than 80	80 or higher	Found in approx. 14% of active cases; usually in infections with related organisms

*From Coleman *In* Diagnostic Procedures and Reagents, 1950, 3rd ed. New York, American Public Health Association.

loopful of a broth culture or saline suspension of an agar slant culture. High concentrations of antibodies often cause almost immediate cessation of motility followed by clumping, but in greater dilution the rate of reaction is retarded and the gradual formation of large aggregates can be observed.

MACROSCOPIC SLIDE AGGLUTINATION

The macroscopic slide agglutination technique is used in the diagnosis of many infectious diseases and in screening tests for the rapid identification of bacteria. It may be conducted on any flat glazed surface, such as a microscope slide or glass plate, ruled with a diamond point or marked with paraffin to keep tests from running together. Special hollow ground slides containing a dozen or more depressions are also available. A loopful or one small drop each of a low dilution of antiserum and a heavy bacterial suspension are used. The slide is rocked and tilted for 1 to 3 minutes by hand or mechanically, and flocculation or granulation is observed with the naked eye. A control containing saline instead of serum is provided for each organism tested. The agglutination of an unknown organism in any number of different antisera is rapidly determined, and often with single factor sera a complete identification can be made. The macroscopic slide technique is used particularly in identifying the gram-negative intestinal bacteria.

HEMAGGLUTINATION

There are various methods for detecting and/or titrating antibodies that agglutinate erythrocytes. Blood cells suspended in 2 to 4 per cent concentration in saline or in their own serum or plasma are usually employed as the test antigen.

In the tube test, which is considered most accurate, a drop of cell suspension is placed in a 10- × 75-mm. test tube, and a drop of serum or serum dilution is added. The tube may then be incubated at room temperature for 1 hour and examined for agglutination; if necessary, a hand lens or magnifying mirror can be used as an aid. Alternatively, the tube may be centrifuged at 1,000 to 2,000 r.p.m. for 1 minute and examined for agglutination. For some purposes tubes are incubated at 37° C. for 15 to 60 minutes and read directly or after centrifugation.

In the slide test, 1 drop of antiserum is placed on a microscope slide or glass plate, followed by 1 drop of the 2 to 4 per cent cell suspension. The reagents are mixed with toothpicks or applicator sticks and spread over an area about 22 mm. in diameter. The slide is tilted and rotated and observed after not more than 2 minutes. In certain tests (e.g., Rh typing) whole blood is used as the source of erythrocytes and the reaction is performed on slides warmed to 40° to 45° C. on a viewing box or microscope substage lamp.

Coombs' Antiglobulin Test. Those anti-erythrocyte antibodies formerly called incomplete or univalent antibodies can be detected by Coombs' antiglobulin test. The procedure is also useful for detection of erythrocyte antigens by use of such antibodies. The basis of the test is the reaction of antibody against γ-globulin with the γ-globulin attached as an antibody to red blood cells. Some anti-erythrocyte antibodies are apparently so constructed that they can react with determinants on only one red blood cell, or else the determinants are deeply situated. In any case, lattice formation does not occur, and hence the cells are not agglutinated. However, if antiglobulin antibody is added, lattice formation promptly takes place and the cells agglutinate.

In some disease conditions, naturally formed anti-red cell antibodies react with red blood cells in vivo but fail to agglutinate until a Coombs-type antiglobulin serum is added; this is the direct antiglobulin test. The indirect test is used to detect "incomplete" antibodies or, by use of known nonagglutinating antibodies, to detect certain antigens. The test cells and "incomplete" or nonagglutinating antibodies are incubated together at 37° C. for 15 to 60 minutes, after which the cells are thoroughly washed and treated with antiglobulin. Agglutination follows promptly if the reagents are homologous.

APPLICATIONS OF SEROLOGIC PRECIPITATION

Serologic precipitation (as well as agglutination) has long been useful in the diagnosis of infectious disease, in the identification of bacteria, proteins, and other antigenic substances, and in studies of animal and plant phylogeny. Techniques based on these reactions are increasingly used to study the structures of enzymes, hormones, and other substances, and immunology is now one of the cornerstones of molecular biology.

Detection of Bacterial Antigens in Tissues

The presence of plague or anthrax bacteria in animal tissue can be indicated by precipitin tests. Plague, for example, is primarily a disease of rats, and during epizootic periods considerable numbers of dead rats may be found. Isolation of the plague organism from carcasses is difficult, but the plague antigen may be detected, even in partly decomposed tissues, by the "thermoprecipitin" test. Organs or tissues are ground, and the finely divided tissue is boiled with five to ten volumes of distilled water and filtered. This constitutes the antigen solution. It is used in a ring test with known antiplague serum. Positive results demonstrate the presence of plague antigen.

Identification and Typing of Bacteria

Pure cultures of certain bacteria are identified or typed by precipitin tests. The usefulness of diagnostic agglutination tests with hemolytic streptococci is diminished by the marked overlapping of antigens within the group and a strong tendency to spontaneous agglutination. However, Lancefield found that strains isolated from the same source or disease condition could be grouped together by the precipitin test. The organisms are extracted with dilute hydrochloric acid (pH 2.0 to 2.4) at 100° C., neutralized, and centrifuged; the clear supernatant liquid constitutes the test antigen. Eleven groups of hemolytic streptococci have been established; the majority of strains from human disease are in Group A. An unknown streptococcus is typed by testing its extract against antisera of the various groups. The ring test is usually employed, and tubes of narrow bore are used to conserve serum.

The Neufeld "Quellungreaktion" may be considered a precipitin test in which the antigen is a specific polysaccharide in the bacterial capsule; the latter increases strikingly in size as a result of union with antibody. This phenomenon occurs quickly and is observable with the microscope. It provides the easiest and most rapid method of determining the type of a capsulated pneumococcus, either in a clinical specimen such as sputum or in a young culture grown in suitable medium. A loopful of sputum or culture is mixed with an equal amount of antiserum on a slide, usually with the addition of methylene blue to facilitate observation of the capsules. In homologous antiserum the capsules become markedly swollen within a few moments. Capsules of type 3 organisms swell more than those of most others because this type produces polysaccharide in greatest abundance. This was formerly an important tool in the diagnosis of lobar pneumonia. Similar procedures are applicable in the identification or typing of certain streptococci, *Klebsiella pneumoniae, Hemophilus influenzae,* and *Neisseria meningitidis.*

Flocculation Tests for Syphilis

Several modifications of the precipitation test are employed in the laboratory diagnosis of syphilis. Blood serum from the patient is examined for the presence of an antibody-like substance, "reagin," produced in response to the infection. Reagin appears within a few weeks after infection and persists in varying concentration throughout the course of the disease, usually disappearing when symptoms disappear.

The syphilis test antigen is a lipid extract of beef heart. Antigens first employed were aqueous or alcoholic extracts of syphilitic tissues, but it was subsequently found that similar extracts of normal tissues possessed equal or better reactivity. The antigen for the Kahn precipitation test is prepared from beef heart powder washed with ether and then extracted with alcohol. The lipid extract is treated with cholesterol, which enhances the sensitivity of the product, and diluted with saline for use in the test. The sensitivity of the antigen must be carefully regulated because supersensitive preparations may give falsely positive reactions with the sera of normal individuals.

The Kahn test is performed with varying amounts of antigen and a constant amount of patient's serum which has been heated at 56° C. for 30 minutes. The tubes are shaken vigorously for 3 minutes, after which saline is added to disperse the floccules, and the degree of particulation is read.

Other precipitation or flocculation tests for syphilis employ antigens prepared by different methods, together with different procedures for setting up, incubating, and reading the reactions. Both test tube and macroscopic and microscopic slide tests are in common use.

Serologic tests for syphilis are of academic as well as diagnostic interest because lipids are essential ingredients of the test antigens. The specifically reactive material was isolated by Pangborn and named *cardiolipin.* This substance has replaced previous lipid extracts in many test antigens. Cardiolipin appears to consist of three glycerol residues joined by two phosphate radicals, with fatty acid molecules esterified to the four available hydroxyl groups of the terminal glycerol molecules. A possible structure is illustrated in Figure 7–6.

Cardiolipin is used in the VDRL (Veneral Disease Research Laboratory) rapid slide microflocculation procedure. In addition to cardiolipin, the test antigen contains cholesterol and lecithin, emulsified in buffered saline. The qualitative test is performed by adding one drop (1/60 ml.) of antigen emulsion to 0.05 ml. of heated (56° C. for 30 minutes) serum in a paraffin ring on a glass slide and rotating the slide, either on a mechanical rotator or by hand, for 4 minutes. Flocculation is read microscopically at 100× magnification. The antigen appears as short rod particles at this magnification and aggregates in the presence of reagin into small or medium to large clumps. A serum that produces small clumps is graded "weakly reactive;" sera that yield medium or large clumps are considered "reactive." Because of possible zonal inhibition reactions, weakly reactive sera should be retested by the quantitative VDRL slide procedure, in which serum dilutions are tested as above.

The fact that supersensitive antigens react with the sera of uninfected individuals indicates that reagin is not produced solely in response to syphilitic infection but may be present in normal persons. Moreover, in certain other diseases, such as malaria,

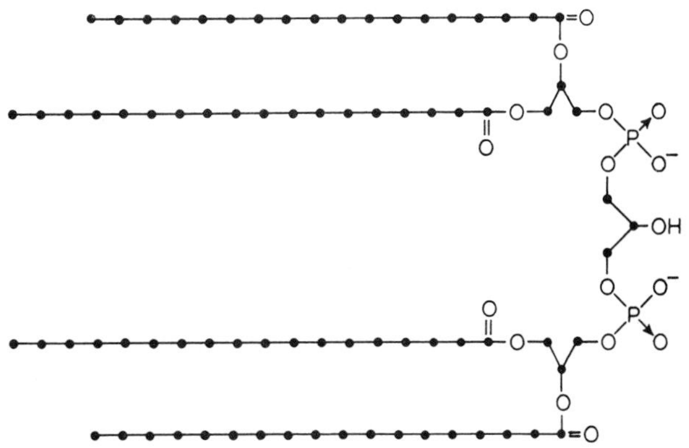

Figure 7-6. Postulated structure of cardiolipin. Four fatty acid residues (chains at the left) are esterified to two glycerol residues, which are joined by a phosphate-glycerol-phosphate link. (From Rapport, 1961. J. Lipid Res., 2: 25.)

leprosy, and infectious mononucleosis, reagin is temporarily increased to such an extent that positive tests for syphilis are often obtained. In syphilis itself the reagin response is marked and remains at a high level until all symptoms of the disease disappear.

Kahn postulated that reagin is an antibody against tissue lipids. Lipids are presumed to be liberated from body tissue in the course of normal wear and tear. These, perhaps with the assistance of some "schleppering" agent in the individual serum, induce the formation of antibodies (reagins) within the same individual. These antibodies are normally low in concentration but may increase in certain disease conditions as a result of increased tissue breakdown. In the final analysis the test for syphilis is quantitative rather than qualitative.

C-Reactive Protein

The sera of patients in the acute phase of various infections and certain other diseases contain a protein not found in normal human serum. Its presence was discovered by Tillett and Francis (1930) in an investigation of antigenic components of the pneumococcus. They found that a nitrogenous polysaccharide, the C substance, from rough pneumococci precipitated with high dilutions of the sera of patients during the acute phase of pneumonia. The serum component was a protein, later designated the *C-reactive protein.* It appears less than 24 hours after the onset of symptoms of pneumonia, remains at a high level during the disease, and decreases sharply 2 or 3 days after the crisis, when the temperature returns to normal. The protein is not type-specific; type-specific agglutinins did not appear in patients' sera *until the crisis* and persisted thereafter during convalescence, after disappearance of the C-reactive protein.

Sera of patients with streptococcal and staphylococcal infections, acute rheumatic fever, Hodgkin's disease, cirrhosis of the liver, certain carcinomata, and other diseases also contain the same abnormal protein, capable of precipitating with the pneumococcus C-substance. The protein has been isolated and crystallized and found to migrate electrophoretically as a β- or γ-globulin. Its S_{20} is 7.5, somewhat greater than that of normal serum γ-globulin (S_{20} = 6.3). It is not an antibody.

Detection of C-reactive protein is widely used in clinical laboratory diagnosis as a possible indication of persisting pathologic activity. It is precipitated specifically by antiserum against C-reactive protein, and, in fact, this method of detection is favored because it is several times as sensitive as precipitation with the C-polysaccharide.

Forensic Precipitin Tests

One of the most dramatic applications of the precipitin test is the forensic identification of blood stains. It is often necessary, as in murder cases, to determine the species origin of blood dried on cloth, paper, a knife, or some other material. The blood need not be fresh but must be thoroughly dried or otherwise well preserved. Positive results have been obtained with blood spots after many years, and Egyptian mummy tissue 5,000 years old gave a detectable reaction.

Antisera should be highly potent, sterile, and crystal clear. Anti-human sera of high titer can be prepared in rabbits by immunizing with human blood, plasma, or serum. Schiff and Boyd recommended a series of intravenous 1- to 2-ml. doses containing approximately 2 per cent protein, or 3- to 6-ml. intraperitoneal doses. If a rabbit is injected too frequently or with too great an amount of protein, or is bled too soon after the last injection, the antiserum will contain both human serum and anti-human precipitins and will be unsuitable for forensic work. Such a serum will react as an antigen against *properly* prepared antiserum and as an antibody against human serum. A forensic antiserum should give a positive ring test within 20 minutes at room temperature with a 1:20,000 dilution of homologous blood.

The stain is extracted with an amount of saline that varies with the size of the stain. The extract is clarified by filtration or centrifugation. If the stain is very small, the solution will contain only a small amount of protein. Extracts representing a serum dilution of about 1:1000 develop a stable foam upon shaking. If only this amount of material is available, the test must be done in this dilution. A more concentrated extract is diluted serially and tested with constant antiserum as in the regular precipitin test. The presence of blood in the stain should be proved by the benzidine, hemin crystal, or other suitable test, because stains of paint and other materials are sometimes indistinguishable from blood stains.

The ring test is always employed, antiserum constituting the lower layer and blood stain extract the upper layer. A positive result is apparent within 5 to 20 minutes at room temperature if the antiserum is of suitable potency.

In view of the importance of the forensic test, numerous controls are necessary to prove the specificity and reactivity of the antiserum. (1) Blood stain extract tested with normal rabbit serum must give a negative reaction. (2) Saline and antiserum must produce no precipitate. (3) An extract of an unstained portion of the material must not react with the antiserum. As an additional control, the extract from unstained material should not inhibit reaction between the antiserum and homologous blood. (4) Bloods from several species other than those involved in the test must be negative to confirm the specificity of the antiserum. (5) Several different specimens of known blood homologous to the antiserum must all react positively in the same test. For example, bloods from a number of humans must be shown to react with an anti-human test serum.

The forensic precipitin test is most widely known for its use in identification of human blood, but it has been employed for other purposes, such as determination of the hosts of blood-sucking insects. Suitably modified, the procedure is also used to identify the animal origin of semen, bones, milk, meat, and other tissues or fluids.

"Cocto-antisera" are often used in the identification of meats and fish products. These antisera are prepared by immunizing rabbits with heated (70° C. for 1 hour) sera of the animals in question or with heated tissue extracts. Cocto-antisera precipitate extracts of meat from the homologous animal sources, whether the meat is raw or cooked. Highly potent, specific antisera are required. They should give positive results with the homologous antigen diluted 1:10,000 to 1:100,000. Antisera that cross-react with other meats are preferably discarded but are sometimes made specific by adsorption with small amounts of the cross-reacting antigen and subsequent removal of the precipitate. The meat specimen to be examined is homogenized with saline in a Waring Blendor and filtered clear. Ring tests with the appropriate antisera and proper controls quickly indicate species sources of the meat or meats composing the specimen. This test is frequently used to detect horse meat in sausage, hamburger, or other processed meat products.

Use of the Precipitin Reaction in Systematic Serology

Morphologic and functional evolution are the results of modifications that confer a selective advantage on the organisms within which they occur. Both morphology and function depend upon chemical structure, which is controlled by the genetic code of the organism. A chance alteration in the genetic code leads to change in the composition of a substance and synthesis of a new structural or functional component.

Proteins undergo gradual changes of this type. Differences have been discovered between homologous proteins such as hemoglobin in various individuals within a species; some of these differences are chemically minor but functionally important. There are at least a dozen different human hemoglobins, most of which differ from one another by only a single amino acid in a chain composed of nearly 300 amino acids (see Table 7–2). If one glutamic acid residue of hemoglobin A, the normal form, is replaced by valine, hemoglobin S is formed. Hemoglobin S is insoluble when it is deoxygenated and distorts the red cells with formation of a crescent shape that gives the name *sickle cell anemia* to the hereditary disease in which it occurs.

Insulin has undergone evolutionary changes in various animal species (see Table 5–9, page 129). The differences involve only one, two, or three amino acids, and in this case they do not impair the functional properties of the chemical. They evidently affect the surface conformation of the molecules, because the different species of insulin can be distinguished by serologic means. It is differences of this type that are significant in systematic serology.

Taxonomic *relationships* are based upon similarities in the chemical structures of homologous substances (e.g., albumins), and they are indicated serologically by cross-reactions. Chemical *differences* may occur between taxonomically different organisms, and the degree of difference (the serologic "distance") between homologous chemicals is correlated with the evolutionary difference between the organisms.

Use of the precipitin test in the study of animal relationships was initiated shortly after discovery of the reaction itself. Early investigators employed simple mixtures of antiserum and antigen and reported the development of cloudiness or a definite precipitate after varying periods of incubation. Usually a constant amount of antiserum,

Table 7–2 *Portions of the Amino Acid Sequences of Normal Human Hemoglobin (A) and Two Abnormal Human Hemoglobins (S and C)*

Hemoglobin	Amino Acid Sequence
A	His.Val.Leu.Leu.Thr.Pro.**Glu.**Glu.Lys.
S	His.Val.Leu.Leu.Thr.Pro.**Val.** Glu.Lys.
C	His.Val.Leu.Leu.Thr.Pro.**Lys.**Glu.Lys.

such as 0.1 ml., was mixed with 0.5 ml. of one or more dilutions of antigen. Nuttall included in some of his observations a record of the time required for visible reaction and also developed a "quantitative" procedure in which the volume of precipitate was measured in a capillary tube. The ring test was subsequently employed in studies of animal and plant relationships.

Although the inhibition of precipitation in simple mixtures by excess antigen was known at that time, many precipitin tests were performed in which a single dilution of antigen was employed. It is therefore surprising that the results of early phylogenetic studies correlated as well as they did with the systematic position of the test materials when classified on morphologic and other grounds.

Nuttall (1904) studied the antigenic relationships of mammalian, bird, and reptile sera (Table 7–3). Antisera against the various mammalian species gave the greatest percentage of positive precipitin reactions when tested with antigens derived from the same or other species of the same order. Thus, anti-ox serum yielded positive results with 72 per cent of the ungulate antigens, and anti-wallaby serum reacted positively with 68 per cent of the marsupial antigens. Birds constituted a distinct group with practically no evidence of relationship to the other animals tested. Reptiles were heterogeneous among themselves and cross-reacted with only one other antiserum. It may be significant that the cross-reaction occurred in the fowl group, of which reptiles were presumably the evolutionary ancestors.

Numerous interesting relationships have been shown by means of the precipitin test. As long ago as 1905 Friedenthal secured weak reactions between blood serum of the frozen Siberian mammoth and antiserum against Indian elephant. Boyden and Noble in 1933 helped to clarify the relationships between certain amphibia. They found that Siren, Necturus, and Amphiuma are closely related to one another but are only distantly related to the primitive form Cryptobranchus. These relationships were represented graphically in a three dimensional model (Figure 7–7). Boyden later demonstrated that the mule and the hinny, hybrids of the horse and ass, possess serum proteins found in the parent animals.

Williams in 1964 reported studies of antigenic relationships among primates using quantitative procedures to evaluate the serologic similarities between the various major groups. The reactivities of serum albumins and globulins with antisera against human serum albumin and gamma-globulin were determined by analyses of precipitin curves and gel diffusion tests; results were expressed as percentages of the homologous reactivity with human reagents. Figure 7–8 presents the ranges of values obtained with a prosimian, the lemur, and various members of the Ceboideae, Cercopithecoideae, and Pongidae, plotted against a time scale indicating postulated times of divergence of the different groups from the main line of descent to man. It is apparent that a fairly marked acceleration in the rate of antigenic evolution occurred about 50,000,000 years ago.

The precipitin reaction has also been applied to the study of plant materials. Antisera are prepared by immunizing rabbits with solutions of dried, macerated plant tissues in saline, water, buffer, or weak alkali. Serologic work with plants is hampered by the presence of nonspecific precipitating substances, such as organic acids, tannins, alkaloids, and glucosides. Many of these substances can be removed by pre-extraction of plant tissues with ether, alcohol, benzene, acetone, or other solvents. Such treatment is, of course, subject to the objection that it may also remove specific antigenic materials. Nevertheless, valuable information has been secured by use of extracted tissues.

Mez and Ziegenspeck in 1926 summarized work of the preceding thirteen years of the Königsberg school in a serologic "Stammbaum" or genealogic tree (Figure 7–9). The serologic relationships discovered correlated well with anatomy, morphology, cytology, and paleontology.

Table 7–3 *Precipitation of Animal Sera by Rabbit Antisera**

Antigens (Sera)	Numbers of Antigens Tested	Rabbit Antisera						
		PRIMATE (MAN)	INSECTIVORE (HEDGEHOG)	CARNIVORE (DOG)	UNGULATE (OX)	MARSUPIAL (WALLABY)	BIRD (FOWL)	REPTILE (TURTLE)
		Per cent positive						
Primates	64–97	90	2	21	11	11	0	0
Insectivores	8–15	13	47	14	0	0	0	0
Carnivores	76–97	27	5	46	4	5	1	0
Ungulates	57–70	43	7	3	72	5	0	0
Marsupials	21–26	4	0	4	0.6	68	0	0
Birds	262–322	0.3	0	0.3	0.6	0	88	0
Reptiles	34–51	0	0	0	0	0	2	18

*From Nuttall, 1904. Blood Immunity and Blood Relationship. Cambridge, Cambridge University Press.

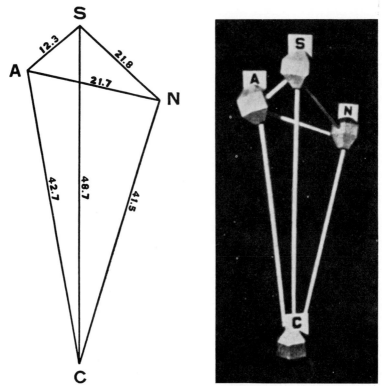

Figure 7–7.   Diagram and three dimensional model showing the interrelationships between Crypto-branchus (*C*), Amphiuma (*A*), Siren (*S*), and Necturus (*N*), based on ring tests with standard antigen dilutions. (From Boyden, 1942. Physiol. Zool., 15:109.)

APPLICATIONS OF THE AGGLUTINATION REACTION

Detection of Agglutinins in Patients' Sera

Antibodies specifically directed against the causative agents of certain infectious diseases appear in the circulating blood a few days after infection. They increase in amount for several weeks, remain relatively constant for varying periods of time, then decrease slowly until little or no titer is detectable. The presence of such antibodies is therefore presumptive evidence for infection by the specific etiologic agent if the patient has not previously been infected or immunized with this organism. Unfortunately, from the diagnostic point of view, many individuals normally possess low or moderate amounts of certain antibodies. These "normal" antibodies, together with anamnestic reactions, complicate the interpretation of a positive agglutination test. In the absence of specific information regarding the history of the patient, two or more tests are performed at weekly intervals and a rising antibody titer is considered evidence of active infection.

Detection of agglutinins in patients' sera is of value in cases of typhoid and paratyphoid fevers and many other infections. The serum is diluted 1:10, 1:20, 1:40, 1:80, 1:160, or higher and tested with appropriate antigens. Enteric fever antigens include *S. typhosa, S. paratyphi A,* and *S. paratyphi B;* usually both H (flagellar) and O (somatic) suspensions are employed. The results of tests for typhoid fever are interpreted as indicated in Table 7–1 (see page 191). Tests for paratyphoid agglutinins have similar significance. A test for Vi agglutinins is also performed. These antibodies are not always found in active cases of typhoid fever but are present so frequently in typhoid carriers that the test for Vi antibody has been used to detect such individuals.

Diagnosis of undulant fever is sometimes aided by the agglutination test. This disease is notoriously difficult to diagnose by clinical methods; it runs a prolonged course, often subacute or chronic, and is easily confused with enteric or other infections. Agglutination tests with Brucella are often performed on the sera of suspected typhoid and paratyphoid patients. Before interpreting agglutination with Brucella antigen it is necessary to know whether the patient has constant opportunity for infection by use of raw milk or by handling infected animals. Such a person is likely to have a relatively high agglutinin titer. A titer of 160 in individuals with infrequent opportunity for infection sometimes indicates active disease. This figure, however, may be within the normal range for persons continuously exposed to Brucella. In any case, a titer of 1000 is rare except in active brucellosis.

Brucella antibodies can be detected also in the blood serum and milk of infected cows or other animals. Whole milk is tested by adding a heavy suspension of Brucella stained with hematoxylin. The milk and antigen are thoroughly mixed and allowed to stand until the cream rises. The mass of agglutinated dyed bacteria is swept upward with the cream and is readily distinguished. This "ring test" is sufficiently delicate to detect agglutinins from a single positive cow in the pooled milk from a large herd.

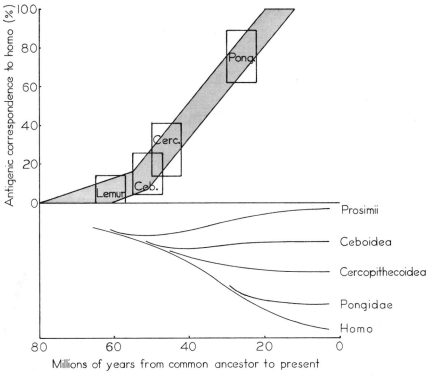

Figure 7–8. Correlation between the antigenic evolution of primates and the divergence of major groups from the line of descent leading to man. *Top,* Boxes indicate cross-reactivities of serum albumins and serum globulins from representatives of the various groups with rabbit antihuman serum albumin and rabbit antihuman gamma globulin (Pongidae: chimpanzee, gorilla, orangutan; Cercopithecoidea: rhesus monkey; Ceboideae: cebus, spider monkey; Lemur: a modern prosimian). Shaded area shows the general trend of antigenic cross-reactivity as a function of time of divergence. *Bottom,* Curves suggesting the times of divergence of the major groups, with internal branches and extinct forms omitted. (Adapted from Williams *In* Beuttner-Janasch, J. (Ed.): Evolutionary and Genetic Biology of Primates, 1964, vol. 2. New York, Academic Press, Inc.)

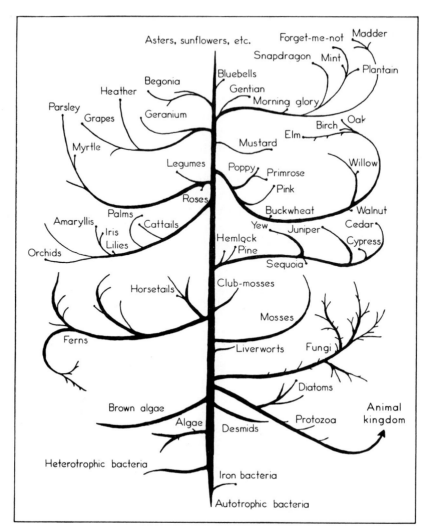

Figure 7–9. Excerpts from the Königsberg "Stammbaum," showing phylogenetic relations of plant species and genera as indicated by serologic reactions. (Modified and redrawn from Gortner, 1929. Outlines of Biochemistry. New York, John Wiley and Sons, Inc.)

Furthermore, the results with pasteurized milk are as satisfactory as with raw milk, which greatly increases its usefulness over methods of examination requiring isolation of the pathogenic agent.

Tularemia, like brucellosis, is prolonged, debilitating, subacute or chronic, and rather difficult to diagnose. A titer of 160 or higher is considered indicative of infection, and titers of 2,560 or 5,120 are not uncommon. Sera agglutinating *Francisella tularensis* may also agglutinate *Br. abortus* because the bacteria contain common antigens. Tularemia agglutinins often persist in low concentration for years.

Agglutination tests in bacillary dysentery and bubonic plague are of limited value, because detectable antibodies do not always develop. Titers of 20 or greater against *Shigella dysenteriae* and *Sh. sonnei* and of 160 or greater against *Sh. paradysenteriae* are suggestive of active infection in areas where these organisms are not endemic. Any positive result is of value in bubonic plague, and the titers may be low (less than 40).

The Weil-Felix test for typhus fever is a heterogenetic reaction of theoretic as well as practical interest. In 1916, Weil and Felix isolated from the urine of a typhus fever patient a strain of Proteus that was agglutinated by the patient's serum and by serum from other typhus fever patients. Serum from normal individuals did not agglutinate the organism. It was soon found that Proteus was not the cause of typhus fever, but the test is a highly useful diagnostic tool. The strain of Proteus, designated *X19*, agglutinated in titers of 50 to 50,000 with typhus fever sera, but never over a titer of 25 with serum from patients without the disease. Since the reaction involves somatic antigens of the organism, only nonmotile strains are used. These are designated by the letter O (e.g., *Proteus OX19*). Two additional strains, *OX2* and *OX-K*, are useful in the diagnosis of various other Rickettsial diseases (Table 7–4). Normal agglutinins for Proteus occur with considerable frequency in man, so an increasing titer in second and third specimens taken at intervals of several days is considered more significant than the magnitude of the titer of a single specimen. *Proteus OX19* and *Rickettsia prowazeki*, the cause of typhus fever, share a common polysaccharide hapten. The three *OX* strains possess similar haptens. There is no direct evidence that *R. orientalis* (the cause of tsutsugamushi fever) shares the polysaccharide of *OX-K*, although they apparently possess some antigen in common.

An interesting diagnostic agglutination test is used in infectious mononucleosis or "glandular fever." Infectious mononucleosis is a benign disease, occurring principally in individuals in the 13 to 25 year age group. It is of uncertain etiology but is thought to be caused by the herpeslike Epstein-Barr virus. It is characterized by sudden onset with fever, usually a sore throat, and pronounced enlargement of the cervical lymph nodes. There is moderate leukocytosis with marked increase in lymphocytes (50 to 90 per cent), which are somewhat atypical. The serologic test is performed by adding a suspension of sheep erythrocytes to dilutions of inactivated patient's serum and incubating at 37° C. for 2 hours. Agglutination titers of 320 or higher are considered significant, and titers of 40,960 have been obtained. The laboratory diagnosis of infectious mononucleosis is complicated by the fact that injection of antitoxin or other horse serum preparations may induce a disease known as serum sickness, in which there is also an increase of sheep red cell agglutinins. Furthermore, normal individuals may possess a Forssman-like antibody that agglutinates sheep cells. These three sheep hemagglutinins can be distinguished from one another by adsorption of the serum with guinea pig kidney emulsion and boiled beef erythrocytes, as indicated in Table 7–5. It is usually sufficient to treat the patient's serum with the kidney preparation; after removal of the tissue by centrifugation, the agglutinin titer is compared with that of the unadsorbed serum. A diagnosis of infectious mononucleosis is confirmed if at least part of the hemagglutinin remains.

"Cold" agglutinins for human erythrocytes are occasionally important in laboratory diagnosis and in the production of disease. These antibodies are sometimes found in primary atypical pneumonia and other diseases and may also be present in normal human serum and in some animal sera. They agglutinate red blood cells at tempera-

Table 7–4 *Agglutination Test for Rickettsial Disease**

Disease Group	Proteus Test Antigen		
	OX19	OX2	OX-K
Typhus fever	++++	0 or +	0
Spotted fever	0 or ++++	++++ or 0	0
Tsutsugamushi fever	0	0	++++
Q fever	0	0	0

*From Sabin et al. *In* Rivers, T. M. (Ed.): Viral and Rickettsial Infections of Man, 1952, 2nd ed. Philadelphia, J. B. Lippincott Company.

Table 7–5 *Differentiation of Sheep Erythrocyte Agglutinins in Human Serum**

Antibody	Antibody Removed from Serum by	
	GUINEA PIG KIDNEY	BOILED BEEF RBC
Infectious mononucleosis	−	+
Serum sickness	+	+
Forssman	+	−

*From Stuart *In* Diagnostic Procedures and Reagents, 1950, 3rd ed. New York, American Public Health Association.

tures below that of the body, but the agglutinated cells redisperse when warmed to 37° C. Cold agglutination titers usually decrease as the test incubation temperature increases, but there is considerable variation between individuals and animals in the thermal range through which agglutination occurs, some sera reacting only below 20° C., others as high as 35° C. The test is performed for diagnostic purposes at 2 to 5° C. Normal titers at this temperature are usually not more than 40. Titers of 160 or greater are not uncommon in atypical pneumonia, and there is some correlation between the severity of the infection and the titer observed. Washed human red cells, usually of blood group O, are employed as test antigen. Serum is obtained from blood allowed to clot and centrifuged at room temperature or preferably 37° C., because cold agglutinins are adsorbed by erythrocytes of the same individual at refrigerator temperature. Serum dilutions plus antigen are incubated overnight in the refrigerator and agglutination is read immediately upon removal. Positive tests are warmed to 37° C. and reread after 2 hours to be sure that aggregation is caused by cold agglutinins, whose action is reversed under such conditions.

Some forms of autoimmune hemolytic anemia are associated with or caused by cold hemagglutinins. The origin of these antibodies is unclear; it has been suggested (1) that they result from a break in tolerance to normal antigens or (2) that modification of cell components by drug therapy or viral infection produces "neoantigens" that incite antibody formation. Cold IgM antibodies may appear against a red cell antigen that forms after birth during maturation of the erythropoietic system. These antibodies agglutinate red blood cells in a chilled extremity, such as a fingertip, toe, nose, or earlobe, and the plugging of the capillaries by the aggregated cells causes local necrosis. Paroxysmal cold hemoglobinuria may be produced by cold autoantibodies of the IgG class. The antibodies bind to red cells at low temperature. A patient who has suffered cold shock has a severe hemolytic episode following return to normal body temperature.

Identification and Classification of Bacteria

Soon after the description of agglutination in 1896, it was found that this procedure could be used to distinguish between bacteria that appeared identical by most other laboratory criteria, e.g., the typhoid and paratyphoid organisms. Although the chemical basis of serologic specificity was not known for many years, especially with reference to bacterial cells, it was quickly learned (1903) that motile bacteria possess antigens lacking in nonmotile bacteria of the same species. These antigens could only be associated with the flagella. It then appeared that different bacterial strains possess different flagellar and nonflagellar (somatic) antigens, and this knowledge became the basis for serologic identification and typing of bacteria as practiced today.

ANTIGENIC ANALYSIS

The serologic type of an organism is determined by its distinctive antigenic components or combination of components. Complete antigenic analysis includes detection of all components possible. Rapid progress is being made in determining the chemical composition of various microbial and animal cellular determinant groups (for example, see Figure 5–9, page 147). No one knows how many different antigenic constituents a cell possesses. A score or more have been detected in *Bordetella pertussis* and in hemolytic streptococci of group A, but these probably are only a small percentage of the total. Bacterial cells contain antigens in their flagella, capsules, cell walls, protoplasmic membranes, and in the cytoplasm. They include structural and enzymic proteins, nucleoproteins, polysaccharides, lipopolysaccharides, and mucopeptides.

It has been traditional, in the absence of specific knowledge of the chemical composition of cellular antigens, to designate the different antigenic determinants by letters and numerals (e.g., A,B,C. . .I,II,III. . .1,2,3. . .). In general, there is a definite system of antigenic nomenclature within each genus or other group of bacteria, but the system within one group usually bears no relationship to that within other groups.

Inasmuch as individual bacterial cells contain numerous antigenic components or determinants, each of which can induce the formation of a separate antibody, the antigenic structure of bacteria has been likened to a mosaic. Four organisms, for example, might possess the following antigenic structures and produce corresponding antisera:

ORGANISM	ANTIGENS	ANTISERUM	ANTIBODIES
I	A B C	1	a b c
II	B C D	2	b c d
III	C D E	3	c d e
IV	D E F	4	d e f

Each organism is related to those that immediately precede and follow it by common possession of one or two antigenic components. Organism I, however, is completely unrelated in its antigenic structure to organism IV, although both are members in a series of related forms. The situation pictured here probably extends throughout the natural world, and if all the "missing links" could be found, each living form would appear as a member of a continuous intergrading series.

Antiserum 1 contains antibodies a, b, and c, and can agglutinate organisms, I, II, and III, but cannot agglutinate IV because the latter possesses no antigen corresponding to an antibody in Antiserum 1. Antisera 2 and 3 can agglutinate all four organisms, and Antiserum 4 can agglutinate II, III, and IV. Adsorption of Antiserum 1 with organism II removes all antibodies except a. This adsorbed serum can therefore be used to detect antigen A in any organism and is a so-called *mono*specific or *single factor serum*. It will agglutinate I but not II. Monospecific sera can be similarly prepared for any of the other antigenic components.

The various serologically different components or antigenic determinants of an organism are detected by use of appropriate unadsorbed and adsorbed antisera. The simplest case is that in which two organisms are compared. The first step is to prepare antisera against each organism. Cross-agglutination tests are conducted by preparing duplicate sets of dilutions of both sera and treating one series of dilutions of each serum with the homologous organism, the other with the heterologous organism. Agglutination results like those in Table 7–6 might be obtained. These two organisms are related, since each agglutinated in each antiserum.

Table 7–6   *Results of a Cross-agglutination Experiment*

Antiserum	Agglutination Titer With Organism	
	A	B
A	5,120	5,120
B	10,240	10,240

Occasionally, one organism agglutinates in both antisera, but the other reacts only in its homologous antiserum. The explanation of this nonreciprocal cross-reaction is not clear. It can be supposed that a given antigenic component, common to both organisms, is so situated in one organism as to be readily accessible to antibody but in the other organism is either more deeply located or is masked by other surface substances; that is, steric hindrance may prevent a given antibody molecule from approaching its homologous determinant site closely enough to react with it. Agglutination is a surface phenomenon in which only superficial antigens participate, because antibody molecules cannot penetrate far into the cell substance.

Cross-agglutination does not tell anything about the antigenic complexity of the two organisms. One or many antigenic determinants may be concerned. Furthermore, there is no indication whether each organism possesses all the determinants of the other. Organism A, for example, might contain antigens X and Y, whereas organism B might contain Y and Z.

The comparative antigenic composition of the two bacteria can be determined by reciprocal adsorptions or the "mirror test." Each antiserum is adsorbed with the heterologous organism, and cross-agglutination tests with the adsorbed antisera indicate whether any antibodies remain uncombined. If, as supposed previously, organism A possesses antigens X and Y, and B possesses Y and Z, results might appear as in Table 7–7.

A problem in antigenic analysis becomes more complicated when additional organisms are compared, but much more information can be gained about each. Table 7–8 presents data from a study of three strains of *Sh. dispar*. Cross-agglutination (lines 1, 4, and 7) indicated that organism 171 was weakly related to 167 and 205 which, in turn, were strongly related to each other. The nature of these relationships was shown by reciprocal adsorption. Antiserum 171 adsorbed with strains 167 or 205 (lines 2 and 3) still agglutinated organism 171 to the original 5,120 titer. This antibody and its corresponding antigenic component were designated by the letter A. Organisms 167 and 205 lacked this component. Adsorption of serum 167 with organism 171 (line 5) re-

Table 7–7   *Results of a Reciprocal Adsorption Experiment*

Antiserum	Adsorbed with Organism	Antibodies Remaining after Adsorption	Tested with Organism	Agglutination Titer
A (x, y)*	B (Y, Z)†	x	A (X, Y)†	5,120
			B (Y, Z)†	0
B (y, z)*	A (X, Y)†	z	A (X, Y)†	0
			B (Y, Z)†	10,240

*Antibodies present in the unadsorbed serum indicated in parentheses.
†Antigenic components indicated in parentheses.

Table 7–8 Antigenic Analysis of Three Strains of Shigella dispar

Line	Antiserum	Adsorbed with Organism	Titer When Tested with Organism			Antibodies in Antisera (and Antigens in Corresponding Organisms)
			171	167	205	
1	171	Unadsorbed	5,120	640	1,280	
2		167	5,120	0	0	A, D
3		205	5,120	0	0	
4	167	Unadsorbed	640	20,480	20,480	
5		171	0	10,240	5,120	B, C, D
6		205	0	2,560	0	
7	205	Unadsorbed	320	10,240	10,240	
8		171	0	10,240	5,120	B, D
9		167	0	0	0	

moved all antibody for 171 as expected, but did not alter the titer for 167 significantly and reduced the titer for 205 slightly. It was not certain that the antibody agglutinating 167 was the same as that agglutinating 205, but at this point it was simplest to consider it so and to designate it B. Adsorption of antiserum 167 with organism 205 (line 6) removed all agglutinins except a portion capable of reacting with 167, which therefore contained an additional antigenic component, C. Adsorption of antiserum 205 with organism 171 (line 8) confirmed the previous finding that strains 167 and 205 shared an antigen (B) lacking in 171, and the final adsorption (line 9) showed that organism 167 had all the antigens possessed by 205. The major antigenic components of these organisms were therefore A, B, and C. The weak cross-reactions indicated by titers of 320, 640, and 1,280 (lines 1, 4, and 7) were not accounted for, so a minor fraction, D, was postulated.

ANTIGENIC STRUCTURE OF BACTERIA

The antigenic structure of a bacterium consists of the sum of its various antigenic components. Capsular antigens are generally polysaccharide (polypeptide in *Bacillus anthracis* and some other Bacillus species), flagellar antigens are protein, and somatic antigens are protein-polysaccharide-phospholipid complexes.

The various antigens are not necessarily separate chemical entities; in fact, many are merely different determinant sites on the same molecule of polysaccharide or protein. As such, they might comprise three to six amino acid or monosaccharide residues. It will be recalled that Staub and her co-workers determined the chemical identity of the terminal sugars and, in some instances, the subterminal sugars of a few Salmonella and Escherichia somatic antigens (see Figure 5–9, page 147). Although *S. paratyphi B* appears to contain four O antigens, two (4 and 5) behave as though joined in a single unit or complex molecule having multiple antigenic determinants. Certain of the somatic antigens of paradysentery bacteria seem to be similarly bound together.

ANTIGENIC VARIATION IN BACTERIA

The antigenic structure of a bacterial isolate is not always constant. Both somatic (O) and flagellar (H) constituents are subject to variation.

The S-R transformation affects bacterial O antigens. This phenomenon, sometimes called dissociation, has usually been described as a change from smooth to rough colony form with accompanying decreased virulence and increased spontaneous agglutinability in physiologic saline. Rough forms possess little or none of the original smooth somatic antigen. Antiserum for one R form of Salmonella may agglutinate the R forms of other Salmonellas or even of Shigellas and more distantly related bacteria. The R antigen is largely polysaccharide (see Figure 5–11) and comprises only a portion of the entire somatic antigen of S cells. The S-R transformation is caused by a mutation; the reverse mutation also occurs, but at a much lower rate.

Flagellar antigens of Salmonella species undergo qualitative changes known as "phase variations." The flagella of certain species exist in two alternative antigenic forms. H antigens of one form appear to be characteristic of the species and are called *specific antigens* (phase 1); those of the other form are found in several species and are designated *group antigens* (phase 2). Cultures possess flagella in one phase or the other or both. When a culture containing both forms is plated and numerous colonies are tested, some are found to possess phase 1 antigens, and the others contain phase 2 antigens. Upon continued subcultivation of the isolates, each eventually undergoes variation and contains both phases again.

Phase variation occurs spontaneously in cultures with a relatively high frequency (e.g., 1 in 100,000 to 1 in 1,000 cell divisions). The variant form can be selectively cultivated by a simple procedure. To secure the specific phase from a group phase culture, the organism is grown in semisolid agar containing antiserum against the group phase. The spreading of group phase cells is inhibited by the antiserum, and motile cells in the specific phase can be isolated at a point distant from the original inoculation (Figure 7–10).

The significant antigens of an organism are customarily listed in an expression known as an *antigenic formula*. The formula of S. *paratyphi B*, for example, is 1,4,5,12:b:1,2. The four somatic antigens are listed first, then the specific flagellar antigen, b, and finally the group flagellar antigens, 1, 2. This formula means that S. *paratyphi B* is diphasic, and that cells in the specific phase possess antigens 1,4,5,12:b, whereas those in the group phase contain 1,4,5,12:1,2. Some Salmonellas appear to be

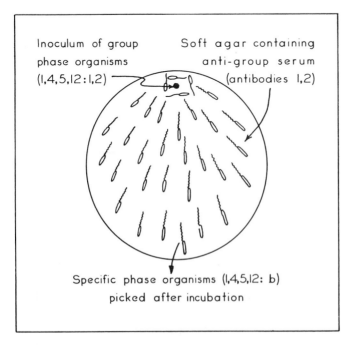

Inoculum of group phase organisms (1,4,5,12:1,2)

Soft agar containing anti-group serum (antibodies 1,2)

Specific phase organisms (1,4,5,12: b) picked after incubation

Figure 7–10. Isolation of a specific phase culture from a group phase culture by use of soft agar containing antiserum against the group antigens. Group phase organisms are prevented from spreading, but specific phase variant organisms will be motile and can be isolated at a point distant from the inoculation.

permanently monophasic with respect to either phase 1 or phase 2 antigens, because the second phase has never been isolated.

Induced Antigenic Variations. Changes in the antigenic structure of a bacterium can sometimes be induced by various laboratory manipulations. One of these is transformation, first demonstrated in 1928 by Griffith. He injected mice subcutaneously with small amounts of noncapsulated type 2 pneumococci in the rough (R) form, and simultaneously introduced heat-killed capsulated pneumococci of type 3. Some of the animals died and were found to be infected with capsulated type 3 pneumococci. Since the type 3 organisms injected had been killed by heat, it was obvious that the 2R organisms had been transformed into type 3 bacteria. The derived type 3 organisms maintained their type specificity through subsequent transfers in the laboratory. Several other similar pneumococcal type transformations were induced. The acquired specificity in each case was that of the dead, capsulated organism injected.

This transformation was carried out in vitro by Dawson and Sia in 1931. They were successful in transforming a rough type 2 pneumococcus into a capsulated type 3 pneumococcus by cultivating the 2R organisms in broth containing anti-R serum and heat-killed capsulated organisms of type 3 or a cell-free extract of them. The capsular substance that induced this transformation was later shown by Avery and his colleagues to be a form of deoxyribonucleic acid.

Specifically directed alterations in serotype were produced by Zinder and Lederberg through the process of transduction, defined as unilateral genetic transfer in which one character at a time is transferred from one bacterium to another. Genetic material was transferred via a filterable agent in phage lysate of the donor organisms; selection of new or different serotypes was facilitated by the antiserum-agar technique. This method was used to produce nine new monophasic serotypes of *S. typhosa*. For example, the transduction from 9,12:d: - - - to 9,12:i: - - - was brought about by the filterable agent of *S. typhimurium* (1,4,5,12:i:1,2).

Induced changes in antigenic structure are of great evolutionary interest because they may indicate the natural mechanism and path by which the various serologic types of bacteria have arisen. They also emphasize the artificiality of species and generic distinctions in such a continuous series of intergrading forms.

Blood Grouping and Typing

The blood groups and types are characterized by the presence on red cells of antigens known as isoantigens (i.e., antigens found in certain individuals of a species but not in others). When these antigens encounter homologous antibodies, either in vivo or in vitro, the cells of which they are a part may be agglutinated. This process is termed isohemagglutination. It first attracted attention as an explanation of transfusion accidents in which hemoglobinuria, jaundice, and occasionally death resulted. Normal antibodies in the serum of the recipient agglutinate the injected erythrocytes within the vascular system, producing embolism, or sensitize them to the hemolytic action of complement.

In addition to normal antibodies, immune isoantibodies may be found in the sera of individuals who have previously received transfusions and of some women who have borne children with blood characteristics other than their own (i.e., as a result of inheritance from the father). There are at least nine blood group systems, listed as follows in order of discovery:

ABO	1900
MNSs	1927

Pp	1927
Rh	1940
Lutheran (Lu^{a}Lu^b)	1946
Kell (Kk)	1946
Lewis (Le^{a}Le^b)	1946
Duffy (Fy^{a}Fy^b)	1950
Kidd (Jk^{a}Jk^b)	1951

THE ABO BLOOD GROUPS

Isohemagglutination was clearly described by Landsteiner in 1900. Within the next 2 years the existence of four human blood groups had been reported. These were differentiated by the presence or absence of one or both of agglutinogens A and B in the erythrocytes, and are usually designated by the letters, A, B, AB, and O.

The normal antibodies corresponding to these agglutinogens are anti-A and anti-B, respectively. In no case did Landsteiner find anti-A in the serum of an individual who possessed antigen A in his cells, nor did anti-B occur in the serum of a person with antigen B. Furthermore, he observed that human serum always contained antibodies corresponding to the A and B agglutinogens missing from the red cells of the same individual. Thus, serum from a person of group O possessed agglutinins anti-A and anti-B, and so forth. Anti-A clumps cells containing agglutinogen A, and anti-B clumps cells containing the B antigen. Sera and cells of the four blood groups agglutinate when mixed in the various combinations indicated by the + signs in Table 7–9.

Human group O cells, as well as A, B, and AB cells, stimulate the production in other animals of antibodies that react with all human red blood cells because they possess common human species antigens. Antisera produced in other animals against A, B, and AB cells contain in addition anti-A and/or anti-B agglutinins.

Blood grouping formerly consisted of testing the erythrocytes for agglutination with normal human sera containing anti-A and anti-B antibodies. The diagnostic reactions are readily determined from Table 7–9. Immune sera are also available and are satisfactory if they have been rendered specific by adsorption. In addition, various plant seed extracts contain globulins called *lectins* that agglutinate human and other animal erythrocytes. Boyd and his colleagues found by extensive trials that lectins can be chosen that react specifically with red cells of certain human blood groups and can be used to identify them. Both test tube and slide methods of grouping are in use.

Subgroups of A and AB.   There are two major subdivisions of groups A and AB based upon the structure of the polysaccharide that determines blood group specificity: A_1 and A_2. Four serotypes therefore occur: A_1, A_2, A_1B, A_2B. Most normal sera of group O and B individuals contain two qualitatively different antibodies capable of reacting with A determinants: (1) anti-A_1 agglutinates only cells containing determinant A_1; (2) anti-A agglutinates cells containing either A_1 or A_2. Monospecific anti-A_1 antibodies can be secured by adsorbing serum from a group B individual with A_2 cells.

The A_1 and A_2 determinants on red blood cells are detected by two tests. First, cells are tested with anti-A antiserum (i.e., serum from a group B individual, which contains anti-A and anti-A_1 antibodies). Agglutination indicates that the cells possess A_1 or A_2. Another sample of the cells is then tested with adsorbed anti-A serum (containing only anti-A_1 antibodies). Agglutination demonstrates the presence of A_1; lack of agglutination indicates that the positive result with anti-A antiserum was due to A_2. A_1 cells are more sensitive than A_2 cells to serum hemolysis with freshly drawn anti-A (group O or B) sera containing complement. Cells of subgroups A_2 and A_2B can also be distin-

Table 7–9   Agglutination in Mixtures of Serum and Red Blood Cells of the Four Principal Human Blood Groups

Blood Group Designations	Agglutinogens in Cells	Human Sera Containing Agglutinins				Per Cent in U.S.A.
		ANTI-A ANTI-B	ANTI-B	ANTI-A	NONE	
		Agglutination				
O	O	–	–	–	–	45
A	A	+	–	+	–	41
B	B	+	+	–	–	10
AB	AB	+	+	+	–	4

guished from those of subgroups A_1 and A_1B by their slower and weaker agglutination in inactivated (56° C. for 15 minutes) anti-A test sera.

The A_1 determinant is five to six times as frequent as A_2. The occurrence of these factors is controlled by inheritance, A_1 being dominant over A_2.

Further subgroups of the A antigen are found. Determinants A_3, A_4, etc., are characterized in part by progressively weaker reactions with anti-A sera.

Inheritance of the ABO Groups.   The lifelong permanence of the blood groups is well confirmed. Agglutinogens A and B are already established in newborn infants and even in fetuses. The normal isohemagglutinins in the serum, however, are not demonstrable at birth but become evident within 3 to 6 months, increase rapidly to a maximum at 5 to 10 years of age, and thereafter decrease gradually.

The A and B characteristics of the erythrocytes are inherited according to Mendelian law by means of four allelic genes, A_1, A_2, B, and O. A child receives one of these genes from each parent, and ten genotypic combinations are possible, as shown in Table 7–10. The six phenotypes recognizable by use of anti-A, anti-A_1, and anti-B sera are also indicated.

It is possible to calculate the average frequency with which individuals of the various groups will result from any mating. A few examples are given in Table 7–11.

Table 7–10   Genotypes and Phenotypes of Human Blood Cells

Genotype	Phenotype	Antigenic Determinants on Erythrocytes	Antibodies in Sera
OO	O	H	anti-A, anti-A_1, anti-B
A_1A_1 A_1A_2 A_1O	A_1	A_1	anti-B, (anti-H)*
A_2A_2 A_2O	A_2	A_2, H	anti-B, (anti-A_1)
BB BO	B	B	anti-A, anti-A_1
A_1B	A_1B	A_1, B	(anti-H)
A_2B	A_2B	A_2, B	(anti-A_1)

*Parentheses indicate antibodies sometimes present.

Table 7–11   *Illustrations of Blood Group Inheritance*

	$BB \times OO$	$A_1B \times OO$	$A_1B \times A_2O$	$A_1A_2 \times BO$
Genotypes of parents				
Genetic combinations	$\begin{array}{c c} & O \quad O \\ B & BO \quad BO \\ B & BO \quad BO \end{array}$	$\begin{array}{c c} & O \quad O \\ A_1 & A_1O \quad A_1O \\ B & BO \quad BO \end{array}$	$\begin{array}{c c} & A_2 \quad O \\ A_1 & A_1A_2 \quad A_1O \\ B & A_2B \quad BO \end{array}$	$\begin{array}{c c} & B \quad O \\ A_1 & A_1B \quad A_1O \\ A_2 & A_2B \quad A_2O \end{array}$
Genotypes of children	BO	$A_1O \quad BO$	$A_1A_2 \quad A_1O \quad A_2B \quad BO$	$A_1B \quad A_2B \quad A_1O \quad A_2O$
Phenotypes of children	B	$A_1 \quad\quad B$	$A_1 \quad\quad A_2B \quad B$	$A_1B \quad A_2B \quad A_1 \quad A_2$
Expected percentage	100	50 50	50 25 25	25 25 25 25

Fifty-five different types of mating are possible. From charts such as those illustrated, it can be ascertained whether a given child could or could not be the offspring of certain parents. These facts are useful in cases of disputed parentage and questioned paternity, as will be discussed later.

Secretors and Nonsecretors. The blood group A and B substances are found not only in the erythrocytes but also in other tissue cells, such as sperm, liver, muscle, spleen, kidney, and lung cells. The blood group substances are also present in various body fluids of 75 to 80 per cent of individuals, including saliva, seminal fluid, gastric juice, and sweat. These persons are known as "secretors." Blood group substances in such fluids can be detected by a precipitin test with anti-A and anti-B sera or by an inhibition test. The blood group substance reacts with the corresponding antibody and inhibits agglutination of homologous erythrocytes subsequently added. Saliva, for example, is mixed with anti-A and anti-B sera; A and B erythrocytes are then added to the respective serum-saliva mixtures. If agglutinogen A is present in the saliva, it combines with anti-A and prevents agglutination of A red cells; likewise, agglutinogen B in the saliva prevents agglutination of B red cells.

The specific substances may be present in aqueous extracts of the organs of secretors, and similar blood group substances are detectable in alcoholic extracts of the organs of nonsecretors as well as secretors. It is therefore possible to determine the blood group of an individual by examination of almost any tissue.

The capacity to secrete water-soluble blood group substance is inherited as a Mendelian dominant character through the agency of a gene *Se*. An individual homozygous for the allelic gene, *se*, does not secrete the blood group substances, but this has no effect on the occurrence of the A and B determinants on the red cells.

Group O(H). It was originally believed that the group O character of the erythrocytes of an individual whose genotype was *OO* indicated the lack of any antigen. Then animal sera were found that agglutinated cells of group O. The agglutinin was called anti-O, and the antigen with which it reacted was designated the O substance. Later a few human sera, many animal sera, and some plant lectins were discovered that agglutinated O and A_2 cells strongly and other human erythrocytes less strongly. Even A_2B and A_1B cells were agglutinated to greater or lesser extent. Since individuals producing these cells do not possess gene *O*, even in the heterozygous condition, it appeared that the antigen in question is more widely distributed than was first thought. It was therefore designated the H substance, a term that has generally replaced the expression O substance.

Almost all human red cells contain H substance, the amount detectable varying according to the ABO group in decreasing order as follows:

$$O>A_2>A_2B>B>A_1>A_1B$$

O cells react most strongly with anti-H agglutinins, and A_1B cells react least strongly. It should be pointed out that the H antigen is different from the common species antigen possessed by erythrocytes of all humans. This is present in relatively constant amount in cells of any group.

H activity is present, along with A and/or B activity, in the saliva of secretors. Individuals of group O secrete only H, but secretions of even A_1B persons may contain some H activity.

THE LEWIS GROUPS

The Lewis system is composed of antigens closely related chemically to the ABH antigens but genetically independent of them; the Lewis antigens differ in the possession of 1 or 2 additional fucose sidechains. Although discovered by means of two antibodies, anti-Le^a and anti-Le^b, which agglutinated the red blood cells of approximately 22 per cent and 72 per cent of Europeans, respectively, the antigens were later found principally in saliva and serum, and their presence on erythrocytes is the result of adsorption from the body fluids. This is indicated by the observation that Le^a substance is present in the saliva of more than 90 per cent of Europeans.

The Lewis antigens are inherited but not in the usual Mendelian fashion. Two gene pairs apparently participate: *Le* controls the presence of Le^a in the body fluids and is dominant over *le*, which causes its absence; *Se* and *se* are the genes that normally regulate secretion of the ABH substances. There is no gene for Le, but production of this antigen depends on interaction of the *Le* and *Se* genes, as indicated in Table 7-12. It is apparent that individuals with red cells of type Le(a−b+) actually produce Le, but that it remains in the saliva.

CHEMICAL NATURE AND ORIGIN OF THE ABH AND L*E* ACTIVITIES

Isolation of the ABH and Le^a substances for chemical analysis is facilitated by their abundance in water-soluble form in the saliva, gastric juice, ovarian cyst, and other fluids of secretors, and by the occurrence of antigens closely related serologically

Table 7–12 Genetic Control of the Lewis Antigens and Secretion of the ABH Substances

Genotypes		Erythrocyte Phenotype	Le Substance in Saliva		Secretion of ABH Substances
			LE^a	LE^b	
LeLe *Lele*	*sese*	Le (a+b−)	+	−	Nonsecretor
LeLe *Lele*	*SeSe* *Sese*	Le (a−b+)	+	+	Secretor
lele	*SeSe* *Sese* *sese*	Le (a−b−)	−	−	Usually secretor

in the stomachs of horses and hogs. Blood group A substance is chemically related to the Forssman hapten; some anti-A rabbit sera lyse sheep erythrocytes, and certain rabbit antisera against sheep erythrocytes agglutinate human cells containing A. The same or a similar substance is also present in numerous bacteria and in widely different members of the animal and plant kingdoms. Blood group active substances have been found in nearly half of a large collection of gram-negative bacteria.

The ABHLe activities are attributed to the presence, location, and orientation of certain hexoses on a branched core polysaccharide, which is in turn associated with a polypeptide backbone (in secreted blood group substances) or lipid (in a cell membrane), as indicated in Figure 7–11. The identity of the hexoses responsible for blood group specificity was determined by use of known sugars and amino sugars in attempts to inhibit reaction between the blood group substance and its specific antibody or a lectin. For example, the reaction between A and anti-A was inhibited by a disaccharide containing N-acetyl-D-galactosamine and D-galactose; the former, in a terminal position, defines A activity.

The postulated branched heterosaccharides with which blood group activities are associated are shown in Figure 7–12. Each consists of a basic tetrasaccharide chain attached to the backbone or lipid and two branches. Branch I comprises Gal-(1→3)-GNAc attached (1→3) to Gal of the tetrasaccharide, and branch II comprises Gal-(1→4)-GNAc attached (1→6) to the same tetrasaccharide Gal. This basic core is the precursor that acquires specific blood group activity upon attachment of N-acetyl-D-galactosamine, D-galactose, or L-fucose at the locations indicated. Steps in the formation of Le^a, H, A, B, and Le^b active sites from the branch I core are shown in Figure 7–13.

Rh BLOOD TYPES

Previous to 1940 there were numerous reports of newborn infants with general edema and more or less marked anemia, a condition called *erythroblastosis fetalis* or *hemolytic disease of the newborn*. In 1939, Levine and Stetson observed a transfusion reaction in a pregnant woman following administration of blood from her husband. Serum from this woman contained an agglutinin that reacted with about 80 per cent of group O bloods examined.

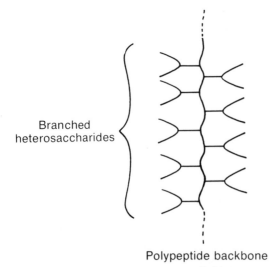

Branched heterosaccharides

Figure 7–11. Proposed structure of the ABHLe megalosaccharide. The branched heterosaccharide side chains are attached to a polypeptide backbone of serine or threonine in secreted blood group substances, or are associated with lipid in nonsecreted cell membrane blood group substances. The structures of the branched heterosaccharides are indicated in Figure 7–12.

Polypeptide backbone
or lipid

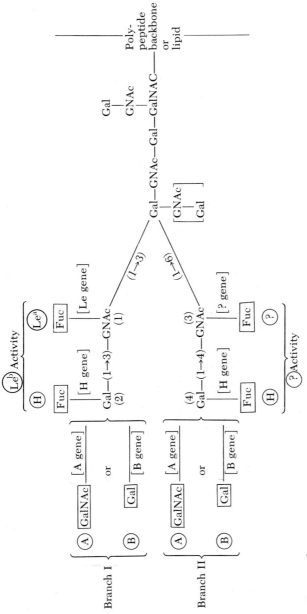

Figure 7–12. Postulated structures of the heterosaccharides that determine the ABHLe blood group activities. The primary gene products are glycosyltransferases that attach sugar residues to the branched core structure at the points indicated (see Figure 7–13). The residues responsible for blood group activities are encircled. The presence of Fuc on Gal (2) and (4) confers H activity. If GalNAc is attached to Gal (2) and (4), the heterosaccharide has A₁ activity and little if any H activity, even though Fuc may be present, since it is masked by the GalNAc. If only Gal (4) has a terminal GalNAc, the heterosaccharide has A₂ activity and retains some H activity. The saccharide produced when Gal is attached to Gal (2) and (4) has B activity. (Modified from Lloyd et al., 1968. Proc. Natl. Acad. Sci. USA, 61:1470; and 1970. Biochemistry, 9:3414.)

Fuc = L-fucose
Gal = D-galactose
GNAc = N-acetyl-D-glucosamine
GalNAc = N-acetyl-D-galactosamine

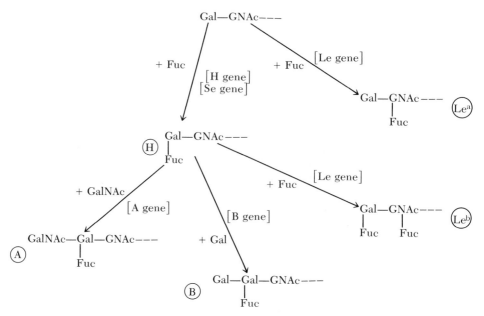

Figure 7–13. Steps in the synthesis of heterosaccharide side chains with A, B, H, and Le specificities (encircled). Glycosyltransferases transfer sugars from activated precursors (guanosine or uridine diphosphohexoses) as indicated. (Modified from Grollman et al., 1970. Ann. N. Y. Acad. Sci., 169:153.)

The following year Landsteiner and Wiener, investigating human and monkey blood group characteristics, found that sera produced in rabbits inoculated with rhesus monkey blood possessed antibodies that agglutinated the erythrocytes of about 85 per cent of humans tested. They named the red cell agglutinogen the *Rh antigen*, because it also occurred in rhesus monkey blood cells, and designated as Rh positive those individuals who possessed it. Wiener and Peters observed that after several transfusions of Rh positive blood into an Rh negative individual, the recipient might show increasing signs of transfusion reaction and that his serum contained agglutinins for the Rh factor.

Levine then found that the patient who had had a transfusion reaction in 1939 possessed Rh antibody in her serum and that her husband's red cells were Rh positive. He suggested that this woman, who was Rh negative, had been isoimmunized by the Rh antigen of the fetus, which was inherited from the Rh positive father. Although only about 15 per cent of the normal population is Rh negative, nearly all mothers of erythroblastotic infants are Rh negative, but the fathers and babies are Rh positive.

The role of Rh in transfusion reactions appears fairly clear. An Rh negative recipient of Rh positive blood produces antibody against the Rh antigen. If sufficient Rh antibody is formed, subsequent transfusions with Rh positive blood provide opportunity for intravascular reaction with the introduced erythrocytes. The Rh factor may be poorly antigenic in some individuals, and consequently several transfusions can often be given before the recipient develops enough antibody to cause complications.

Present explanations of erythroblastosis fetalis closely follow the original suggestion of Levine and Stetson. The child of an Rh positive father and Rh negative mother may possess Rh positive red blood cells. Erythrocytes may pass from the fetal to the maternal circulation and stimulate formation of Rh antibodies by the mother. If these are IgG, they may cross the placenta into the fetus, where they react with the Rh positive red cells, producing anemia and jaundice. The anemic condition causes the fetus to produce immature red blood cells (erythroblasts) at a high rate.

If the antigenic stimulation is not great, only IgM may be produced, and since this does not cross the placenta it does not cause an immediate problem. This is usually the situation in a first pregnancy. However, at the time of delivery a small amount of fetal blood often enters the maternal circulation, and this may initiate Rh sensitization of the mother. In a subsequent pregnancy with an Rh positive fetus, she produces a higher concentration of Rh antibodies, including IgG, due to the anamnestic reaction, so erythroblastosis is increasingly common with succeeding pregnancies.

Rh disease can be prevented by a simple procedure, which was introduced in 1967. Inasmuch as most cases of maternal sensitization are attributable to fetal red cells acquired at the time of delivery, passive immunization of the mother with anti-Rh serum during the first 72 hours results in clearance of the Rh+ cells from her circulation and also suppresses antibody formation by negative feedback. Her next Rh positive baby should therefore have no greater risk of erythroblastosis than a first-born. This preventive measure must be repeated after delivery of each Rh positive child.

Erythroblastosis fetalis does not occur in all cases in which it appears theoretically possible. The percentage distribution of Rh positive and Rh negative individuals in the general population (85 and 15 per cent, respectively) indicates that approximately 13 per cent of matings involve an Rh positive father and an Rh negative mother. Actually, erythroblastosis occurs in only one of every 200 to 400 births, or less than 5 per cent of cases in which it might be expected. Many factors contribute to this low percentage. Only about 50 per cent of Rh positive persons are homozygous for Rh antigen. Half the children of heterozygous fathers and Rh negative mothers are therefore Rh negative. Moreover, fetal red blood cells cross the placenta or get into the maternal circulation at delivery in only one-third of pregnancies.

More than 30 Rh determinants or factors are now known, and these occur in various combinations on the erythrocytes of different individuals. There are three different systems of nomenclature, two of which are in common use. The comparative terminology applied to the six most important Rh determinants is shown in Table 7–13. According to the Wiener system, the determinants or blood factors are designated Rh_0, rh′, rh″, etc., and in the Fisher-Race terminology they are indicated by the letters D, C, E, etc. These systems are so commonly used that the report of a laboratory test usually includes both (e.g., Rh_0(D)). Rosenfield et al. (1962) proposed a simple numerical classification that avoids the subscripts, superscripts, capitals, lower case letters, and other symbols that characterize the Wiener and Fisher-Race systems; it is not yet widely used.

In the Wiener system, Rh_0 is capitalized because it is clinically the most important factor of the Rh series by virtue of its great antigenicity. The determinants hr′ (c) and hr″ (e) are reciprocally related to rh′ (C) and rh″ (E), respectively; that is, the cells of an

Table 7–13   Systems of Rh Nomenclature (Abridged)

Rh Determinants (Blood Factors) [Wiener System]	Rh Agglutinogens [Fisher-Race System]	Rh Agglutinogens [Rosenfield et al.]
Rh_0	D	Rh1
rh′	C	Rh2
rh″	E	Rh3
[Hr_0]*	[d]*	
hr′	c	Rh4
hr″	e	Rh5
hr	f	Rh6

*Hypothetical; reports of its existence unconfirmed.

individual contain either rh′ (C) or hr′ (c) or both, and also either rh″ (E) or hr″ (e) or both. A blood factor Hr_0(d), related in the same way to Rh_0(D) was postulated, but early reports of its existence have not been adequately confirmed. Determinant hr (f) is regularly present in cells of types Rh_0 and rh (see Table 7–14).

The antigenic composition of the red cells of an individual is determined by agglutination tests with appropriate antisera, as indicated in Table 7–14. The first three sera (anti-Rh_0, anti-rh′, and anti-rh″) indicate the major Rh types and are often the only ones used in routine Rh typing. The three hr sera provide serologic and, indirectly, genetic information and permit recognition of occasional variant antigens that may be clinically or medicolegally important.

The differences between the Fisher-Race and Wiener terminologies reflect fundamental differences in concept of the nature and genetic control of the Rh antigenic specificities. Fisher and Race postulated that the individual Rh antigens are separate molecules, formed under the control of closely linked, allelic pairs of genes (Cc, Dc, Ee). As additional antigenic specificities were discovered, it became difficult or impossible to accommodate them. Wiener's view is that each Rh antigen is a molecule on which numerous factors or determinant sites are distributed, formation of which is regulated by many allelic genes. Although the Fisher-Race system is simpler than that of Wiener and has been used widely by clinicians in the United States and generally in Europe, evidence is accumulating that the latter is more nearly correct. However, blood typing reagents sold commercially in the United States bear both designations on their labels; e.g., anti-Rh_0 (anti-D).

Rh *testing* consists of determining whether an individual's erythrocytes contain the classical and clinically most important Rh factor, Rh_0. Such a person is said to be Rh positive. The Caucasoid population of New York City consists of about 85 per cent of Rh_0 positive people. Rh *typing*, with sera containing anti-rh′ and anti-rh″, as well as anti-Rh_0, detects the additional individuals who possess factors rh′ and rh″. Rh antisera for diagnostic use are secured from humans sensitized naturally or deliberately with appropriate erythrocytes. For example, pure anti-Rh_0 serum can be obtained from the Rh negative (i.e., type rh) mother of an erythroblastotic infant with Rh_0 blood cells or from an Rh negative individual immunized by injection of Rh_0 cells.

Several different kinds of antibody may be present in the sera of individuals isoimmunized against Rh antigens (Table 7–15). Classic agglutinating antibodies

Table 7–14　　*Rh Types Distinguished by the Principal Rh and Hr Antisera*

	Agglutination with						Rh Type	Incidence in Caucasoids (N.Y.C.)
	ANTI-Rh_0 (ANTI-D)	ANTI-rh′ (ANTI-C)	ANTI-rh″ (ANTI-E)	ANTI-hr′ (ANTI-c)	ANTI-hr″ (ANTI-e)	ANTI-hr (ANTI-f)		
	+	−	−	+	+	+	Rh_0	2.1%
Rh	+	+	−	+	+	+	Rh_1rh	35.0%
	+	+	−	−	+	−	Rh_1Rh_1	19.0%
Positive	+	−	+	+	+	+	Rh_2rh	12.2%
(84.6%)	+	−	+	+	−	−	Rh_2Rh_2	2.4%
	+	+	+	+	+	−	Rh_1Rh_2	13.5%
	+	+	+	+	+	+	Rh_zrh	0.2%
	+	+	+	−	+	−	Rh_zRh_1	0.2%
Rh	−	−	−	+	+	+	rh	14.4%
Negative	−	+	−	+	+	+	rh′rh	0.5%
(15.3%)	−	−	+	+	+	+	rh″rh	0.4%

Modified from Weiner and Wexler, 1966. Immunogenetics. Woodbury, N.Y., Certified Blood Donor Service, Inc.

Table 7–15   Types and Methods of Detecting Rh Antibodies

Synonyms	1	2	3	4
	"Complete" Antibody	"Incomplete" Antibodies		
	Saline Agglutinin	Conglutinating Antibodies (Albumin Agglutinins)		
		Blocking Antibody	Cryptagglutinoids	
Agglutination of RBC in saline	+	–	–	–
Agglutination of RBC in protein, etc.	+*	+	+	–
Blocking test	–*	+	–	–
Coombs' test	+*	+	+	+
Agglutination of trypsinized RBC in saline	+*	+	+	–

*Not ordinarily tested because these antibodies are readily detected by agglutination of saline suspensions of RBC.

aggregate homologous red blood cells suspended in saline. These are known as "complete antibodies" or "saline agglutinins." "Incomplete" antibodies do not agglutinate saline suspensions of homologous erythrocytes and were formerly thought to be univalent. However, they may agglutinate red cells suspended in a high concentration of serum albumin or treated with the proteolytic enzyme trypsin, so they are evidently bivalent.

One kind of antibody can be demonstrated by the "blocking test." Saline suspensions of erythrocytes mixed with certain Rh antisera containing "incomplete" antibodies do not agglutinate when subsequently mixed with homologous saline agglutinin. "Blocking antibodies" combine with the corresponding agglutinogens and specifically prevent later reaction with saline agglutinins.

The Coombs test is a sensitive method of detecting either complete or incomplete antibodies. In the indirect test, saline suspensions of Rh positive red cells are incubated with Rh antiserum, washed with saline, and mixed with antihuman globulin serum. Rh antibody first combines specifically with its homologous agglutinogen and then, as a globulin, reacts with the antiglobulin, which agglutinates the erythrocytes. In vivo sensitization of the red cells of an erythroblastotic infant by passively acquired maternal Rh antibodies is detected by the direct Coombs (antiglobulin) test. Thoroughly washed cells from the baby are suspended in saline, and antihuman globulin serum is added. Agglutination always occurs in typical erythroblastosis caused by Rh or hr antibodies.

Most typing sera in use today contain blocking antibodies, so saline must not be used as a diluent. Fresh whole blood or blood taken into a tube containing dry oxalate as anticoagulant is employed in the slide test. The test serum and blood are mixed on a microscope slide or glass plate and rocked slowly over a lamp or other source of heat which maintains a temperature of about 40° C. Agglutination should be seen within 30 to 60 seconds, and at the end of 2 minutes nearly all red cells should be clumped into large masses. These tests are observed without the aid of the microscope and are discarded after 2 or 3 minutes to avoid errors in reading caused by drying or rouleaux formation.

OTHER BLOOD GROUPS

The MNSs System.   In 1927 Landsteiner and Levine immunized rabbits with the cells of a number of different group O individuals. Adsorption of the antisera with some group O erythrocytes removed all agglutinins; adsorption with other group O cells left agglutinins that reacted with cells of certain individuals. The rabbit immune sera identified two agglutinogens, M and N, independent of A and B. All human red blood cells contain either M or N or both. They are inherited according to Mendelian principles. Consequently, there are three genotypes, *MM, NN, MN,* and corresponding phenotypes, M, N, MN. Blood specimens are classified as AM, BM, ON, ABN, ABMN,. . ., depending on the presence in the cells of the A, B, M, and N factors.

The M and N agglutinogens are detected with rabbit immune sera because normal isoagglutinins for M and N do not occur in humans. Rabbits are immunized with OM and ON cells, and the antisera are adsorbed with cells containing N and M (e.g., AN and AM), respectively, to remove human species agglutinins.

A related pair of antigens, S and s, was later discovered. Erythrocytes contain either or both, but none have been found lacking both. Their association with the MN system was indicated by the fact that S is present in over three-quarters of individuals possessing antigen M.

Minor Systems.   Several minor blood group systems, in addition to the Lewis, MNSs, and Pp systems, are listed in Table 7–16. The commonest phenotypic varieties of erythrocytes are shown, together with approximate incidence in Caucasian populations.

APPLICATIONS OF BLOOD GROUPING

Preparation for Transfusion.   One of the most important applications of blood grouping is that concerned with preparation for transfusion. It is advisable always to employ blood of the same ABO group as that of the recipient. This means that the bloods of the recipient and of the prospective donors must be tested. Ideally, not only are the agglutinogens in the cells determined but also the agglutinins in the sera, although the latter tests are often omitted. The importance of Rh isoimmunization also makes it necessary to determine the Rh type of recipient and donor, lest Rh positive blood be introduced into an Rh negative recipient and induce sensitivity. Presence of the other blood factors is not usually determined, because they are not strongly antigenic in man. However, complications may arise in repeated transfusions as a result of immunization against any of the blood cell agglutinogens. Natural and immune agglutinins can be detected by "cross-match" tests, which are always performed. Serum from the patient is tested for its power to agglutinate cells of the donor (see Table 7–17). The reverse cross-match is also recommended if time permits.

The chief danger from incompatible transfusions lies in the fate of the injected cells. The patient may suffer a transfusion reaction if there is sufficient antibody in his circulation to cause agglutination or hemolysis of the donor's erythrocytes. Despite the presence of anti-A and anti-B agglutinins in the sera of group O individuals, their blood can often be given to persons of any group. The titer of normal isohemagglutinins is ordinarily low, and they are diluted by the blood of the recipient to such an extent that they do not agglutinate or hemolyze the patient's cells. Members of group O are called "universal donors." Group AB individuals, or "universal recipients," can accept blood of any group because their serum does not contain anti-A or anti-B, and any introduced

Table 7–16   Incidence of Various Minor Blood Group Types in Caucasian Populations

Blood Group System	Blood Type	Incidence (approximate per cent)
Lewis	Le (a+b−)	22
	Le (a−b+)	72
	Le (a−b−)	6
MNSs	MS	6
	Ms	8
	MSs	14
	MNS	4
	MNSs	24
	MNs	22
	NS	1
	Ns	15
	NSs	6
Pp	P_1	79
	P_2	21
	p	<0.1
Duffy	Fy (a+b−)	17
	Fy (a+b+)	49
	Fy (a−b+)	34
Kell	K+k−	0.2
	K+k+	9.1
	K−k+	90.1
	K−k−	<0.1
Kidd	Jk (a+b−)	27
	Jk (a+b+)	51
	Jk (a−b+)	22
Lutheran	Lu (a+b−)	0.1
	Lu (a+b+)	7.5
	Lu (a−b+)	92.4

agglutinins are diluted within the vascular system. Heterologous transfusions of these kinds are not recommended when homologous blood can be obtained without too much difficulty.

The hemagglutination reaction is used to determine the survival time of transfused blood. For this purpose the donor and recipient must be of different types. Group O blood, for example, is transfused into a group A recipient. The group O cells mingle with those of the patient and persist in the blood for some time. Samples of the recipient's blood are mixed with anti-A serum, and only his own cells are agglutinated; the type O cells from the donor remain dispersed. The test is observed microscopically, and the agglutinated and unagglutinated cells are counted. Other blood types may be used in the same manner. Tests of this sort indicate that the survival time of introduced cells is as great as 80 to 120 days. Blood cells stored for 21 days before transfusion survive only about 24 hours in the circulation of the recipient.

Medicolegal Applications.   Problems of relationship, including disputed paternity, can sometimes be solved by isohemagglutination because blood group characteristics are inherited in a known manner (Table 7–11). This method has been used in the past to identify babies born at the same time in a hospital and accidentally given to the wrong parents, although present practices almost certainly obviate this chance of confusion. One of the best known cases of this kind occurred when Mrs. B., on

Table 7-17   *Two-tube Cross-match Test with Patient's Serum and Donor's Cells to Detect Major and Minor Incompatible Antibodies**

Tube 1	Tube 2
Patient's serum + donor's cells in own serum + bovine albumin	Patient's serum + donor's cells in own serum

Centrifuge immediately and read

Agglutination or hemolysis indicates

Most Rh-Hr incompatibilities	ABO incompatibility

Incubate at 37° C. for 15 minutes

Centrifuge and read	Wash 3 or 4 times with saline, add anti-human serum, centrifuge and read
Agglutination indicates low-titered anti-Rh, certain Rh albumin antibodies, other "warm" agglutinins	Agglutination indicates Rh cryptagglutinoids, anti-K, anti-Fy^a, anti-Jk^a, anti-Le^a, etc.

*Adapted from Levine, 1960. Blood Group Antigens and Antibodies. Raritan, N.J., Ortho Pharmaceutical Corporation.

returning home from the hospital, found that her baby had a piece of adhesive tape on its back with the name W. Mrs. W. likewise found her baby to be labeled B. Blood tests of the two babies and four parents showed the following results:

	Group		*Group*
Mr. W	O	Mr. B	AB
Mrs. W	O	Mrs. B........	O
Baby B	A	Baby W	O

Obviously Baby B. could not have been the child of Mr. and Mrs. W. nor could Mr. and Mrs. B. have been the parents of Baby W. The children had been accidentally switched before the mothers took them home, and the labels they bore were correct.

The known information in cases of disputed paternity consists of the blood characteristics of the mother and of the child. The A, B, M, N, Rh, and other factors are used. The rules of genetics sometimes permit exclusion of certain men as fathers of the child in question. It is never possible to state that the putative father is in fact the real father. It can only be stated that he may be or cannot be the father. Table 7–18 shows the AB blood groups possible or impossible from any mating combination. Similar tables can readily be prepared for the MNSs, Rh, and other systems. The use of such tables is self-apparent. Taking into account the frequency distribution of the various blood groups in this country, an innocent man has, on the average, one chance in six of proving nonpaternity by the ABO groups alone. Addition of the MNSs and Rh systems increases his chance of establishing nonpaternity to about one in two.

There are many other forensic applications of hemagglutination in the solution of violent crimes, such as murder and rape, and in the identification of individuals concerned in inheritance suits and other legal proceedings. Under suitable conditions and by use of extremely careful technique, it is possible to determine the blood type of an individual from almost any kind of specimen: blood stain, tissue fragment, saliva (e.g., a cigarette stub), semen, and even from a corpse.

Stains should first be proved to be blood by chemical tests and to be human blood by the precipitin test. There are two chief methods for typing a blood stain. The first is by detection of isoagglutinins in relatively fresh specimens. A small flake of the dried smear or some of the powdered material is placed on a slide and near it a suspension of group A erythrocytes. A similar preparation is made with group B cells. Cover glasses are put in position and adjusted so that the specimen and cells make contact, and the preparations are observed for agglutination of the known erythrocytes near the region of contact. A second method, suitable for older stains, is to detect agglutinogens in the specimen by the inhibition test.

It is imperative that numerous controls be included in these tests, using all blood types and including an extract of the substrate (cloth, etc.) from which the blood stain was taken. Fresh blood stains are most satisfactory, but fairly reliable results have been obtained with stains as old as 40 years.

The blood type of a corpse can be determined quite readily, if it is not too old, from examination of the clotted blood. After partial decomposition, it may still be possible to secure pericardial fluid that is satisfactory for typing. Muscles, various organs, and even bones can also be employed. Agglutinogens have been detected in corpses of considerable age. Several Egyptian mummies were claimed to possess group A or B substances after about 5,000 years of preservation.

Phylogeny of Primates. The occurrence of human blood group substances in apes and monkeys is of interest to students of evolution. As might be anticipated, the higher an animal is in the primate scale, the more closely its blood characteristics resemble those of man. Substances indistinguishable from A and B are widely distributed among the higher primates, and in some of the lower members of the group there are substances that resemble A and B closely but are distinguishable from them.

Table 7–18   Blood Groups of Offspring Possible or Impossible from Any Combination of Parents*

Alleged Father	Known Mother	Possible Children	Children Not Possible (decisive for nonpaternity)
O	O	O	A, B, (AB)†
O	A	O, A	B, AB
O	B	O, B	A, AB
O	AB	A, B	AB, (O)
A	O	O, A	B, (AB)
A	A	O, A	B, AB
A	B	O, A, B, AB	
A	AB	A, B, AB	(O)
B	O	O, B	A, (AB)
B	A	O, A, B, AB	
B	B	O, B	A, AB
B	AB	A, B, AB	(O)
AB	O	A, B	O, (AB)
AB	A	A, B, AB	O
AB	B	A, B, AB	O
AB	AB	A, B, AB	(O)

*From Schiff and Boyd, 1942. Blood Grouping Technic. New York, Interscience Publishers, Inc.

†Blood groups in parentheses represent individuals who could not be children of the corresponding mothers.

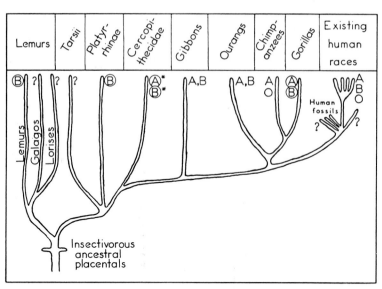

Figure 7–14. Distribution of blood factors A, B, and O in man and other primates. Antigens within circles are similar to A and B, respectively. Asterisks designate antigens present in tissues and secretions. (Adapted from Landsteiner, 1945. The Specificity of Serological Reactions, Rev. ed. Cambridge, Harvard University Press.)

*Table 7–19   Distribution of the ABO Blood Groups Among Selected Human Populations**

	Per Cent of Blood Group			
	O	A	B	AB
American Indians				
Blackfoot and Blood (pure)	22.8	76.7	0.0	1.0
Navajo	69.1	30.6	0.0	0.0
Peru (pure)	100.0	0.0	0.0	0.0
Yucatan (pure)	97.7	1.3	0.5	0.5
Arabs	34.1	30.8	28.9	6.2
Australian aborigines	53.1	44.7	2.1	0.0
Bushmen	56.1	29.6	7.5	6.8
Chinese (Peking)	30.0	25.0	35.0	10.0
Danes	42.0	43.6	10.4	3.9
Egypt (Moslems, Cairo)	26.9	36.9	26.4	9.8
English (London)	40.4	46.8	9.6	3.2
Eskimos (Baffin Land)	55.4	43.6	0.6	0.6
French	43.2	42.6	11.2	3.0
Germans	39.1	43.5	12.5	4.9
Hindus	30.2	24.5	37.2	8.1
Japanese	31.1	36.7	22.7	9.5
Negroes (Congo)	45.6	22.2	24.2	8.0
(North America)	47.0	28.0	20.0	5.0
North Africans (Algiers)	39.0	37.6	18.6	4.6
Norwegians	39.2	48.7	8.5	3.5
Russians	32.9	35.6	23.2	8.1
Spanish	43.6	51.2	3.9	1.1
United States	45.0	41.0	10.0	4.0

*From Wiener, 1943. Blood Groups and Transfusion, 3rd ed. Springfield, Ill., Charles C Thomas, Publisher.

Likewise, a substance capable of reacting with anti-M sera has been found in certain primates. Some of the work with monkeys and anthropoids is summarized in Figure 7–14.

Blood group determinations have provided anthropologists with an objective tool for the study of various racial and other groups. It is noted, for example, that the factor B occurs with unusual frequency in central Asia, whereas A is especially prominent in the Spanish peninsula, Scandinavia, and certain isolated areas of North America. A few figures illustrating the distribution of the various groups are presented in Table 7–19.

ANTIGENIC INDIVIDUALITY

Blood Groups. It is evident that human and animal bloods display marked individuality. In addition to the six combinations of human blood group antigens in the ABO system, including subgroups A_1 and A_2, there are 28 or more Rh groups, two categories based upon secreting ability, and $3 \times 9 \times 3 \times 3 \times 4 \times 3 \times 3$ groups involving the antigens listed in Table 7–16. This makes a total of 2,939,328 different possible combinations. Several other types, including the "public" and "private" groups, have been studied in only small populations. It can readily be calculated that the blood types now known indicate the potential existence of many million different kinds of persons according to their blood cell antigen characteristics, and it has been postulated that each has his own peculiar blood type.

Additional Sources of Information

Day, E. D.: Foundations of Immunochemistry. 1966. Baltimore, The Williams and Wilkins Company.
Roitt, I.: Essential Immunology. 1971. Oxford, Blackwell Scientific Publications.
Rose, N. R., F. Milgrom, and C. J. van Oss (Eds.): Principles of Immunology. 1973. New York, Macmillan Publishing Company, Inc.

CHAPTER EIGHT

IN VITRO ANTIGEN-ANTIBODY REACTIONS: CYTOTOXICITY AND NEUTRALIZATION

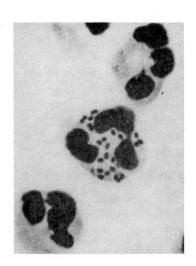

The reactions to be discussed in this chapter can be shown to take place in vitro, but the fact that reaction has occurred is best demonstrated in vivo. Most of the types of reaction also occur in the living animal body under normal conditions.

COMPLEMENT-MEDIATED CYTOTOXICITY

Cytotoxicity is the general term applied to cell damage or death caused by an immunologic reaction. Destruction and dissolution of cells is called *cytolysis* (*hemolysis* in the case of erythrocytes, *bacteriolysis* in the case of bacteria.). Cytotoxicity due to the action of humoral antibody usually also requires complement, whereas that due to the direct action of lymphoid cells or soluble mediators (lymphokines) liberated from them does not. Complement-mediated cytotoxicity, including bacteriolysis and hemolysis, will be discussed in this chapter; cell-mediated cytotoxicity will be deferred to Chapter 10.

Complement

Complement is a collection of 11 proteins in fresh blood serum that participate in various immunologic reactions. Although it is not produced as a result of immunization, it combines with antigen-antibody aggregates under suitable conditions and may lyse, kill, or immobilize the sensitized cells, or promote their immune adherence and/or phagocytosis and the formation of anaphylatoxin. Complement is normally present in the blood of most vertebrate animals. Even cold-blooded animals, such as the frog and the carp, contain complement similar to that of the guinea pig. However, the complement of one species or even of one individual may differ from that of another species or individual. These differences are due, at least partly, to differences in the percentages of the components present in the various animals.

PHYSICAL AND CHEMICAL NATURE OF COMPLEMENT

Instability. Complement is highly unstable. Inactivation by mild heat is its most distinctive property. The inverse correlation between temperature and the time re-

Table 8–1   Time Required for Thermal Inactivation of Complement*

Temperature	Time
51° C.	35 minutes
53° C.	14 minutes
55° C.	12 minutes
57° C.	8 minutes
59° C.	4 minutes
61° C.	2 minutes

*From Manwaring, 1906. Trans. Chicago Pathol. Soc., 6:425.

quired for complete loss of activity is shown in Table 8–1. Although less than 15 minutes is necessary to inactivate at 53° C., in routine work sera are heated for 30 minutes at 56° C. to deprive them of complement activity.

Aging, especially at room temperature or higher, leads to almost complete deterioration within a day or two, and even in the refrigerator considerable loss of activity occurs within 3 or 4 days.

Violent agitation, such as shaking a 1:10 dilution of fresh serum for 20 to 25 minutes, also inactivates complement. Moreover, complement is destroyed or inactivated by acids and alkalies, proteolytic enzymes, ether, chloroform, alcohol, bile salts, soaps, particulate or colloidal substances, tissue cells or extracts, yeast cells, and many kinds of unsensitized bacteria. The latter are particularly important when they occur as contaminants of antisera employed in complement fixation, as in the Wassermann test for syphilis, because their anticomplementary action (nonspecific adsorption of complement) may give falsely positive results that escape notice unless proper controls are included in the test.

Complement that has been inactivated by heat may regain part of its activity upon standing at temperatures between 7° and 37° C. Highest activity is reacquired in about 24 hours (Table 8–2). Spontaneous reactivation is important in the repeated testing of clinical and other serum specimens and necessitates reinactivation. Heated complement may also be completely reactivated by adding about 10 per cent of fresh complement.

The lability of complement and its inactivation by so many diverse agents are undoubtedly due to the fact that each of its many protein components must be present in proper concentration and in undenatured condition for the entire complex to be active. Denaturation of a single component suffices to inactivate the entire mixture. It may be presumed that spontaneous reactivation is due to slow renaturation of a denatured component. Likewise, reactivation by addition of a small amount of fresh serum may actually consist of replacement of a denatured component by use of a normal serum in which that component is abundant.

Table 8–2   Spontaneous Reactivation of Complement*†

Interval Between Inactivation and Test	Hemolysis after			
	10 MIN.	20 MIN.	30 MIN.	40 MIN.
None	0%	20%	40%	70%
1.5 hours	0	30	60	80
24 hours	20	70	80	100
48 hours	10	40	70	–

*From Gramenitzki, 1912. Biochem. Z., 38:501.

†Complement diluted 1:10 was heated to 56° C. for 7 minutes and was then tested at intervals for hemolytic activity against beef erythrocytes sensitized with homologous amboceptor.

The lability of complement necessitates extreme care to maintain it as highly active as possible. Routine use of complement requires bleeding animals almost daily to provide a fresh supply of normal serum. Bleeding and subsequent operations are performed carefully to avoid tissue damage and hemolysis, which introduce anticomplementary effects. Serum is removed from the clot and stored at a temperature near 0° C. Dilutions are made in ice-cold saline with a minimum of vigorous agitation. All glassware must be chemically clean, although not necessarily sterile.

Complement is preserved for long periods by lyophilization and for lesser intervals by freezing and storing at low temperature. The lower the temperature, the longer the activity remains high. Serum can be kept without appreciable loss of activity for 1 month at −20° C. and for at least 6 months at −40° C.

Complement Components.   A hint of the complexity of complement was given by early experiments in which fresh normal serum was dialyzed against distilled water until a precipitate formed. Neither the precipitate, redissolved in saline, nor the remaining liquid possessed complement activity when tested separately. Full activity was restored, however, when the two fractions were recombined. It appeared that the simple process of removing salts split complement into two fractions, both of which were necessary for activity. The precipitate, insoluble in water but soluble in saline, was considered to be a globulin, and the water-soluble fraction in the supernate was thought to be an albumin. Further investigation revealed that the "albumin" could not combine with a sensitized antigen until the globulin had reacted. The globulin was therefore called *midpiece* and the "albumin," *endpiece.* In cytolysis reactions midpiece appears to combine with the sensitized cells first, after which endpiece reacts with midpiece and catalyzes dissolution of the cells. The water-soluble material was later found to be a mucoeuglobulin rather than an albumin.

Midpiece and endpiece are highly thermolabile, being inactivated within a few minutes at 56° C. These fractions are not pure chemical entities. Other methods of separation and inactivation indicated that each consists of one or more components, which have been designated C1, C2, . . . C9, and subfractions of some of these have been identified, e.g., C1q, C1r, C1s. The major components and some of their properties are listed in Figure 8–1.

Prior to development of methods for purification of the various components, only the crude fractions (C′1, C′2, . . .) obtainable by dialysis and inactivation with heat, zymosan, or ammonia were available. Mixtures of these fractions prepared in various combinations lacking one or another of the fractions were employed as reagents for the assay of the various fractions in sera of different animal species, by adding dilutions of the unknown. Results such as those in Table 8–3 demonstrate the superiority of guinea pig serum as source of complement for hemolysis of sensitized sheep erythrocytes. C′2 and C′3 were the critical or limiting components in guinea pig sera. C′2 was the smallest fraction in the human, hamster, and rat sera tested. The complement activity of swine and rabbit sera was limited by their C′2 and C′4 content. Sera of several species were poorly hemolytic for sheep cells but nevertheless possessed considerable amounts of one or more complement components.

THE COMPLEMENT CASCADE

The complement cascade is a series of enzymatic reactions leading to death or lysis of a cell or to some other significant and usually damaging event (Figure 8–2). The classic sequence is initiated by union of C1 with an antigen-antibody complex. C1 consists of the three proteins, C1q, C1r, C1s, held together by Ca^{++} as ligand. The effect of antigen on antibody (IgM, IgG1, IgG2, or IgG3) is a conformational or allosteric change that makes accessible a C1q receptor site in the Fc region. In order to

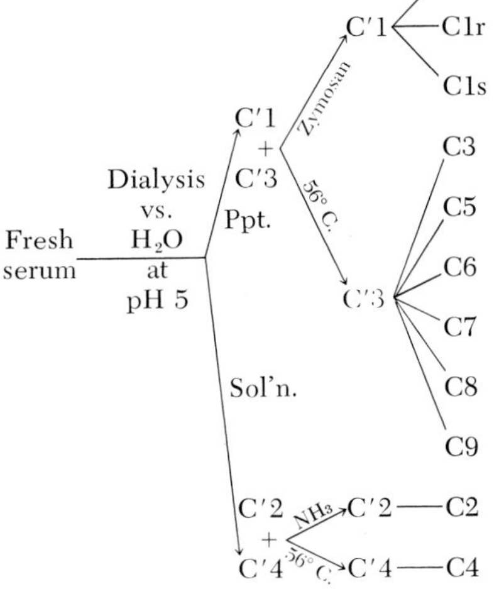

		PURIFIED COMPONENTS				
CRUDE FRACTIONS	COMPONENT	ELECTRO-PHORETIC MOBILITY	MOLECULAR WEIGHT	CARBO-HYDRATE (%)	THERMOLABILITY (56° C., 30 m.)	SERUM CONCENTRATION (μg/ml.)
	C1q	γ_2	400,000	17	+	190
	C1r	β	168,000		+	?
	C1s	α_2	80,000		+	22
	C3	β_1	180,000	2.7	−	1,200
	C5	β_1	185,000	19	+	75
	C6	β_2	125,000		−	60
	C7	β_2	?		−	?
	C8	γ_1	150,000		+	<10
	C9	α	70,000	+	+	1-2
	C2	β_2	130,000		+	30
	C4	β_1	240,000	14	−	430

Crude fractions diagram at left: Fresh serum → Dialysis vs. H₂O at pH 5 → C'1, C'3, C'2 + C'4. C'1 (zymosan, 56° C.) → Ppt. and C'3; Ppt. → Sol'n. C'2 (NH₃) + C'4 (56° C.) → C'2—C2, C'4—C4.

Figure 8–1. Some characteristics of human complement components. Crude fractions secured by dialysis against water at pH 5, followed by treatment with zymosan, ammonia, and heat at 56° C., are designated C'1, C'2, C'3, and C'4. C'1 and C'2 are thermolabile; C'3 and C'4 are thermostable. C'3 is inactivated by yeast or zymosan, a yeast component. C'4 is inactivated by ammonia.

activate complement, the polyvalent C1q must attach to at least two Fc sites; that is, two sites on a single IgM molecule or sites on two closely situated IgG molecules that have reacted with the antigen. C1q then appears to undergo a conformational change that modifies C1r so that it activates the proenzyme, C1s.

The substrates of C1s are C4 and C2. C4 splits to C4a and C4b, the latter of which binds to $\overline{C1}$. ($\overline{C1}$ is the activated form of C1). In the presence of Mg^{++} ions, C2 splits to C2a and C2b. C2a joins C14b to form $\overline{C14b2a}$, an active peptidase known as C3

Table 8–3   *Titers of the Components of Complement in Various Animal Sera**†

Species	C'‡	C'1	C'2	C'3	C'4
Guinea pig	625	3750	750	1000	8000
Human	100	4000	225	500	1750
Hamster	225	1750	210	325	625
Swine	153	1720	120	3670	95
Rabbit	60	150	68	625	55
Rat	150	600	110	1600	210
Mouse	10	390	10	50	10
Horse	10	500	18	125	10
Beef	15	500	10	175	10
Sheep	10	1380	10	20	10
Deer	10	100	15	250	50

*From Rice and Crowson, 1950. J. Immunol., 65:201.

†Results are expressed as mean titers (units per ml.) of four or more samples or pools of serum from each animal species. Sera were tested with sheep red blood cells and rabbit anti-sheep amboceptor.

‡Hemolytic titer of whole complement for sensitized sheep RBC.

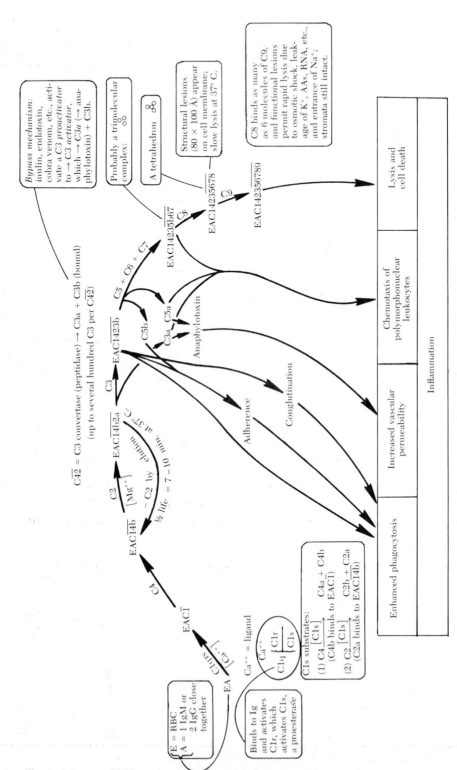

Figure 8–2. The complement cascade.

convertase. It splits C3 into a small fraction, C3a, and C3b, which binds to the C4b2a complex or to other sites on the cell membrane. Each C3 convertase molecule splits several hundred C3 molecules.

The activated C$\overline{\text{4b2a3b}}$ portion of the complex attached to the cell membrane enzymatically cleaves C5, yielding a small fragment, C5a, with anaphylatoxic and chemotactic activity (like C3a), and a larger fragment, C5b, which joins C3b on the cell membrane and forms a ternary complex with C6 and C7. C8 then unites with the complex, and the resulting phospholipase initiates formation of circular lesions about 100 Å in diameter that may lead to slow lysis at 37° C. This is greatly accelerated when C9 adds to the complex.

The lesions may be caused by hydrolytic enzymes or by the surface tension depressing activity of groups of hydrophobic radicals on the activated C$\overline{89}$ complex. They are not to be considered as holes but rather as circumscribed areas of increased permeability ("leaky" sites), through which K^+ ions, small organic molecules (e.g., AMP), and finally macromolecules, such as RNA and proteins, escape and through which Na^+ ions enter. The result is that the osmotic pressure inside the cell increases, water enters, and the cell swells.

In the case of erythrocytes, hemoglobin leaves the cells; nucleated eukaryotic cells undergo structural damage affecting their organelles (e.g., mitochondria, endoplasmic reticulum, lysosomes).

There is an alternative pathway for activation of complement that bypasses C142. It is initiated by various plant polysaccharides, such as inulin, or by zymosan, bacterial endotoxin, or aggregated immunoglobulins (IgG4, IgA, and IgE, which cannot bind C1q and hence do not initiate the classic complement sequence). The initiator substance acts upon C3 and cleaves it to C3a and C3b, which may then perform their usual functions. The principal activities of activated complement components are listed in Table 8–4.

Bacteriolysis

Bacteriolysis is limited to some of the gram-negative bacteria, apparently because the greater thickness of the cell wall of gram-positive bacteria and its concentration of mucopeptides reduce access of antibody and complement to the cytoplasmic membrane. The first reported example of bacteriolysis was Pfeiffer's (1894) observation that

Table 8–4 *Activities of Complement Components or Fragments*

Components	Activity
C3a; C5a	Anaphylactic release of histamine from mast cells and increase in capillary permeability
C5a; C$\overline{\text{5b,6,7}}$; ?C3a	Chemotactic attraction of polymorphonuclear leukocytes
C3b; C5b	Immune adherence of Ag-Ab-C complexes to leukocytes, platelets, etc., and increased susceptibility to phagocytosis by leukocytes and macrophages
C8; C9	Membrane damage and lysis of erythrocytes and some gram-negative bacteria, leakiness of plasma membrane of nucleated cells

Vibrio cholerae injected intraperitoneally into immunized guinea pigs disappeared from the peritoneal fluid within one hour, whereas the bacteria injected into nonimmune guinea pigs multiplied and soon killed the animals. The Pfeiffer reaction was then demonstrated in hanging drop preparations. Cholera vibrios mixed with anticholera serum were lysed promptly if the serum was fresh or if fresh normal guinea pig serum was added. Normal serum alone did not lyse the bacteria, and the agent in normal (and immune) serum that was necessary to cooperate with the antibody was found to be labile at 56° C., whereas antibody was stable.

Not all gram-negative bacteria are suitable for bacteriolysis demonstrations. Others that are susceptible include *Salmonella typhosa* and *Borrelia recurrentis*. *Treponema pallidum* is not lysed, but it is immobilized by antibody and complement.

Hemolysis

Immune hemolysis was discovered soon after bacteriolysis, and since it could be observed readily without use of the microscope, most of the theoretic work on the mechanism of complement reactions has been conducted with this model.

The first step in the reaction is binding of the antibody to an antigen on the surface membrane of the red blood cell. The antigen does not need to be a membrane constituent; it may be a chemical, such as a hapten, or a bacterial polysaccharide or somatic antigen coupled to the membrane. Union with its homologous antibody then initiates the complement sequence that produces the lytic lesion.

Optimal sensitization of an erythrocyte seems to require about 1,000 molecules of antibody, but the *minimal* requirement is a single IgM molecule or two closely spaced IgG molecules. It has long been observed that the amount of complement needed for complete hemolysis of a given number of cells is inversely related to the amount of antibody provided; results of a quantitative experiment are presented in Table 8–5. This relationship is important to the clinical serologist, because it necessitates careful preliminary titration of reagents used in diagnostic procedures such as the Wassermann test.

The degree to which an erythrocyte suspension is hemolyzed is easily measured colorimetrically. This method can be used to determine the effect of various amounts of complement upon red cells sensitized with a constant quantity of amboceptor, and of various amounts of amboceptor in the presence of a constant dose of complement. The results of such experiments yield an S-shaped curve in which the central portion (between 30 and 70 per cent lysis) is nearly linear (see Figure 8–3). Above this range each added increment of complement or amboceptor produces less effect, and relatively enormous doses are required for complete hemolysis. It was customary for many years to use 100 per cent hemolysis as the end point in titrations and, in fact, this is still the situation in many laboratories. Greater precision is obtained with a 50 per cent end

Table 8–5   *Relationship between Amounts of Amboceptor and Complement Required for Complete Lysis of Sheep Erythrocytes**

Amboceptor Nitrogen	Complement (C′1) Nitrogen
0.008 μg.	0.30 μg.
0.015 μg.	0.20 μg.
0.020 μg.	0.13 μg.

*From Heidelberger, Weil, and Treffers, 1941. J. Exp. Med., 73:695.

Figure 8–3. S-shaped curve showing the relationship between amount of complement and per cent hemolysis of sensitized red blood cells. Between 30 per cent and 70 per cent hemolysis the curve is almost linear. (Redrawn from Wadsworth, 1947. Standard Methods, 3rd ed. Baltimore, The Williams and Wilkins Company.)

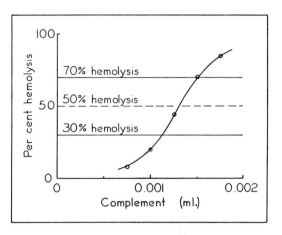

point, because the curve of hemolysis is steeper in this region. Simple procedures are available to estimate the 50 per cent end point and are gradually being adopted.

The speed of hemolysis depends on the amounts of the various reagents, the total volume of the test, the temperature of incubation, and other factors. Complete hemolysis usually occurs within 15 to 60 minutes. Increasing the volume of liquid reduces the apparent titer of the reagents. Slightly higher titers are obtained at 33° to 35° C. than at 37° C. The presence and concentration of Mg^{++} ions is very important. Addition of only 0.005 per cent $MgCl_2$ to normal saline almost doubles complement titers. A barbital buffered saline at pH 7.3 to 7.4, containing 47.6 mg. of $MgCl_2$ and 16.6 mg. of $CaCl_2$ per liter, gives excellent results.

Complement Fixation

It was indicated previously that only a few gram-negative bacteria and no gram-positive bacteria lyse when mixed with homologous antibody and complement. However, even though lysis does not occur, it can be demonstrated that complement does combine with the sensitized bacteria. The process is called complement fixation. It also occurs with soluble antigens such as egg albumin or bovine serum albumin mixed with homologous antiserum in optimal proportions.

As in bacteriolysis and hemolysis, the initial step, prerequisite to fixation of C1q, is the reaction of antigen with antibody. After this has occurred, C1q can react with the complement combining site of the antibody. The amount of complement employed in the test is carefully regulated by preliminary titration so that all will be fixed when equivalent amounts of antibody and antigen are employed. If one or the other of these two reagents is lacking, complement will not be fixed. At this point, another antigen-antibody system—the hemolytic system—is added: ordinarily sheep red blood cells (SRBC) and rabbit antiserum against SRBC called *amboceptor* or *hemolysin*. Any complement that remains unfixed by the primary antigen-antibody system reacts with and hemolyzes the sensitized red cells. Hemolysis therefore occurs in a negative complement fixation test and does not occur in a positive test.

All reagents are used in constant amounts except one, the unknown, of which a series of dilutions is employed. The highest dilution of this reagent that produces a given degree of complement fixation represents the unit or titer. The success of the test depends upon complete fixation of complement in the presence of adequate amounts of all reagents and complete hemolysis in the absence of the unknown. The known reagents must therefore be carefully prepared and titrated in order to balance one another. For example, there must be just sufficient amboceptor to sensitize the cells and just enough complement to lyse the sensitized erythrocytes. Quantitative details of the procedure vary from one laboratory to another, but certain general principles are usually followed.

PREPARATION OF REAGENTS FOR COMPLEMENT FIXATION

Amboceptor is prepared by injecting rabbits with thoroughly washed red blood cells until a sufficiently high titer has been developed. The rabbit serum contains amboceptor. It is often preserved by adding an equal volume of neutral glycerin. Amboceptor is very stable and will keep for years.

Guinea pig serum is the usual source of complement, although other species may be used for special purposes. Complement from each of several animals should be titrated individually, and sera of high titer may be pooled. Complement should not be kept more than 24 hours because of loss of titer.

Erythrocytes from the sheep are most widely used. Blood is taken into citrate or other anticoagulant or is defibrinated by shaking with glass beads. The cells should be fresh or preserved in such manner as not to be too fragile lest they lyse spontaneously. Each day the cells to be used are washed three or more times by centrifuging with five to ten volumes of saline (until the washings are no longer pink). Measured amounts of the sedimented cells are suspended in saline for titration of the other reagents and for the final test. Two per cent or 5 per cent suspensions are commonly employed.

Amboceptor is titrated by mixing various dilutions with constant amounts of red cell suspension and a more or less arbitrary dose of complement selected by trial and error or by experience. Mixtures are incubated in a waterbath at 37° C. for 30 minutes. The highest dilution of amboceptor producing complete hemolysis is called *one unit*. One to four units are usually employed in subsequent titrations and tests, according to the procedure being followed. The amboceptor solution is prepared to contain the required dose in a constant definite volume (e.g., 0.1 or 0.5 ml.). Amboceptor needs to be titrated only occasionally because of its stability.

Complement must be titrated each day. Closely spaced volumes of a moderate dilution (1:10 to 1:40) of guinea pig serum are pipetted into a series of tubes, together with sufficient saline to make a constant volume. The tubes are incubated at 37° C. for 30 minutes, after which sensitized red cells are added. (Sensitized red cells are prepared by mixing equal volumes of cell suspension and the predetermined dilution of amboceptor.) After secondary incubation at 37° C. for 30 minutes the smallest amount of complement that produces complete hemolysis is noted. This constitutes *one unit* of complement. Preincubation of complement alone is important because this reagent is so readily inactivated by heat and because two periods of incubation are required in the final test. The complement titration should therefore be performed in a similar manner.

The dose of complement employed in a complement fixation test varies according to the particular application of the reaction in question and the experience of the investigator. For research it is advisable to use approximately one unit, but in this case careful work is required. More precise results can be obtained than by use of greater quantities of complement, but occasionally tests have to be repeated because the controls do not react properly. Diagnostic techniques, such as the Wassermann reaction, often employ two or more units and thus allow a greater margin of error.

Soluble antigens (e.g., crystalline ovalbumin) may require no more preparation than dissolving in saline. Bacterial antigens are often prepared by extracting mass cultures, heating, and aging.

With some systems, such as bacterial antigens and lipoid extracts of tissues, which are highly anticomplementary, both antigenicity and anticomplementary titrations are necessary to define the upper and lower limits of antigen dosage to employ in complement fixation tests. The antigenic titration is performed if a known positive homologous antiserum is available. An amount of antigen is determined which, combined with antiserum, just completely fixes the dose of complement and therefore inhibits hemolysis. This represents the smallest quantity of antigen that can be expected to give satisfactory results in the final test.

The anticomplementary titration of antigen is performed by incubating various amounts of antigen with the dose of complement and subsequently adding the hemolytic system. The anticomplementary unit is the smallest amount of antigen that slightly inhibits hemolysis. The dose employed in the final test is some amount between the antigenic unit and the anticomplementary unit.

The preceding discussion has been based upon the 100 per cent hemolysis or inhibition end point, but the same general principles apply to the 50 per cent end point, although the details of technique differ. Exactly 50 per cent hemolysis is rarely encountered, but two or three determinations bracketing this value permit it to be calculated by interpolation.

TITRATION OF AN ANTIGEN OR AN ANTISERUM

Complement fixation tests are sometimes performed with dilutions of antiserum, sometimes with dilutions of antigen. In general, soluble antigens such as egg albumin are diluted serially and tested against antiserum either undiluted or diluted only slightly (e.g., 1:5). Bacterial antigens and lipoid tissue extracts are usually employed in constant amounts and mixed with serial dilutions of patient's serum or rabbit antiserum. In either case, the serum is inactivated by heating at 56° C. for 30 minutes to destroy normal complement, which might upset the balance of reagents and yield falsely negative results.

The experimental procedure and results of a complement fixation test with egg albumin antigen are indicated in Table 8–6. Dilutions of the antigen are prepared, and 0.1 ml. of each is placed in the tubes indicated. Rabbit anti-egg albumin serum

Table 8–6   Complement Fixation by Egg Albumin and Homologous Rabbit Antibody

Tube	Egg Albumin (0.1 ml.)	Anti-Egg Albumin Serum (undil.)	Complement Dilution	Saline	Primary incubation: 37° C. waterbath, 30–60 min.	Amboceptor Dilution	Sheep RBC	Secondary incubation: 37° C. waterbath, 15–30 min.	Results: Complement Fixation†
1	1:100	0.1 ml.	0.1 ml.	—		0.1 ml.	0.1 ml.		++++
2	1:1,000	0.1	0.1	—		0.1	0.1		++++
3	1:10,000	0.1	0.1	—		0.1	0.1		++++
4	1:100,000	0.1	0.1	—		0.1	0.1		+
5	1:1,000,000	0.1	0.1	—		0.1	0.1		−
6*	—	0.1	0.1	0.1 ml.		0.1	0.1		−
7*	1:100	—	0.1	0.1		0.1	0.1		−
8*	—	—	0.1	0.2		0.1	0.1		−
9*	—	—	—	0.4		—	0.1		++++

*Controls:
  Tube 6 = Antiserum control
  Tube 7 = Antigen control
  Tube 8 = Hemolytic control
  Tube 9 = Corpuscle control

†++++ = Complete fixation of complement
    (i.e., no hemolysis)
  − = No fixation of complement
    (i.e., complete hemolysis)

(inactivated) and complement are then added. The control tubes (6 to 9) lack one or more reagents, so sufficient saline is employed to give a constant final volume. All tubes are incubated for one-half to one hour at 37° C. or overnight in the refrigerator. The hemolytic system is added and the tubes reincubated at 37° C. The duration of secondary incubation may be judged by observation of the hemolytic control tube. Five to 10 minutes after this is completely lysed the tests may be read.

Results are recorded in terms of fixation of complement. A tube showing no hemolysis indicates complete fixation, which is recorded as ++++. The anti-egg albumin serum illustrated fixed complement partially after reaction with egg albumin diluted 1:100,000, which may be considered the complement fixing titer of the serum.

The four controls are absolutely essential. The *antiserum control* is used to show that the antiserum under test is not anticomplementary. When serial dilutions of antiserum are tested, a single serum control containing the largest amount of serum employed in any of the tubes usually suffices, although occasionally a control is necessary for each dilution. The *antigen control* is required to demonstrate that the antigen is not anticomplementary. As in the case of the serum control, this tube usually receives the largest amount of antigen employed in any of the actual tests. The *hemolytic control* indicates that the complement and amboceptor are active in the dosages employed. The *corpuscle control* shows that the red cells are not too fragile and that hemolysis in the test proper actually indicates a deficiency of the reagent being titrated. The first three controls should be completely hemolyzed, and the fourth should be unhemolyzed. When reacting correctly, the controls prove that the results of the test are significant insofar as the preparation of the reagents is concerned.

APPLICATIONS OF COMPLEMENT FIXATION

Complement fixation is used in the laboratory diagnosis of viral and rickettsial infections, and has been employed experimentally in some bacterial, parasitic, protozoan, and helminthic diseases. Its most widely publicized application is the Wassermann test for syphilis. The antibody-like substance or "reagin" detected in patients' sera is the same as that which reacts in the Kahn, VDRL, and other flocculation tests. The test antigen, formerly prepared from beef heart, has been replaced by cardiolipin (see page 195) in most laboratories.

The Kolmer modification of the Wassermann test is performed with one to seven dilutions of patient's serum or spinal fluid and a constant amount of antigen and guinea pig complement. After primary incubation in the refrigerator overnight, the hemolytic system is added and secondary incubation is at 37° C. for not longer than 1 hour. Definite inhibition of hemolysis is interpreted as evidence of fixation of complement. A tube is graded 4+ if there is 50 per cent hemolysis (judged by comparison with a standard hemoglobin solution representing the laked cells of one-half the dose of erythrocytes used in the test), and so forth.

The concentration of syphilitic reagin in the serum or spinal fluid varies according to the number and severity of the lesions. It appears within 4 or 5 weeks after infection, increases rapidly during the next 5 to 6 weeks to a maximum at the time when secondary lesions appear. It stabilizes at a high level for about 2 years and then tends to decrease during and after the latent period, but in about 75 per cent of cases it can be detected throughout the remainder of life. Reagin disappears when individuals are clinically cured, either spontaneously or as a result of treatment.

The nonspecific nature of reagin is indicated by the fact that it is also present in many other disease conditions. It will be recalled that Kahn postulated that it is an autoantibody to lipid released normally in the course of tissue wear and tear and formed in greater amounts during generalized diseases like syphilis and some of those listed in Table 8–7.

The occurrence of "biologic false-positive" reactions in the standard serologic tests for syphilis led inevitably to search for other tests that would be more highly specific. One of these is the *Treponema pallidum* immobilization (TPI) test. The TPI test has become one of the major reference procedures because it is based upon an anti-treponemal antibody rather than upon reagin and is therefore much more specific for syphilis. The Nichols strain of *T. pallidum* is grown in rabbit testes and harvested, and mixtures in a special medium with dilutions of patient's serum and complement are incubated 18 hours at 35° C. under anaerobic conditions. Microscopic preparations of each mixture are examined, and the percentage of cells that remain motile is determined. From a semilogarithmic plot of the results the serum dilution that immobilizes 50 per cent of the cells is ascertained; this represents the TPI antibody titer. Unfortunately, cultivation and preparation of *T. pallidum* for the test is so complex and the procedures so elaborate that few laboratories are equipped to perform the test. Moreover, it is expensive and is usually done only on a weekly or even less frequent basis.

Anti-treponemal antibodies appear in the sera of patients at about the same time as reagin; they persist longer, perhaps throughout the remainder of life, and in high titer, whereas reagins disappear at the time of clinical cure. The TPI test is therefore often used in cases in which complement fixation and flocculation tests give conflicting results.

Cytotoxicity of Nucleated Mammalian Cells

Most of the experimental work on complement-mediated cytotoxicity of cells other than bacteria and erythrocytes has been conducted with mammalian cells cultivated in vitro. Cells from a given host possess surface antigens that are characteristic of all cells of the animal, such as species antigens, Forssman antigens, and genetically controlled isoantigens (histocompatability antigens). In addition, cells from different organs may possess organ-specific antigens (e.g., kidney, adrenal, and thyroid antigens).

The mechanism of cytotoxicity of mammalian cells is very similar to that of cytolysis. Antibody, produced either naturally in the course of an autoimmune disease or by artificial immunization with tissue cells or cell constituents, is necessary, together

Table 8–7   *Biologic False-positive Tests for Syphilis Reagin in Nonsyphilitic Diseases**

Disease	Per Cent
Malaria	100
Leprosy	60
Typhus fever	20
Vaccinia	20
Atypical pneumonia	20
Infectious mononucleosis	20
Lupus erythematosus	20
Trypanosomiasis	10
Infectious hepatitis	10
Subacute bacterial endocarditis	5
Rheumatoid arthritis	5
Tuberculosis (advanced)	3–5
Pneumococcal pneumonia	2–5

*From Moore and Mohr, 1952. J.A.M.A., 150:467.

with complement. Within minutes after adding these reagents to a monolayer of the cells on a glass or plastic surface, the cells become rounded, prominent cytoplasmic granules appear, the cytoplasm swells, and translucent blisters form; in less than an hour the cytoplasmic membrane ruptures, the nucleus and other organelles degenerate, cell "ghosts" form, and the cell detaches from the substrate.

As in cytolysis, the classic sequence from C1 through C9 yields lesions or functional "holes," through which K^+ and Na^+ pass freely, leading to increased intracellular osmotic pressure, swelling, enlargement of the lesions so that macromolecules are lost, and severe structural damage. Cytotoxicity can be observed by direct microscopic examination of either unstained or supravitally stained preparations (i.e., dead cells take up trypan blue but not neutral red), by attempted cultivation of cell clones from individual cells, or by release of ^{51}Cr from injured cells.

Usually the antigenic sites that react are on the cell surface, readily accessible to antibody. Occasionally serum antibodies enter the cells by pinocytosis and react with internal components, causing vacuoles and damaging the cytoplasm directly. In the absence of complement, antibody causes the cells to become rounded and to agglutinate (see Figures 8–4 and 8–5). The surface membrane undergoes structural alteration, developing folds and exposing lipid components, and the lysosomal membranes become fragile and permeable. Complement is necessary for blister formation and lysis (Figure 8–6).

The role of complement-mediated cytotoxicity in the body is not known in detail, since conditions in vitro are far different from those in vivo. Antibodies to leukocyte antigens have been detected after multiple transfusions, concurrent with a marked decrease in the number of circulating granulocytes. Cytotoxic antibodies may also be significant in some types of human cancer, preventing metastasis of tumors. Cytotoxic antibodies are also found in autoimmune diseases, but it is not certain that they actually cause the diseases.

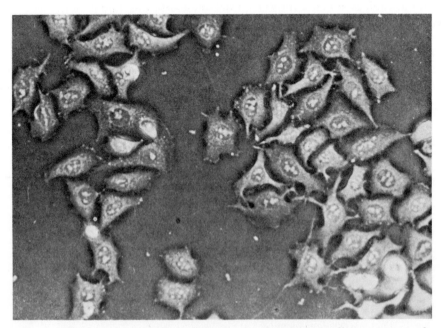

Figure 8–4. Normal appearance of HeLa (human cervical carcinoma) cells growing on a glass surface in the presence of normal rabbit serum. (From Rose et al., 1973. Principles of Immunology. New York, Macmillan Publishing Company, Inc.)

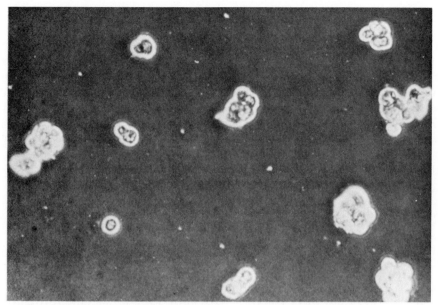

Figure 8–5. Rounding and agglutination of HeLa cells by treatment with rabbit anti-HeLa serum. (From Rose et al., 1973. Principles of Immunology. New York, Macmillan Publishing Company, Inc.)

PHAGOCYTOSIS

The body response to microbial infection includes inflammation, which is induced by irritation caused by the organisms or their products. Examination of an inflamed area reveals an accumulation of microorganisms and phagocytic cells. Some substance or

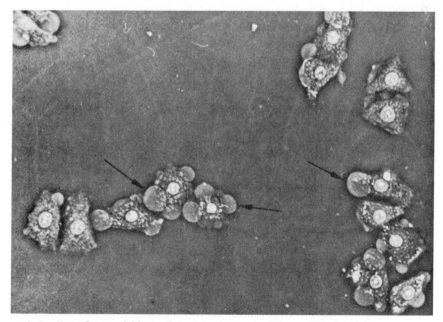

Figure 8–6. Rounding and blister formation (arrows) of HeLa cells treated with rabbit anti-HeLa serum plus fresh guinea pig serum (complement). (From Rose et al., 1973. Principles of Immunology. New York, Macmillan Publishing Company, Inc.)

condition retards the flow of blood through the regional capillaries so that polymorphonuclear leukocytes can adhere to the walls and migrate by diapedesis (an ameboid type of mobility between the capillary wall cells) into the infected tissue. They then ingest the bacteria if conditions are favorable. This is the process of phagocytosis.

Phagocytosis is the most important body defense against infectious agents and other foreign substances; it also provides a means for disposal of effete or worn out blood cells and other body cells. It is phylogenetically the most primitive defense mechanism and appears to be an outgrowth of the ameboid method of ingestion of food particles. Metchnikoff (1887) recognized this in connection with his studies of digestion in the water flea, Daphnia. This organism, being transparent, provided an excellent subject for microscopic study. Metchnikoff observed ameboid cells within Daphnia that could ingest small numbers of the yeast, *Monospora bicuspidata.* Large numbers of the yeast cells, however, injured the ameboid cells, and the water flea itself might be killed. Metchnikoff proposed that these *phagocytic cells,* as he called them, were a defense of the animal against fatal infection.

This primitive digestion-defense mechanism is nonspecific; it cannot distinguish between "self" constituents and invading microorganisms. The specific affinity of phagocytic cells for microorganisms, and hence the defense function, depends upon the immunologic system and participation of antibodies as specific recognition substances. Complement or its components may participate, subject to the triggering action of antibody, and accelerate or promote more efficient operation of the phagocytic system.

Phagocytic Cells

There are two chief varieties of phagocytic cells in the mammalian body: cells of the polymorphonuclear system, sometimes called microphages, and cells of the mononuclear system.

POLYMORPHONUCLEAR PHAGOCYTIC SYSTEM

Cells of the polymorphonuclear phagocytic system comprise the first line of defense against infectious agents. These are the circulating leukocytes or white blood cells that are characterized by a lobular nucleus and cytoplasmic granules of various staining properties. Neutrophiles are the most abundant and comprise about 70 per cent of the normal white blood cell population. They are the principal cells in the inflammatory response to infection. Eosinophiles and basophiles possess less phagocytic activity, although they participate in other ways in the immune response. Cells of the polymorphonuclear system increase drastically in response to many types of infection.

MONONUCLEAR PHAGOCYTIC SYSTEM

The active cells of the mononuclear system include monocytes of the peripheral blood and macrophages, either "fixed" or "wandering," which comprise the cells often known as the reticuloendothelial system (R.E.S.). Fixed macrophages line the endothelium of capillaries and of the sinuses of organs such as the spleen, bone marrow, and lymph nodes. Reticular or supporting cells of various organs, especially the liver, also possess phagocytic properties. Fixed macrophages normally appear to participate in the disposal of worn out and fragmented red blood cells. Wandering macrophages, including monocytes, migrate through tissues and assist in the repair of damage by destroying and absorbing dead materials and by aiding in the disposal of erythrocytes and other blood cells that have passed out of blood vessels.

Macrophages are much larger than granulocytes and contain a single nucleus, often kidney-shaped. They constitute the second line of defense against invading microorganisms. Their distribution throughout the vascular system and other tissues bathed by blood and lymph ensures that foreign particles encounter macrophages readily. Although there is a steady influx of macrophages from the monocytes of the circulation, the population of macrophages is partly maintained by self-propagation. Macrophages can be "activated" by lymphokines liberated by T cells that have reacted with homologous antigens. These "angry" macrophages are more strongly phagocytic than normal macrophages. They develop greater numbers of enzyme-secreting lysosomal granules and display exaggerated bactericidal activity.

Steps in Phagocytosis

The various phagocytic cells of both systems continuously police the blood, lymph, and the respiratory and gastrointestinal tracts and keep these free from foreign particles. There are, however, sequestered locations or unusual situations (e.g., an infected splinter in the skin) in which phagocytic cells are not normally plentiful. Mobile granulocytes and macrophages therefore use a "search and destroy" mechanism to track down these infectious agents. They also possess a system for distinguishing "nonself" from "self," so that they can concentrate on "nonself" agents.

CHEMOTAXIS

The physical act of damaging tissue, either by trauma alone or by microbial multiplication, releases substances that are attractive to phagocytic cells, which then migrate toward the source of these substances. This process, *chemotaxis*, concentrates phagocytic cells in the area where they are needed. If the host possesses antibodies, either natural or immune, that can react with the surface of the foreign particle, complement components unite with the sensitized antigen. Complement complexes and fractions that attract leukocytes and enhance phagocytosis are formed (see Table 8–4). Even in the absence of the early stages of the complement sequence, the bypass mechanism may be called into play by the presence of endotoxin or other microbial constituents or tissue ingredients and yield the chemotactic fraction C3a.

Chemotactic attraction induces typical ameboid migration. The phagocytic cells pass through the walls of the small blood vessels by diapedesis, insinuating themselves through the intercellular junctions.

The principal factor that determines whether phagocytosis of a particle can occur is the physical nature of the surface of the particle in comparison with that of the phagocyte. Phagocytosis takes place when the interfacial tension between the surface of the phagocyte and water is lower than the interfacial tension between the particle and water; that is, the particle must be more hydrophobic than the phagocyte. Most nonpathogenic bacteria are hydrophobic and are readily ingested by phagocytes. Bacteria that are highly hydrophobic, such as *Mycobacterium tuberculosis*, are spontaneously ingested by phagocytic cells. These organisms owe their pathogenicity to their resistance to digestion by phagocytic enzymes. Bacteria like *Diplococcus pneumoniae* that possess a hydrophilic carbohydrate capsule are not normally subject to phagocytosis.

OPSONIZATION

After antibody against the pneumococcal polysaccharide has been produced, it reacts with the capsule surface antigens via its Fab portions and makes the cell hydrophobic, whereupon ingestion can occur. The hydrophobic character of the antibody-coated capsule is attributable to the Fc portion of the immunoglobulin molecule. The specificity of immune phagocytosis is a function solely of the antibody that opsonizes the bacteria.

Complement is not necessary for phagocytosis, but if it is present in conjunction with antibody, it increases the hydrophobic nature of bacterial cells to which it is attached and increases the rate and extent of phagocytic ingestion.

INGESTION AND DIGESTION

When the hydrophobic particle has been brought into direct contact with the phagocytic cell, whose surface is comparatively hydrophilic and hence has a lower surface tension than that of the particle, the phagocytic cell membrane invaginates and the particle is gradually enveloped. A vacuole forms around the particle and soon fuses with one or more lysosomal granules that contain bactericidal agents and hydrolytic enzymes, including lysozyme, phagocytin, and various lipases, nucleases, proteases, and phosphatases, which quickly kill and digest most bacteria. A few, such as *M. tuberculosis*, *Listeria monocytogenes*, and Brucella species, resist digestion and tend to produce prolonged, chronic infections. As hydrolytic digestion of the ingested bacterium takes place, the contents of the phagocytic vacuole liquefies, the process often requiring no more than 15 minutes.

SURFACE PHAGOCYTOSIS

Wood and his associates discovered a mechanism by which encapsulated bacteria are ingested prior to the formation of antibody. This process, *surface phagocytosis*, depends upon the roughness of surfaces adjacent to phagocytic cells and the bacteria, such as the surfaces of tissues or fibrin clots. Phagocytic cells trap microorganisms against rough surfaces or against each other and then engulf the encapsulated organisms (see Figure 8–7).

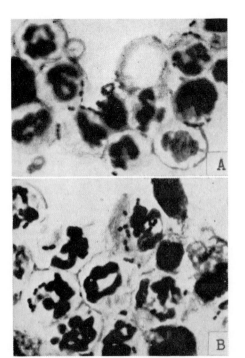

Figure 8–7. A, Failure of phagocytes to engulf encapsulated pneumococci on glass surface. Many pneumococci are in contact with the surfaces of the cells, but none has been ingested.

B, Phagocytosis of pneumococci on surface of moistened filter paper. Many organisms are within the cytoplasm of the phagocytes. (From Wood et al., 1946. J. Exp. Med., 84:387.)

Demonstration of Phagocytosis and Opsonizing Activity in vitro

Phagocytosis can be shown by the simple technique employed by Wright and Douglas (1903). Leukocytes, either in whole blood or in peritoneal or pleural exudate, are washed repeatedly with saline by centrifugation to remove plasma constituents. They are then mixed with test bacteria such as staphylococci, incubated for 30 minutes at 37° C., smeared on a microscope slide, and stained by any appropriate blood stain. One hundred polymorphonuclear cells in the smear are examined, and the number of bacteria ingested per cell is counted. Mixtures can be prepared with specific antiserum instead of saline as a diluent to demonstrate the opsonizing effect of natural or immune antibodies. A typical experiment might give results such as the following:

Mixtures	Average Number of Bacteria per Leukocyte
1. Washed leukocytes + saline + staphylococci	1.2
2. Washed leukocytes + normal serum + staphylococci	10.0
3. Washed leukocytes + immune serum + staphylococci	40.0

The saline control (1) demonstrates minimal spontaneous phagocytosis. The average number of bacteria per leukocyte in each serum mixture is called the *phagocytic index*. The ratio of the phagocytic index obtained with immune serum (3) to that obtained with normal serum (2) is the *opsonic index*; in the example cited, the opsonic index of the immune serum was 40/10 = 4.0.

Phagocytosis in Relation to Disease

Bordet and other early investigators maintained that the ability of an animal to resist or overcome infection is closely paralleled by the phagocytic vigor of the animal's cells. If complete phagocytosis and destruction of the parasite occur, infection is averted or cured, but if some organisms escape ingestion or intracellular killing, they can multiply and produce fatal disease. Depression of phagocytic activity lowers resistance to infection—for example, paralysis by anesthesia or by raising or lowering the body temperature, or reduction in number by chemical or physical agents. On the other hand, pathogens are less likely to produce fatal disease when introduced into an area rich in phagocytic cells, and a favorable turn in an infection often follows an increase in the number of circulating leukocytes.

Wood described in detail the role of phagocytosis in recovery from pneumonia. Against a well established infection in the lung, three areas of cellular defense become active. First is the primary pneumonic lesion. Edema fluid in the peripheral zone supports a large population of rapidly multiplying pneumococci. Within this zone is a region of early consolidation containing numerous leukocytes with ingested bacteria, then a zone of pus cells in which very few intact organisms can be found, and finally a central area of resolution where macrophages predominate and the exudate is clearing. In the region of early consolidation, surface phagocytosis takes place as polymorphonuclear leukocytes trap pneumococci against the alveolar walls, against each other, and against strands of fibrin in the alveolar exudate.

The second area of defense consists of the tracheobronchial lymph nodes, which drain the site of primary infection. Uningested bacteria reach these nodes, where secondary inflammation is quickly established and large numbers of polymorphonuclear leukocytes accumulate. The leukocytes in the nodes efficiently remove most bacteria from the lymph and keep them from entering the subclavian veins and the bloodstream.

Bacteria that escape phagocytic destruction in the lymph nodes and invade the circulation establish a bacteremic state, which may be fatal if the third line of cellular defense, capillary phagocytosis, is inadequate. Polymorphonuclear leukocytes, which normally roll freely along blood vessel walls, apparently attach to the walls of capillaries and small veins and arteries when there are large numbers of bacteria in the blood. They become motile and may be phagocytic, trapping bacteria against the walls, adjacent leukocytes, or small thrombi. This occurs in the liver, spleen, and lungs and, to a lesser extent, elsewhere in the body.

A large proportion of the bacterial population may be destroyed in these three sites by surface phagocytosis, at a time when antibody has not yet appeared. Later, after antibody has been formed, immune phagocytosis can complete the removal of the bacteria.

The pneumococci are typical of the group of extracellular pathogens that do not survive within phagocytic cells. They produce acute infections, inciting a violent inflammatory response, which leads to a fairly prompt recovery by phagocytic action. Bacteria such as M. tuberculosis survive and multiply intracellularly within polymorphonuclear leukocytes, where they are protected from bacteriolytic antibodies, and produce chronic infections that persist for months or years. Eventually, the polymorphonuclear cells are damaged and ingested, together with the surviving bacteria, by mononuclear cells. These, in turn, may be damaged by toxic substances from the bacteria, but their eventual fate depends on the immune state of the individual. Elberg found least monocytic degeneration when cells and serum from an animal immunized with BCG were used in in vitro experiments. Degeneration was greater with normal cells and immune serum or with immune cells and normal serum. Bacteria released from degenerative monocytes are free to multiply and perpetuate the infectious process.

Phagocytosis is an important means of combating pyogenic infections. Hemolytic streptococci are phagocyted and then destroyed within the phagocytic cells. Urethral smears in gonorrhea and spinal fluids in meningitis often show large numbers of bacteria ingested by neutrophiles (see Figure 8–8). Some strains of bacteria are less susceptible to ingestion than others. Coagulase-positive staphylococci are ingested less easily than coagulase-negative strains in the presence of coagulable plasma. It has been suggested that formation of a fibrin envelope around the organisms prevents phagocytosis by clumping the cocci or by hindering their union with antibody.

Certain types of antibody are necessary for opsonization of some bacteria, such as the typhoid organism. Phagocytosis of *Salmonella typhosa* is enhanced by O antibody but not by H antibody, and Vi antigen-containing strains highly resist ingestion unless Vi antibody is present.

IMMUNOLOGIC REACTIONS OF VIRUSES

Physical and Chemical Nature of Viruses

Viruses are submicroscopic, obligate, intracellular parasites consisting essentially of DNA or RNA and a protein coat, which protects the block of nucleic acid genetic material from the environment, assists in its transmission from one host cell to another, and initiates its replication. Individual types of virus may contain additional constituents (e.g., lipids, carbohydrates, a few enzymes), but the basic structure of a virus particle or *virion* consists of the nucleic acid core with its protein, which is called a *capsid.* Some virions also possess an outer envelope, usually lipid, acquired from the host cell membrane when the particle is liberated from its site of replication and

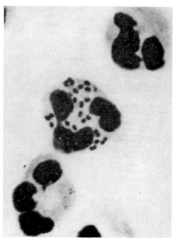

Figure 8–8. Phagocytosis of *Neisseria meningitidis*. The center polymorphonuclear leukocyte has ingested nearly two dozen of the paired cocci. × 1,200. (From Ruch and Fulton, 1960. Medical Physiology and Biophysics. Philadelphia, W. B. Saunders Company.)

assembly. Viruses lack organelles and enzyme systems necessary for synthesizing protein and generating ATP and hence depend on their host cells for these essential bits of machinery.

Replication of Viruses

Virus replication, unlike that of eukaryotic cells or even of prokaryotes, does not occur by synthesis of protoplasm, cell enlargement, and division. Instead, the virion components are synthesized separately and are then assembled. Preexisting virus supplies the DNA or RNA pattern, according to which the host cell puts together protein enzymes used in making virus nucleic acid and structural (e.g., capsid) proteins.

Steps in the replication of virus are illustrated diagrammatically in Figure 8–9.

Figure 8–9. Diagrammatic representation of the steps in replication of a deoxyribovirus. (From Fenner and White, 1970. Medical Virology. New York, Academic Press, Inc.)

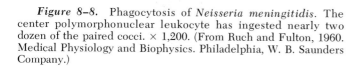

1 Attachment

2 Penetration

3 Uncoating

4 Transcription of mRNA

5 Translation of early proteins

6 Replication of viral DNA

7 Transcription of mRNA

8 Translation of late proteins

9 Assembly of virions

10 Release

When random collision brings the virion into contact with a host cell possessing on its plasma membrane an appropriate complementary receptor site, attachment occurs, followed by engulfment, in which the virion penetrates by a process similar to phagocytosis. It loses its protein coat as it passes through the cell membrane or within the phagocytic vacuole. The next steps depend upon whether the nucleic acid is DNA or RNA. In Figure 8–9 a DNA virus is illustrated, so the uncoated DNA is transcribed to RNA, which is translated to early enzyme proteins that assist in the subsequent steps of synthesis of viral DNA and protein. When all constituents have been synthesized, they are assembled and finally released.

Effects of Viruses on Host Cells

The effects produced by viruses vary greatly. (1) Cytocidal viruses (e.g., the poliovirus) kill the host cell by interfering with cellular macromolecular synthetic reactions or by inducing the release of lysosomal enzymes that autolyze the cell. Many viruses alter the host cell membrane, some causing it to fuse with that of other cells and produce giant, multinucleate cells (as in measles, mumps and herpes), some producing new virus-specified plasma membrane antigens. Some stimulate the formation of "inclusion bodies," which are either sites of virus synthesis, aggregates of virions, or degenerative bodies. (2) Steady-state, noncytocidal viruses, such as the virus that produces lymphocytic choriomeningitis in congenitally infected mice, multiply without any apparent adverse effect on their host cell. In these latent infections, cellular DNA, RNA, and protein synthesis may be hardly affected; viral RNA is only 1 per cent of cellular RNA, and there is little cell damage, even though large numbers of virions are produced. (3) Transformation occurs in many cells infected by potentially oncogenic viruses. Transformed cells are not killed, but their growth characteristics are permanently altered. They lose the property of contact inhibition, so their growth in vitro is piled up instead of forming a monolayer. They also show chromosomal abnormalities and produce new surface and intracellular antigens (neoantigens).

Virus-Associated Antigens

The capsid proteins of viruses are foreign to the animal within which the virus is replicating and hence incite the formation of antibodies. Antibodies may also form against envelopes and virion subunits and other macromolecules such as enzymes that are synthesized during virus replication.

The surface antigens are responsible for serotype specificity of various groups of viruses. There is only one serotype of each of the viruses that cause smallpox, chickenpox, measles, and mumps, and this fact contributes in part to the relatively good state of immunity against these diseases. On the other hand, three serologically different viruses cause poliomyelitis, and immunity against one serotype confers protection only against itself, so it is necessary to immunize against each. Unfortunately there are over 100 rhinoviruses, which means that the chance of a satisfactory immunization against the common cold is very remote.

The cell transformation that occurs during replication of oncogenic viruses is often accompanied by the formation of new antigens, both intracellularly and on the cell surface. T (tumor) antigens are situated in the nucleus, as demonstrated by immunofluorescence. They appear to be proteins encoded by virus DNA and synthesized early in the replication cycle. They are found in all cells infected by a given virus, no matter what the species of animal may be or whether oncogenesis occurs. Tumor-specific transplantation antigens (TSTA) are cell surface neoantigens that appear on transformed cells. They also are proteins formed by the cell according to the code specified by the viral genes and hence they are characteristic of the virus rather than the host cell. The immunologic response to these antigens is responsible for rejection of the tumor when it is transplanted into another animal.

Serologic Reactions of Viral Antibodies

Neutralization, protection and complement fixation tests have long been used in the study of viral diseases. Serologic reactions are employed for detection of viral antibodies in normal populations and in the sera of patients for study of the response to prophylactic immunization and for identification and classification of viruses. In vitro tests are more rapid and less expensive than in vivo methods. Attempts are usually made to correlate test tube reactions with neutralization or immunity tests, which better indicate actual resistance to disease.

The serologic investigation of viruses received a great impetus when it was discovered that many could be cultivated in the developing chick embryo. Previously it had been necessary to employ animals, some of them expensive (e.g., monkeys). The technique of egg inoculation is relatively simple. Fertile eggs (Figure 8–10) that have been incubated for a suitable length of time are cleansed and disinfected, an opening is made through the shell with a dental drill or small grinding wheel, and the desired site is inoculated by hypodermic needle. The opening is then closed with sterile paraffin, Scotch tape, or a cover glass sealed with paraffin. Embryonated eggs provide adequate quantities of virus material for serologic as well as animal inoculation experiments.

Another technical advance of importance to virology was the development of methods for routine in vitro cultivation of animal tissues and cells. Although tissue cultures had been used in research since 1907, and the ability of viruses to multiply in such cultures was proved in 1925, it was not until 1950 that the technique assumed major importance in the virus laboratory. Interest was stimulated by the discovery that many viruses damage the cultured cells in which they grow, producing characteristic cytopathogenic effects; moreover, cytopathogenicity can often be prevented by addition of specific antiserum, which neutralizes the virus. Tissue cultures can therefore replace the slower and more expensive animal inoculation procedures for isolating and

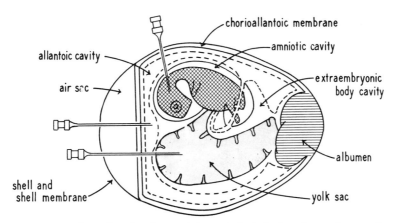

Figure 8–10. Section through a developing (10- to 12-day) chick embryo, showing how inoculation can be made into the head of the embryo, the allantoic cavity, and the yolk sac. (From Burrows, 1959. Textbook of Microbiology, 17th ed. Philadelphia, W. B. Saunders Company.)

identifying viruses and studying their immunologic properties. A further advance that enhanced the usefulness of the method was a revival of an earlier procedure for preparing suspensions of tissue cells by trypsin digestion. These suspensions can be used to inoculate an agar nutrient medium uniformly so that the cells establish a continuous sheet or monolayer. In such a culture inoculated with virus, cytopathogenicity is revealed by the appearance of clear areas or plaques, within which virus particles are concentrated and from which they can be isolated by use of an inoculating needle (see Figure 8–11). Neutralization of the virus by antibody prevents plaque formation. This technique provides a rapid and inexpensive means of titrating neutralizing antibody.

COMPLEMENT FIXATION WITH VIRAL ANTIGENS

Complement fixation is one of the most widely employed in vitro tests used with viruses. Preparation of satisfactory antigens is the major problem because virus is necessarily secured from living tissue, which is likely to contribute anticomplementary and nonspecific properties to the reagent. These properties are removed by extraction of infected tissues with benzene, acetone-ether, and other lipid solvents, by precipitation of nonspecific proteins with protamine, and by ultracentrifugation and Seitz filtration.

The complement fixation test is inherently less sensitive than most other tests used with viruses (see Table 4–1), so there often appear to be discrepancies between the results of various serologic tests for virus antibodies. Neutralizing antibodies for many viruses appear within 2 weeks of clinical onset and remain in the circulation for years. Complement fixing antibodies appear later and often disappear within a few weeks or months.

AGGLUTINATION AND PRECIPITATION

Agglutination is restricted to some of the larger viruses like psittacosis, lymphogranuloma venereum, vaccinia, herpes zoster, varicella, and fowlpox. Tests can be

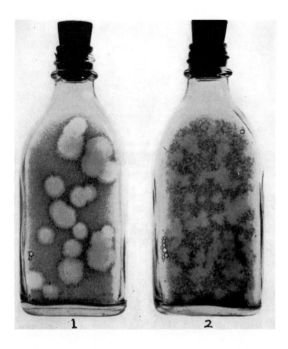

Figure 8–11. Plaques of (1) type III poliovirus and (2) type 6 ECHO virus in a thin layer of monkey epithelial cells growing on a special nutrient medium solidified with agar. (From Frobisher, 1957. Fundamentals of Microbiology, 6th ed. Philadelphia, W. B. Saunders Company.)

performed as usual in test tubes or, with dense antigen suspensions, by a slide technique observed by darkfield microscopy.

The antigen for vaccinia agglutination consists of elementary bodies from the skin of rabbits inoculated with the virus. The viral particles are purified by differential centrifugation and washed in dilute buffer. In the agglutination tests either the antigen or the antiserum is kept constant and the other reagent varied, depending upon whether the antibody or antigen titer is desired. Tubes are incubated at 50° C. overnight.

Inert or nonspecific particulate agents have been employed to adsorb viruses from crude suspensions for use as test antigens in agglutination. Such materials include bacteria, blood cells, collodion, and insoluble dyes.

Precipitation or flocculation tests performed in narrow serologic tubes give positive results with the soluble antigens of pox viruses, herpes, influenza, mumps, Newcastle disease, and poliomyelitis viruses and antisera containing homologous antibodies. Gel diffusion techniques afford striking demonstrations of serologic relationships between certain of these viruses. Both the Oudin single diffusion method and the Ouchterlony double diffusion procedure give excellent results.

FLUORESCENT ANTIBODY IN THE DETECTION OF VIRUS

The various methods of using antibodies labeled with fluorescent dyes are applied to routine diagnosis and to research on virus diseases. Specifically, viruses can be detected by use of appropriate labeled antisera in pathologic specimens, infected tissue or cell cultures, embryonated eggs, and laboratory animals. Influenza virus has been detected in epithelial cells from the nasal membranes. Poliovirus can be detected and its serologic type determined in monkey kidney cells. Fluorescent antibodies were used to demonstrate that the soluble antigens of certain viruses are formed first in the host cell nucleus and the protein capsomeres are later produced in the cytoplasm, where the intact virus particle is then assembled.

HEMAGGLUTINATION (HA) AND HEMAGGLUTINATION INHIBITION (HI)

Many viruses contain virus-coded proteins in their outer coat that can bind to complementary receptor sites in the outer membrane of certain species of erythrocyte. Red blood cells usually possess many receptor sites, and if a virion attaches to two red cells simultaneously, a framework of alternating cells and virions can form, yielding an aggregate. This phenomenon, discovered by Hirst (1941), is called viral hemagglutination. It is caused by myxoviruses (influenza), paramyxoviruses, and viruses of many other groups. Specific conditions must often be provided, including the species of red cell, pH, and incubation temperature.

Inasmuch as the viral hemagglutinin is a foreign protein, it is immunogenic, and an infected host produces antihemagglutinin that prevents viral hemagglutination. This antibody can be titrated by relatively simple procedures. The hemagglutination inhibition test is an important diagnostic tool for detection of antibodies in patients' sera and for identification of viruses.

Dilutions of the inactivated test serum are mixed with virus suspension and washed erythrocytes. Test tubes containing the mixtures are observed without agitation after 1 to 2 hours at room temperature, the time of incubation depending upon the virus. Failure of hemagglutination constitutes a positive test for antibody in the various serum dilutions. Unagglutinated cells slide down the sides of the tube or settle directly to the bottom and form a compact circular "button" with smooth, sharply defined edges. Agglutinated cells stick to the sides of the bowl at the bottom of the tube or form a ragged edge around the "button" of unagglutinated cells. Tests can also be performed in plastic trays or plates containing several rows of depressions.

VIRUS NEUTRALIZATION

Serum neutralization of viruses was first demonstrated in animal experiments by Sternberg in 1892 in a study of vaccinia, and for years it was considered the best method of demonstrating the immunologic relationships of viruses and the amount of protective antibody in antiserum. Mixtures of serum and infectious material were inoculated into susceptible animals, and the host response was compared with that of control animals that received only the virus. Antibody titrations of this kind are very expensive, because many animals are required for each test. Consequently, when chick embryo and tissue culture techniques were developed, they were quickly adapted for titration of virus neutralizing antibody.

A significant evidence of virus activity in chick embryos and tissue cultures is cytopathogenicity, demonstrated by the formation of pocks or other visible lesions on the egg membranes or by clear areas or plaques in the sheet of cells cultivated as a monolayer. These cytopathogenic effects are prevented by mixing neutralizing serum with the virus before inoculating the embryonated egg or cell culture. Neutralizing antibody is assayed by using various dilutions of serum with a constant dose of virus. The end point is the highest dilution of antiserum that causes an arbitrarily chosen percentage reduction in cytopathogenic effect.

The virus neutralization test is the most specific and sensitive diagnostic procedure available for titrating protective antibodies and for identifying virus serotypes. The antigens are those surface components by which the virion attaches to the host cell. Inasmuch as surface antigens are peculiarly susceptible to change due to evolutionary pressures, it is these antigens that distinguish one serologic type of virus from another. The neutralization test is therefore especially useful when it is necessary to decide which virus type is the cause of an epidemic (e.g., poliomyelitis, influenza) so that the most effective preventive or therapeutic measures may be instituted.

The mechanism of neutralization by antibody is not known with certainty. Inactivation of virus is not irreversible, and both active virus and active antibody can be recovered from neutral mixtures by simple dissociation procedures, such as dilution, change in pH, and sonication. It is presumed that the most important action of antibody is to prevent attachment of the virion to the host cell receptor site, probably by steric hindrance or some other allosteric mechanism. Since attachment of virus is a necessary prerequisite for replication, this effectively prevents its activity. It should be noted that intracellular virus is protected from antibody present in the external environment, and viruses that pass directly from cell to cell without encountering the surrounding plasma or tissue fluids (e.g., vaccinia, herpes simplex) produce expanding lesions even in the presence of a high concentration of serum antibody. Other viruses, such as influenza and poliomyelitis, are released to the saliva or the intestinal contents, where they may immediately encounter antibody (IgA) and be prevented from further spread.

Cell-Mediated Immunologic Reactions of Viruses

Cell-mediated immunity or delayed-type hypersensitivity plays a role in the response to certain viral infections, notably smallpox, measles, and mumps. It has already been noted that children with Bruton's agammaglobulinemia possess little or no γ-globulin, they survive most infections only through the aid of antibiotics and antisera, and they do not respond to active immunization with bacterial vaccines. However, they recover uneventfully from measles and mumps and respond normally to smallpox vaccination, exhibiting an immediate (hypersensitivity) reaction upon revaccination.

Passive immunization, either by maternal antibody or by injection of γ-globulin, has long been known to prevent or decrease the likelihood of infection in individuals exposed to viruses such as smallpox, measles, and mumps. It has been suggested that the roles of antibody and hypersensitivity differ. The former prevents infection, and delayed hypersensitivity or cell-mediated immunity aids in recovery from established infection. This hypothesis is supported by experiments with a rabbit fibroma, which indicate that antibody neutralizes circulating virus and inhibits its spread about the body, while delayed hypersensitivity causes regression of any local tumors that may develop.

NEUTRALIZATION OF TOXINS

Toxins

The components of bacteria that are toxic to higher forms of life include exotoxins, endotoxins, and certain hydrolytic and other enzymes. A typical bacterial exotoxin is released into the medium during the life of the cell, whereas an endotoxin remains a part of the cell until death and autolysis occur. The enzymes referred to are also released from living cells and, in fact, are sometimes listed as exotoxins. They include (a) hemolysins and leukocidins, which attack red and white blood cells, respectively; (b) coagulases, which produce fibrin clots, and fibrinolysins, which dissolve them; (c) hyaluronidases, which increase tissue permeability; and (d) proteolytic and lipolytic enzymes. One of the exotoxins of *Clostridium perfringens* is a collagenase and another is a lecithinase.

EXOTOXINS AND ENDOTOXINS

The chief characteristic that distinguishes exotoxins (and toxic enzymes) from endotoxins is their chemical nature. The former are proteins, whereas endotoxins are complexes containing polysaccharide and phospholipid in addition to protein. Endotoxins are also known by other names: somatic or O antigens, Boivin antigens, etc.

Some characteristics of exo- and endotoxins are listed in Table 8–8. It should be emphasized that, aside from the difference in chemical composition, there is no sharp distinction between the two classes of toxic substance. As proteins, exotoxins are nondialyzable and are denatured at 60 to 80° C. with loss of toxicity. Most endotoxins remain toxic, even when heated at 100° C. or higher; this indicates that their toxic properties are associated with the polysaccharide or phospholipid portion of the complex. However, the α-toxin of *Cl. perfringens* retains three-quarters of its activity after 5 minutes at 100° C. and one-fifth after 30 minutes, and one type of staphylococcus enterotoxin remains toxic in culture filtrates or in infected foods after boiling for 30 minutes.

The differences between the lethal doses of exotoxins and endotoxins are not so marked as was once believed, and there is great variation among exotoxins. This is illustrated in Table 8–9, which lists two snake venoms and a plant poison, ricin, in addition to various bacterial toxins. Other plants and animals also produce substances with properties similar to those of bacterial exotoxins: Indian licorice (abrin), spiders,

Table 8–8   Properties of Exotoxins and Endotoxins

	Exotoxins	**Endotoxins**
Source	Principally living, gram-positive bacterial cells	Cell walls of gram-negative bacteria, liberated by autolysis of dead cells
Chemical composition	Proteins	Polysaccharide-phospholipid-protein complexes
Effect of formaldehyde	Destroys toxicity (producing toxoid)	None
Thermostability	Most are inactivated at 60 to 80° C.	May resist 120° C. for 1 hour
Lethal dose	Small	Large
Pharmacologic action	Usually specific	Nonspecific
Antigenicity	High	Moderate to high
Neutralizing power of antitoxin	High (complete neutralization of toxicity)	Low (partial neutralization of toxicity)

scorpions, etc. Although *Yersinia pestis* is gram-negative, its toxin is probably not an endotoxin, inasmuch as it is composed of protein.

Specificity of site of action is characteristic of most exotoxins. Tetanus and botulinum exotoxins affect only nerve tissues. Tetanus exotoxin acts upon the neuromuscular junctions of voluntary muscles and may also damage the anterior horn cells of the central nervous system, and botulinum toxin is specifically toxic to certain peripheral motor nerves. Hemolytic streptococcus filtrates attack vascular endothelium, and *Shigella dysenteriae* produces a neurotoxin. Diphtheria toxin damages a wider variety of cells than many other exotoxins, including the skin, heart muscle, adrenals, liver, and nerves.

The response to endotoxin is relatively uniform, no matter from what organism derived. A minute (thousandths of a microgram), sublethal dose injected intravenously into a rabbit produces a sharp rise in temperature after 15 to 30 minutes; an hour later the fever abates. There is also initial leukopenia, and the white cell count then

Table 8–9   Toxicity of Various Bacterial, Animal, and Plant Toxins for the Mouse*

Toxin	Lethal Dose (mg.)
Salmonella typhosa endotoxin	0.1
Shigella dysenteriae endotoxin	0.1
Rattlesnake venom	0.007
Diphtheria exotoxin	0.006
Ricin (from castor bean)	0.002
Yersinia pestis toxin	0.000,7
Clostridium perfringens α-toxin	0.000,05
Cobra venom	0.000,02
Tetanus exotoxin	0.000,000,1
Botulinum A exotoxin	0.000,000,03

*Based upon data in van Heyningen, 1950. *Bacterial Toxins.* Oxford, Blackwell Scientific Publications.

increases as the body temperature drops. A larger dose of endotoxin may induce two fever episodes, the second occurring shortly after the first peak and persisting another 4 to 6 hours. This has been attributed to release of a pyrogen from leukocytes damaged by the endotoxin. A lethal dose of endotoxin produces irreversible shock, which is fatal within 24 hours. The animal becomes weak and lethargic, refuses food and water, may have profound hypothermia or continued high fever, and profuse diarrhea. Intestinal hemorrhage is evident at autopsy, but no other noteworthy damage is apparent. Endotoxin produces similar effects in many animal species, including man.

The "classic" exotoxin, such as that of diphtheria, tetanus, and botulism, is highly antigenic, inducing the formation of antitoxin that neutralizes toxin according to the so-called law of multiple proportions; that is, if x units of antitoxin neutralize y units of toxin, $10x$ units of antitoxin will neutralize $10y$ units of toxin.

Endotoxin is moderately to highly antigenic, and the antibody produced can combine with the endotoxin, probably with the polysaccharide moiety, but does not completely neutralize the toxicity, which is associated with the lipid portion. A mixture of endotoxin with any amount of homologous antibody is therefore somewhat toxic for experimental animals. The same antibody solution, however, may strongly agglutinate the bacteria from which the endotoxin was secured.

CHEMICAL PROPERTIES OF EXOTOXINS

Most toxins lose their toxicity when heated to 60° C. for a few minutes but do not necessarily lose their ability to induce antitoxin formation. Detoxified but still antigenic toxin is called *toxoid*.

Toxoid formation results from simple aging of most toxin solutions in the refrigerator and occurs more rapidly at room temperature. Formaldehyde also converts exotoxins into toxoids. Only toxic groups are affected by this conversion; the ability to produce antibodies and to unite with antitoxin remains unaltered. Diphtheria toxin can be detoxified by ketene, an acetylating agent that combines with free amino groups, and by iodine, diazo compounds, ascorbic acid, and various other compounds. The chemical and physical changes that accompany toxoid formation are not known, nor have unusual radicals or configurations that might account for the extreme toxicity of botulinum or of any other toxin been found.

MODE OF ACTION OF TOXINS

It was formerly believed, probably because investigations were carried out with crude impure materials, that injections of exotoxins produced toxic symptoms only after several hours, no matter how large the dose of toxin. The incubation period following injection of tetanus toxin into mice was stated to be at least 8 hours, during which toxin was bound by susceptible cells. However, with a highly purified crystalline tetanus toxin, the incubation period can be varied almost at will by regulating the size of the dose (Table 8–10).

Toxins combine with some constituent of susceptible tissue. Lipid extracts neutralize certain toxins, so lipids are believed to play a role in susceptibility to those agents. The affinity of tetanus toxin for nerve tissue was very early demonstrated. When a mixture of toxin and toxoid is stirred with brain tissue and filtered, only toxoid is present in the filtrate. The active substance in brain tissue is a ganglioside.

A lethal dose of diphtheria toxin is neutralized by a small amount of antitoxin if the two are mixed before injection. If the toxin is injected first and the antitoxin a few minutes later, many thousand times as much antitoxin may be insufficient to prevent death. This shows that toxin is neutralized in vivo in the blood or body fluids and not in the cells, and it demonstrates the affinity of diphtheria toxin for susceptible tissue.

Table 8–10   *Relationship between the Dose of Crystalline Tetanus Toxin*
and the Time Required for Onset of Symptoms and Death
of White Swiss Mice*

M.L.D.	Onset of Symptoms	Death
500,000	35 min.	1 hr.
100,000	1 hr.	2 hrs.
10,000	4 hrs.	10–15 hrs.
10	15 hrs.	30–48 hrs.
1	30 hrs.	90–96 hrs.

*From Pillemer and Wartman, 1937. J. Immunol., 55:277.

There is no single mechanism by which exotoxins exert their destructive effects. Botulinum toxin appears to affect peripheral motor nerve endings by interfering with the formation and/or release of acetylcholine; death is attributed to respiratory paralysis. The peripheral action of tetanus toxin seems to be twofold: (a) spasm caused by stimulation of the neuromuscular junctions in voluntary muscles and (b) paralysis similar to that caused by botulinum toxin. Brain and spinal cord tissues of animals injected with tetanus toxin display no significant histologic changes. Diphtheria exotoxin causes local necrosis at the site where it is produced (in disease) or injected, congestion and acute inflammation of heart muscle fibers, inflammation of the adrenals, and degeneration of certain nerves with resulting paralysis. Cell death is attributed to impaired protein synthesis.

Cl. perfringens exotoxin acts directly on the central nervous system and on peripheral arterioles and liberates histamine, adenyl compounds, and a substance that causes slow contraction of involuntary muscles. The α-toxin of this organism was the first exotoxin shown to be an enzyme. It is a lecithinase and is more thermostable than most exotoxins. Its hemolytic, necrotizing, and lethal properties result from its power of splitting lecithin and lecithoprotein complexes, which are important constituents of nearly all animal and vegetable tissues. *Cl. perfringens* lecithinase hydrolyzes lecithin to phosphorylcholine and a diglyceride. It acts more rapidly than most other exotoxins and is neutralized by specific antitoxin. Certain snake venoms, such as cobra venom, contain a different lecithinase whose products of hydrolysis include an unsaturated fatty acid and lysolecithin.

One milligram of type A botulinum toxin contains about 31,000,000 minimal lethal doses for the mouse. It can readily be calculated that one lethal dose consists of 20,000,000 molecules. The mouse possesses about 2,500,000 nerve cells (van Heyningen), which are believed to constitute the susceptible cells. Evidently, therefore, a fatal result is obtained at a concentration of about eight exotoxin molecules per nerve cell. Similar calculations indicate that the fatal dose for the guinea pig is about four molecules per nerve cell.

DETERMINATION OF POTENCY OF EXOTOXINS

The importance of the species of animal in which an exotoxin is assayed is indicated in Table 8–11. The mouse and guinea pig differ in their susceptibility to diphtheria, tetanus, and botulinum toxins, even when the results are expressed on the basis of equal weights of the animals. Some animals, such as dogs and chickens, are extremely resistant to tetanus toxin, whereas humans, guinea pigs, and horses are highly susceptible. Within a species, larger individuals usually tolerate greater amounts of exotoxin. In consequence of the variation between breeds and even individual animals, it is often necessary to inoculate several animals with each dose of

*Table 8–11   Number of Minimum Lethal Doses per Kilogram Body
Weight Contained in 1 mg. Toxin**

Test Animal	Diphtheria Toxin	Tetanus Toxin	Botulinum Toxin
Guinea pig	3,500	1,200,000	1,200,000
Mouse	3.5	200,000	620,000

*From Dubos (Ed.), 1952. Bacterial and Mycotic Infections of Man, 2nd ed. Philadelphia, J. B. Lippincott Company.

toxin. The average outcome may be analyzed and the degree of statistical confidence to be placed in the results can be ascertained.

The route of administration of toxins is often important. Unlike most other exotoxins, botulinum toxin is highly toxic by mouth, partly because the toxicity is not destroyed by proteolytic enzymes. Tetanus toxin is often introduced intramuscularly in animal experimentation, diphtheria toxin is usually administered by subcutaneous injection, and certain other toxins are given intravenously.

The reactions produced by exotoxin depend upon the kind of toxin, dosage, and route of inoculation. The time at which symptoms appear usually varies inversely with the dosage. The relationship between dosage of tetanus toxin and the time of death of mice is illustrated in Table 8–12. Very small doses may produce only local symptoms or no clinical signs whatever. Ipsen derived an equation and curve that relate the death times of mice with the dosage of tetanus toxin injected (Figure 8–12).

The results presented in Table 8–12 and Figures 8–12 and 8–13 illustrate "graded responses" to a toxic agent. Graded response may also be expressed in terms of areas of necrosis, degrees of paralysis, or other measurable reactions. Evaluation of a graded response requires the establishment of some arbitrary limit or end point. Most mice injected with fatal doses of tetanus toxin die within 5 days. This is a convenient time interval, feasible in ordinary laboratory practice, and it has been widely adopted as the period of observation. Shorter or longer periods of observation are used with other animals and other toxins. A common unit determined at such an end point is the *minimum lethal dose* (M.L.D.), defined as the smallest amount of toxin that will kill a given animal species within a certain interval after inoculation. The route of injection and weight of the animal are usually specified. If more than one animal is tested with each dose, all should die in the group that receives the M.L.D.

The tetanus toxin tested in the experiment shown in Table 8–12 and Figure 8–13 had a lethal dose at the 5-day (120-hour) observation between 0.01 mg. and 0.02 mg. The value of injecting several animals instead of only one or two with each dose is

*Table 8–12   Death Times of Mice Injected with Various
Amounts of Tetanus Toxin**

Toxin per 20-gram Mouse	Death Times (hours)
0.0025 mg.	S, S, S, S, S, S, S, S†
0.0050 mg.	66, 114, 138, 138, S, S, S, S,
0.0100 mg.	53, 66, 66, 66, 66, 87, 119, S
0.0200 mg.	42, 42, 58, 58, 58, 58, 58, 66
0.0400 mg.	42, 42, 42, 42, 42, 42, 42, 66
0.0800 mg.	31, 31, 31, 31, 31, 31, 42, 42

*Eight mice injected intramuscularly with each dose of toxin.
†S = survived.

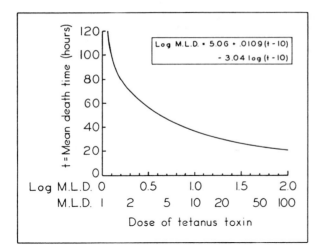

Figure 8–12. Correlation between dose of tetanus toxin and mean death times of mice. (Adapted from Ipsen, 1951. J. Immunol., 66:687.)

obvious, because the variation in times of death among animals that received the same dose was greater than 100 per cent in some cases.

Many investigators prefer to express toxicity in LD_{50} units. The LD_{50} is the dose of toxin required to kill 50 per cent of a group of animals within a specified period. The experimental results often do not contain a group in which exactly half the animals died, but the dosage that would be expected to produce this result can be estimated or calculated by various methods. The simplest procedure is to estimate the 50 per cent end point from a graph of the experimental results. If the data are plotted on semilogarithmic paper, with amounts of toxins on the logarithmic scale, it is often possible to read the LD_{50} to two significant figures. In the experiment recorded in Figure 8–13, the LD_{50} of the tetanus toxin appeared to be 0.0066 mg.

A method that gives a moderately accurate estimate of the LD_{50} is based upon data smoothed by cumulation of survivals and deaths before calculation of percentage mortality. Often attributed to Reed and Muench, who devised a similar procedure, the method was actually worked out by Dragstedt and Behrens. It is illustrated in Table 8–13. On the assumption that animals surviving the largest dose of toxic agent will also survive smaller doses, the survivors are cumulated successively, beginning with the largest dose. Likewise, based on the opposite assumption, deaths are cumulated successively, beginning with the smallest dose. The percentage mortality produced by

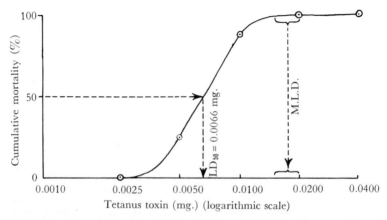

Figure 8–13. Sigmoid "graded response" curve showing the relation between dose of tetanus toxin and cumulative percentage mortality of mice at 120 hours (data from Table 8–12).

Table 8–13 *Calculation of LD$_{50}$ of Tetanus Toxin by the Dragstedt-Behrens Method**

Dose (mg.)	Results in 5 Days		Cumulative		Per Cent Mortality
	LIVED	DIED	LIVED	DIED	
0.0025	8	0	15	0	0
0.0050	6	2	7	2	22
0.0100	1	7	1	9	90
0.0200	0	8	0	17	100
0.0400	0	8	0	25	100
0.0800	0	8	0	32	100

$$\log \text{LD}_{50} = \log 0.0050 + \left(\frac{50 - 22}{90 - 22}\right) \times \log 2$$

$$= \overline{3}.699 + (0.412)(0.301)$$

$$= \overline{3}.823$$

$$\text{LD}_{50} = 0.0067 \text{ mg.}$$

*Data from Table 8–12.

each dose is then calculated from these figures. The LD$_{50}$ of the toxin illustrated is obviously between 0.0050 mg. and 0.0100 mg., and since a logarithmic series of doses was used, it is appropriate to use logarithmic calculation. The factor log 2 is employed because each dose was double the one before. If succeeding doses had increased by a factor of five, log 5 would have been used. The result obtained, 0.0067 mg., is almost identical with that derived from the graphical method. These data are unusually favorable for this type of calculation, because the dose-response curve is nearly symmetrical. With poorer data there is likely to be considerable discrepancy between the results of various methods of estimation or calculation.

The relative numerical values of the M.L.D. and LD$_{50}$ depend upon the steepness of the dose-response curve, that is, the range of dosages through which only a fraction of the animals in a group die. The LD$_{50}$ is usually favored because it gives a sharper end point. It is more expensive, however, because more animals are required, although after sufficient experience with a given type of toxic material the investigator may be able to determine the LD$_{50}$ by testing only three dosages that bracket this end point, if the results fall on a straight line when plotted graphically. Workers involved in preparation of biologic products for human use find that the M.L.D. or 100 per cent end point is as satisfactory for their purposes and in some applications provides an additional slight margin of safety. It is usually recommended that critical tests be made with at least two animals per dosage to reduce the chance of misleading results caused by faulty injections or animal variation.

Antitoxins

PREPARATION AND PURIFICATION

Antitoxin is produced by immunizing animals with toxin or toxoid. The procedure for preparing toxin is, in part, determined by the nature of the organism, that is, its nutrient, temperature, and other cultural requirements. The conditions for toxin formation are sometimes more rigorous than those for bacterial growth. The diphtheria organism, for example, produces toxin only in a neutral or alkaline medium and in the presence of a *very small* amount of iron; moreover, the strain of *C. diphtheriae* must be lysogenic—that is, harbor a temperate bacteriophage growing in an essentially commensal relationship. Synthetic media that yield toxin of high titer offer the important advantage that less purification of the toxin is necessary to reduce undesirable side reactions.

After maximum development of toxin, the bacterial cells are removed by centrifugation or filtration. The toxin may be concentrated by precipitation and is titrated so that sublethal doses can be given during the early injections. Toxin is also converted into toxoid by incubation with 0.2 to 0.5 per cent formaldehyde for several days or weeks at 35 to 37° C.

The choice of animal for production of antitoxin to be used in humans is dictated by several factors. The horse is often used commercially, because large amounts of serum can be obtained, but rabbits, guinea pigs, and other laboratory animals can be used for experimental work. An important factor is the possibility of a dangerous reaction in the recipient. Any antitoxic preparation possesses the specific serum proteins of the animal from which it is derived. An individual receiving antitoxin prepared in horses may become sensitized to horse serum proteins, so that subsequent injection of horse antitoxin induces anaphylactic shock. Purification of antitoxin greatly reduces the possibility of untoward reactions. Antisera from animals other than the horse are sometimes given to individuals sensitive to horse proteins. Cattle and goat sera have been employed, and even rabbit serum, although the latter is very expensive to manufacture.

Among individuals of any given species there is wide variation in antibody producing power. Some laboratories select animals by preliminary trial. Each of a considerable group of animals is given a single injection of toxin or toxoid or a short course of injections. Several weeks or months later an additional injection is given, and blood samples are taken after another 10 to 14 days. The antitoxic potency of these samples is determined, and only those animals are selected for further injection whose sera possess the highest titers.

Diphtheria antitoxin is usually produced by injections of diphtheria toxoid; tetanus and botulinum antitoxins are produced by injections of the corresponding toxins and/or toxoids. Toxoids are preferred if they yield satisfactory antitoxin because larger doses of antigenic material can be administered with safety. Early injections of certain toxins, such as type B botulinum, produce severe reactions. In these cases immunization begins with a series of toxoid injections, followed by toxin when the animal has developed some antitoxin.

Tetanus antitoxin is produced in relatively young horses. These are first given injections of tetanus toxoid, followed later by increasing amounts of toxin at 3-day intervals, until a dose of 100,000 guinea pig M.L.D. is reached. After a rest period, toxin containing aluminum potassium sulfate is administered, beginning with 5,000 M.L.D. and increasing rapidly at 4-day intervals. Trial titrations are made, and large bleedings are started when the serum contains 700 to 800 antitoxic units per ml. Blood is drawn 7 days after the last injection, and 9 L. may be secured at a time. Four or five additional injections of toxin at 4-day intervals are followed by further bleeding. This process is repeated until the titer drops below 500 units per ml. Horses have been known to continue producing potent antitoxin for years.

Blood is collected in citrate and stored in a cold room, and the supernatant plasma is removed after the cells have settled. This crude antitoxin contains nonantitoxic proteins, such as fibrinogen and albumins, together with salts, lipids, and other materials. The antitoxin is principally pseudoglobulin. Fibrinogen and euglobulin are precipitated by 29 per cent saturation with ammonium sulfate and heat. The precipitate is removed, and the solution is treated with additional ammonium sulfate to 48 per cent saturation, whereupon pseudoglobulins precipitate, leaving albumins and other materials in solution. The precipitate containing antitoxin is dialyzed in cellophane bags against running water to remove ammonium sulfate, made isotonic with sodium chloride, treated with a preservative, and stored. During the first few months in the refrigerator some loss of potency occurs, but the final product is relatively stable. It is then filtered to remove any bacteria, tested for sterility, and its antitoxic activity is titrated.

Pepsin digestion of plasma proteins sometimes precedes ammonium sulfate fractionation. This treatment does not affect the antitoxic power of the plasma but greatly reduces its ability to produce undesirable side reactions. Pepsin removes a major portion of the Fc region of the antitoxin molecule, leaving the Fab, which contains the specific antitoxin combining sites.

STANDARDIZATION OF ANTITOXINS

If antitoxin is mixed with toxin in suitable proportions, the toxicity of the latter is neutralized, and the mixture is harmless when injected into an experimental animal. However, exotoxins are so unstable that they cannot be used as permanent standards for the assay of antitoxins. Antitoxins, on the contrary, are extremely stable under proper conditions of storage (see Table 8–14). A standard diphtheria antitoxin has been maintained in the National Institutes of Health since 1905, and a preparation of tetanus antitoxin since 1907. Standardized antitoxins are supplied to qualified laboratories for use as reference in determining the potency of new lots of antitoxin and for control purposes by governmental agencies.

The strength of antitoxins is expressed in arbitrary units whose value differs from one kind of antitoxin to another. The official unit of diphtheria antitoxin in the United States is the amount contained in 1/6000 g. of a certain dried unconcentrated horse serum antitoxin. The official standard unit of tetanus antitoxin in this country is the amount contained in 0.00015 g. of a particular horse serum antitoxin. The international unit of tetanus antitoxin is one-half the amount of the American unit.

The response of animals to injection of mixtures of toxin and antitoxin depends upon the proportions in which the two reagents are mixed. Excess toxin causes characteristic symptoms and death, whereas excess antitoxin completely protects against visible reaction. The most convenient end point is the same as that employed in titrating the corresponding exotoxins: for example, death of all or a certain percentage of the animals within a specified period. Parallel tests employing a constant amount of a given exotoxin preparation and varying amounts of standard and unknown antitoxins permit determination of the antitoxic potency of the unknown.

Titration of a tetanus antitoxin in mice is illustrated in Table 8–15. The observation

Table 8–14   Effect of Storage Temperature on Potency of Antitoxin*†

Temperature	Loss of Potency in 12 Months
0–5° C.	0%
15° C.	9%
22° C.	11%
30° C.	20%
37° C.	60%

*From Glenny: Active immunization with toxin. In A System of Bacteriology in Relation to Medicine (Medical Research Council), 1931, Vol. 6, p. 106. London, H. M. Stationery Office. By permission of the Controller of Her Britannic Majesty's Stationery Office.

†Antitoxin preserved with 0.3% cresol.

Table 8–15   *Comparison of Standard and Unknown Tetanus*
Antitoxins in Mice*†

	Antitoxin (1:10)	Toxin	Results			
			1 day	2 days	3 days	4 days
Standard	0.12 ml.	0.14 mg.	−	−	?	±‡
antitoxin	0.11 ml.	0.14 mg.	−	±	+	++
(10 units/ml.)	**0.10 ml.**	**0.14 mg.**	±	+	+++	**D**
	0.09 ml.	0.14 mg.	+	++	D	
	0.08 ml.	0.14 mg.	++	D		

	Antitoxin (1:400)	Toxin	Results			
			1 day	2 days	3 days	4 days
Antitoxin 3903	0.12 ml.	0.14 mg.	−	−	−	−
(x units/ml.)	0.11 ml.	0.14 mg.	−	−	−	±
	0.10 ml.	0.14 mg.	−	±	+	++
	0.09 ml.	**0.14 mg.**	±	++	+++	**D**
	0.08 ml.	0.14 mg.	+	+++	D	

Calculation:
    Standard antitoxin diluted 1:10 contains 1 unit/ml.
    0.09 ml. antitoxin 3903 diluted 1:400 ≡ 0.10 unit
    0.09 ml. antitoxin 3903 undiluted ≡ 400 × 0.10 = 40 units
    1.0 ml. antitoxin 3903 undiluted ≡ 40/0.09 = 444 units

*From Regamey, 1947. Bull. Serv. Féd. Hyg. Publ., 17:1.

†Toxin-antitoxin mixtures were diluted with buffer to a total volume of 0.4 ml. After one-half hour, mice were injected subcutaneously. The end point in this experiment was death on the fourth day.

‡+ signs indicate severity of symptoms; D indicates death.

period in this experiment was limited to 4 days, and dosages of antitoxin that protected against death until the fourth day were compared in order to calculate the number of units per milliliter contained in the unknown antitoxin No. 3903. The standard antitoxin diluted 1:10 contained 1 unit per ml., and 0.10 unit protected against 0.14 mg. of toxin. Equal protection was afforded by 0.09 ml. of antitoxin 3903 diluted 1:400. Undiluted antitoxin 3903, therefore, contained 444 units per ml.

The *test dose* of tetanus toxin is the least amount that, when combined with 0.1 unit of antitoxin, kills a 20-gram mouse within 5 days. It may be a few hundred to a few thousand times greater than the minimum lethal dose. An amount of diphtheria toxin, called the L+ dose, employed for a similar purpose, is defined as the smallest amount of toxin that, when combined with one unit of diphtheria antitoxin, kills a 250-gram guinea pig in 4 to 5 days.

The official test animal for final titration of both tetanus and diphtheria antitoxins in the United States is the guinea pig. Mouse titrations of tetanus toxin and antitoxin are increasingly used, particularly abroad, because they appear to give equivalent results and are somewhat less expensive.

Römer observed in 1909 that a very small dose (1/500 to 1/250 M.L.D.) of diphtheria toxin inoculated intracutaneously into guinea pigs produced a mild local reaction consisting of swelling and erythema. Slightly larger doses induced definite necrosis within 48 hours. Mixture of the toxin with an adequate amount of antitoxin before injection prevented any sign of local reaction. When insufficient antitoxin was employed, the area of erythematous swelling and necrosis was directly proportional to the amount of free toxin in the mixture. These principles form the basis of the Römer titration of diphtheria antitoxin. The amount of toxin employed (L_r dose) produces a minimal skin reaction when mixed with 1/20 or 1/500 unit of antitoxin and injected intracutaneously into a guinea pig or rabbit. Standard and unknown antitoxic sera are compared in the same animal, a procedure that reduces the variation inherent in the use of several animals for a biologic titration. The test is highly sensitive and has been used to titrate minute amounts of either antitoxin or toxin in blood, milk, and other secretions. As little as 1/50,000 unit of diphtheria antitoxin can be detected in 0.1 ml. of serum.

Inasmuch as exotoxins are proteins, it is not surprising that it was reported very early (Danysz, 1902) that flocculation occurs in nearly neutral mixtures with homologous antitoxin. The Ramon (1922) method of titrating antitoxin consists of mixing varying amounts of antitoxin and a constant amount of toxin and incubating in a waterbath at 44 to 46° C., with frequent observation. The mixture that flocculates first is approximately neutral when tested by animal inoculation. Mixtures containing less antitoxin are toxic to animals, and those containing more antitoxin produce no symptoms.

The antitoxin titer of an unknown serum is determined with reference to a known antitoxin. Homologous toxin is standardized against the known antitoxin by flocculation, and this standardized toxin is then tested with the unknown serum. A sample protocol illustrating the flocculation of tetanus toxin and antitoxin is shown in Table 8–16. Flocculation appeared first in the tube containing 0.15 ml. of antitoxin, the strength of which was 500 units per ml. The unit of toxin measured by this procedure is called the *Lf dose*, which is the amount of toxin flocculating most rapidly with one unit of antitoxin. The Lf content of a toxin is calculated as follows:

$$\text{Lf/ml. toxin} = \frac{\text{Antitoxin units/ml.} \times \text{ml. of antitoxin}}{\text{ml. of toxin}}$$

Flocculation of toxin and antitoxin is analogous to precipitation of a protein antigen by its antibody. It is a test of combining power and is independent of toxicity. The Lf value of a toxin solution does not decrease as its toxicity diminishes with age or with chemical conversion to the toxoid state. The Lf value is therefore more directly related to antigenicity than is the M.L.D. and is useful as an in vitro indication of the potency of toxoids employed in immunization.

An interesting application of optimal proportions in the precipitation of toxin by antitoxin is the Elek in vitro virulence test for diphtheria bacteria. A narrow strip of sterile filter paper soaked in diphtheria antitoxin is covered with agar medium in a Petri dish. The hardened agar is streaked at a 90° angle to the length of the paper strip with

Table 8–16 Flocculation of Tetanus Toxin and Antitoxin*

Antitoxin (500 u./ml.)	0.13 ml.	0.14 ml.	0.15 ml.	0.16 ml.	0.17 ml.
Toxin	2.0 ml.	2.0 ml.	2.0 ml.	2.0 ml.	2.0 ml.
4 min.	Op†	Op	Cl	Cl	Op
8 min.	Cl	Cl	Cl	Cl	Cl
12 min.	Cl	Cl	Fl	Cl	Cl
14 min.	Fl	Fl	Fl	Fl	Fl

Calculation:
    500 × 0.15 ÷ 2.0 = 37.5 Lf/ml. toxin
    1 Lf toxin = 1/37.5 = 0.0267 ml.

*Incubation at 46° C.
†Op = opalescent; Cl = cloudy; Fl = flocculent.

the cultures under test. Antitoxin diffusing from the paper encounters toxin diffusing at a right angle to it from the streak of growth. A narrow line of precipitate forms where the ratio of antitoxin to toxin is optimal (Figure 8–14).

Mechanism of Reaction Between Toxin and Antitoxin

THE DANYSZ PHENOMENON

Danysz (1902) discovered that the toxicity for animals of a mixture of toxin and antitoxin depends upon the manner in which the reagents are mixed as well as upon their relative final concentrations. An amount of toxin can be determined that is just completely neutralized by a given quantity of antitoxin if the toxin is added in a single dose. This mixture produces no symptoms in an experimental animal. A mixture composed of the same amount of toxin added to the antitoxin in two or more portions at intervals of 15 minutes is highly toxic when injected. This toxic mixture, after standing several days, reverts to a nontoxic condition, evidently by dissociation and recombination. Toxin and antitoxin combine in varying proportions, depending upon the ratio in which they are mixed. The resulting complexes slowly dissociate. The first portion of toxin added to antitoxin in the Danysz experiment combines with more antitoxin than would be expected from its proportion in a neutral mixture. Therefore, insufficient free antitoxin remains to combine with all the toxin added a short time later, so the mixture is toxic. It has also been found that a neutral mixture containing equivalent amounts of toxin and antitoxin (TA) can combine with another equivalent of antitoxin during subsequent incubation.

Quantitative data clearly demonstrating combination in variable proportions are presented in Table 8–17. A constant amount of antitoxin was mixed with various amounts of toxin, and the precipitates were analyzed for nitrogen. Tests of the supernates indicated whether all of each reagent had combined and which was in excess. The precipitated antitoxin nitrogen was calculated by difference, and the ratios of antitoxin nitrogen to toxin nitrogen were determined. No precipitate formed in the

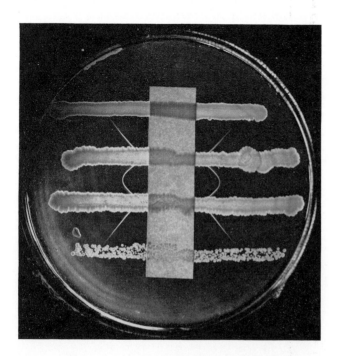

Figure 8–14. In vitro test for virulence. Serum agar covers a strip of filter paper saturated with diphtheria antitoxin. The agar was then inoculated at a right angle to the paper with strains of Corynebacterium. A thin line of precipitate formed when antitoxin diffusing from the paper met toxin diffusing from the growth in proper concentration. (From specimens prepared by Miss Elizabeth O. King. Photo courtesy U. S. Public Health Service, Communicable Disease Center, Atlanta, Ga.)

Table 8–17 Quantitative Analyses of Diphtheria Toxin-Antitoxin Precipitates*†

Toxin		Nitrogen Ppted.		Ratio: Antitoxin N Toxin N	Excess in Supernate
LF UNITS	NITROGEN (MG.)	TOTAL (MG.)	ANTITOXIN (MG.)		
50	0.023	0.000			Antitoxin (63%)
100	0.046	0.000			Antitoxin (32%)
150	0.069	0.386			Antitoxin
175	0.081	0.554	0.473	5.8	Antitoxin‡
200	0.092	0.564	0.472	5.1	Neither
225	0.103	0.579	0.476	4.6	Neither
300	0.138	0.612	0.474	3.4	Neither
400	0.184	0.661	0.477	2.6	Toxin‡
450	0.207	0.652			Toxin‡
500	0.230	0.359			Toxin (20%)
600	0.276	0.000			Toxin (40%)

*From Pappenheimer and Robinson, 1937. J. Immunol., 32:291.
†Antitoxin: 1 ml. containing 300 units.
‡Traces, detectable by the rabbit intracutaneous test.

region of great antitoxin excess. Partial combination was indicated by flocculation tests of the supernates, which showed the presence of 32 to 63 per cent of the antitoxin originally provided. Mixtures in the region of great toxin excess likewise did not precipitate completely and contained uncombined toxin amounting to 20 to 40 per cent of the quantity employed.

The precipitated antitoxin nitrogen was constant at about 0.474 mg. throughout most of the zone of complete precipitation, although the toxin in the precipitates varied from 175 to nearly 400 Lf units. The ratios of antitoxin nitrogen to toxin nitrogen in the precipitates therefore varied from about 6.0 to 2.5.

RELATION BETWEEN L+ AND L_0 DOSES OF TOXIN

Ehrlich designated as the L_0 dose of toxin the largest amount that, when combined with one unit of antitoxin, fails to produce a toxic reaction in the test animal. The L+ dose of toxin is the smallest amount that, when mixed with one unit of antitoxin, kills the test animal in a specified time interval. It might be anticipated that the difference between the L+ and L_0 doses is 1 M.L.D. Actually, however, it is usually between 10 and 100 M.L.D. It is evident that complexes form containing a higher proportion of toxin than at the neutral point. Although these complexes dissociate slowly to yield traces of free toxin, considerable excess of toxin must be added before there will be sufficient free toxin to kill the test animal within the usual 4- to 5-day observation period.

NEUTRALIZATION OF TOXINS BY ANTITOXINS

The fact that antitoxins neutralize homologous toxins is undisputed. The mechanism by which they do so is not known. Union with antitoxin does not permanently change toxin, as demonstrated by the recovery of diphtheria toxin from toxin-antitoxin floccules in a high state of purity and with high toxicity and combining power. It has been suggested that antitoxin "covers the toxin," and steric hindrance prevents it from coming into contact with susceptible tissue. It may also be postulated that antitoxin induces a reversible allosteric effect that inhibits the usual pharmacologic activity of the toxin. This hypothesis is especially attractive with reference to toxins whose mode of action is enzymatic or anti-enzymatic.

In Vivo Uses of Toxins, Toxoids, and Antitoxins

TESTS OF ANTITOXIC IMMUNITY

Schick discovered that a minute amount of diphtheria toxin injected intracutaneously into nonimmune persons caused erythema and edema around the site of inoculation, whereas immune individuals usually gave no reaction. The Schick test employs 0.1 ml. of toxin containing 1/50 of a guinea pig M.L.D. The reaction is read after 24 to 48 hours and at the end of a week. A positive zone of erythema and edema is sometimes as large as 3 cm. in diameter. A control injection of toxin heated at 60° C. for 15 minutes is used to detect allergic sensitization to diphtheria cellular proteins. Slight inflammation, no more than 3.0 mm. in diameter, may appear at the control site. No reaction at either site constitutes a negative test. Diluted toxoid substituted for the heated toxin control (Moloney test) detects sensitivity to toxoid that might cause severe reactions in routine immunization. These reactions are more common in adults than in children up to the age of 15 years.

A positive Schick test indicates lack of immunity to diphtheria. A negative test shows the presence of antitoxin that combines with the injected toxin. The "Schick level" of immunity is considered to represent between 1/100 and 1/30 unit of antitoxin per milliliter of blood and appears to be sufficient to protect the great majority of individuals. The disease usually runs a milder course in the small percentage of Schick negatives who do contract diphtheria than in Schick positives.

The Dick test of immunity to scarlet fever is similar to the Schick test. One-tenth milliliter of properly diluted scarlet fever toxin is injected intracutaneously. A positive reaction, indicating lack of immunity, consists of a circumscribed area of erythema at least 1 cm. in diameter, developing within 16 to 24 hours and fading rather rapidly. Heated toxin is injected as a control.

A positive Dick reaction does not develop in nonimmune persons injected with a mixture of Dick toxin and serum from convalescent scarlet fever patients. Schultz and Charlton found that convalescent serum injected intradermally into a scarlet fever patient caused local blanching of the typical red rash of the disease. This became the basis of the Schultz-Charlton test, sometimes used to distinguish scarlet fever from German measles and other rash-producing infections with which it may be confused. Convalescent serum or horse antitoxin is injected into an area with a bright red rash, and blanching occurs in most positive cases between 6 and 14 hours later over an area from one-half inch to several inches in diameter. The reaction usually persists throughout the duration of the rash. It is considered to be a true toxin-antitoxin reaction in vivo.

ACTIVE IMMUNIZATION

Toxoid is the most widely employed immunizing agent against diphtheria. It is especially useful in young children, in whom it usually produces no severe reactions. Individuals beyond the age of 10 or 12 years may be hypersensitive to other diphtheria bacterial constituents or to toxoid itself. Immunization of such persons poses a problem that is met only in part by the use of highly purified materials. Toxoid has the advantages that it is nontoxic and cannot revert to a toxic condition, is unaffected by aging or by heat to a temperature of 65° C., and can be used in relatively high concentrations. Three injections are desirable, consisting of 0.5-, 1.0- and 1.0-ml. amounts at intervals of 2 to 3 weeks. About 95 per cent of individuals become Schick-negative after the usual course of injections.

Precipitation by alum is generally considered to yield a more highly immunogenic agent. Toxoid is precipitated by 1 to 2 per cent alum, and the precipitate, washed and resuspended in saline (A.P.T.), is administered subcutaneously. Two doses a month apart usually produce an adequate response. Alum-precipitated toxoid is retained in the tissues longer than fluid toxoid, the antigenic component being released slowly over a period of weeks. The alum incites an inflammatory response at the site of injection, which is believed to induce more effective antitoxin formation. Alum-precipitated toxoid, either alone or combined with pertussis vaccine and tetanus toxoid, is employed in infants and young children, in whom the advantage of reducing the number of injections is obvious.

Toxin-antitoxin mixtures are sometimes used for active immunization and may cause less severe reactions than toxoid. Three injections of 1.0 ml. are given at intervals of 1 to 2 weeks. Antitoxin develops gradually, and the Schick reaction may remain positive for 6 months or longer. Slow dissociation within the body releases toxin, which stimulates active immunization. An important disadvantage of toxin-antitoxin is the possible development of hypersensitivity to the horse serum components of the antitoxin.

The duration of immunity against diphtheria following artificial active immunization is considered to be less than 5 years. Although circulating antitoxin may disappear, the capacity of such an individual to respond to further antigenic stimulus may remain high for years or for life. Even the small amount of toxin used in the Schick test often constitutes an effective "booster" dose for previously immunized persons. Inapparent infections in previously immunized persons also constitute important secondary stimuli to antitoxin production and assist in maintenance of a satisfactory state of resistance.

It is to be expected that some cases will occur in artificially immunized individuals who, according to the results of all known tests, should be immune. The size of the infecting dose, the virulence and serologic properties of the organisms, and factors associated with the host may outweigh the results of the immunization procedure. On the whole, however, fewer cases occur in immunized persons, and those that do occur are usually less severe.

Immunity against tetanus is almost entirely associated with circulating antitoxin and with the heightened tissue reactivity resulting from active immunization. Individuals are born with no more than a weak, temporary, passive immunity to tetanus, and they do not acquire active immunity naturally. Subclinical immunizing infections do not occur, as they do in diphtheria. A case of the disease from which the patient recovers does not necessarily lead to immunity; second and even third attacks have been reported. Spontaneous recovery appears to be caused by light infection and fortuitous circumstances rather than by active immunization.

The only recommended immunizing agent against tetanus is toxoid. Tetanus toxoid is even less irritating than diphtheria toxoid and can be used in relatively enormous amounts equivalent to several thousand guinea pig M.L.D. of toxin. The practice of the United States Army during World War II was to administer three doses of 1.0 ml. each at intervals of 3 to 4 weeks, followed by a single stimulating dose of 1.0 ml. after 1 year and an emergency booster dose upon the occurrence of a wound or other injury that might result in tetanus. The effectiveness of this procedure is indicated by the occurrence of only 15 cases of tetanus among over 2,500,000 wounded men in the U.S. armed forces—and 9 of these had not received the scheduled full immunization. The case rate during World War I was 13.4 per 100,000 wounded men.

Two to 3 weeks after the first three injections of tetanus toxoid, the majority of individuals possess a protective level of circulating antitoxin. A stimulating dose some months later increases the titer to far higher levels, which are maintained longer, and repeated booster injections induce more striking responses. Periodic injections of toxoid at intervals of 5 to 10 years thereafter maintain a protective antitoxic level.

Table 8–18   *Diphtheria Antitoxin Necessary to Save Rabbits Given 10 Fatal Doses of Toxin Intravenously**

Interval Between Administration of Toxin and Antitoxin	Therapeutic Dose of Antitoxin
10 min.	5 A. U.
20 min.	200 A. U.
30 min.	2000 A. U.
45 min.	4000 A. U.
60 min.	5000 A. U.
90 min.	No amount

*From Park and Schroder, 1932. Am. J. Public Health, 22:7.

As a general rule, it is advisable to administer tetanus toxoid in cases of injury and major surgery. If there is doubt that the patient has previously been immunized with toxoid, or if the injury is near or within the central nervous system, tetanus antitoxin should also be given.

PASSIVE IMMUNIZATION

Passive immunization with antitoxin formed in another individual or species is employed prophylactically following exposure to infection and therapeutically if disease is apparent. Prophylactic doses are relatively small, but therapeutic doses must be very large. Antitoxin is more or less effective against diphtheria, tetanus, botulism, gas gangrene, and certain other diseases.

It is important in treating diagnosed cases of disease to administer adequate amounts of antitoxin as quickly as possible. The union between toxins and body cells is firm and undissociable, and tissue damage may be rapidly initiated and irreversible. Nerve destruction is practically irreparable because nerves have much less regenerating capacity than most other tissues. The speed with which diphtheria toxin combines with tissues is indicated by Table 8–18, in which it is shown that a delay of only 50 minutes increased a thousandfold the amount of antitoxin required to save the life of an experimentally injected rabbit, and that after another half hour no amount of antitoxin sufficed. Delay of only a few hours in treating human cases of diphtheria, tetanus, or botulism may make the difference between life and death. Prevention of diphtheria in exposed humans requires only 500 to 2,000 units of antitoxin. After symptoms of disease appear in unprotected individuals, 5,000 units on the first day are more effective than 100,000 units on the fourth or fifth day.

It should be pointed out that almost any immunization procedure, whether passive or active, entails certain elements of risk. Passive immunization with foreign serum subjects the patient to the possibility of allergic reactions, particularly if he has previously received injections of serum from the same species. An intradermal test with diluted serum will indicate whether the antiserum can be safely administered.

Additional Sources of Information

Cowan, K. M.: Antibody response to viral antigens. *In* Dixon, F. J., and H. G. Kunkel (Eds.): Advances in Immunology, vol. 17, pp. 195–253, 1973. New York, Academic Press, Inc.

Humphrey, J. H., and R. R. Dourmashkin: The lesions in cell membranes caused by complement. *In* Dixon, F. J., and H. G. Kunkel (Eds.): Advances in Immunology, vol. 11, pp. 75–115, 1969. New York, Academic Press, Inc.

Nelson, D. S.: Macrophages and Immunity. 1969. Amsterdam, North-Holland Publishing Company.

Wheelock, E. F., and S. T. Toy: Participation of lymphocytes in viral infections. *In* Dixon, F. J., and H. G. Kunkel (Eds.): Advanced in Immunology, vol. 16, pp. 124–184, 1973. New York, Academic Press, Inc.

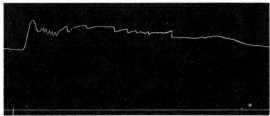

CHAPTER NINE

IN VIVO IMMUNOLOGIC REACTIONS: ANTIBODY-MEDIATED

In vivo reactions between antigen and antibody are difficult to observe directly, particularly with any degree of confidence that lymphoid cells do not also participate in some way. Whereas the process of agglutination in vitro can readily be watched with the microscope and the results of agglutination in the test tube can be observed with the naked eye, it is only assumed that the same reaction occurs in the body—in secretions, blood, lymph, or other fluids. It is postulated that agglutinated bacteria are more rapidly and efficiently ingested by phagocytic cells, but there is little experimental proof that this is actually so.

Similarly, it is assumed that soluble antigenic substances are precipitated when they encounter homologous antibodies in blood, lymph, or various body secretions and that the precipitates are ingested by macrophages or other phagocytic cells. Evidence supporting this hypothesis may be secured by use of antigen or antibody containing radioactive or fluorescent labels whose presence and location in the body can be determined by microscopic or other methods.

The Pfeiffer phenomenon was one of the first antigen-antibody reactions to be studied in vivo. Guinea pigs immunized either actively or passively against *Vibrio cholerae* were challenged by intraperitoneal injection of the organism. Peritoneal fluid was then withdrawn at intervals and examined microscopically; the bacteria soon disappeared from immune but not from control animals.

CYTOTOXICITY

Transfusion Reactions

Transfusion reactions involving the ABH system have been a problem since long before their scientific basis was known (see page 210). In this instance, the presence of the antibodies responsible for intravascular reaction with the donor's erythrocytes is genetically controlled. The consequence of an incompatible transfusion is hemolysis if complement participates; otherwise it is agglutination and possible formation of thrombi and overloading of the reticuloendothelial system.

A comparable situation arises in an Rh negative mother of an Rh positive baby; the mother who becomes immunized against the Rh factor acquires the immunity from fetal erythrocytes that enter her circulation at the time of delivery. If she subsequently bears another Rh positive fetus, placental transfer of Rh antibody may cause hemolytic destruction of fetal blood cells and their replacement by microscopically identifiable immature cells called erythroblasts (see page 214).

Drug Reactions

The essential conditions for antibody-mediated cytotoxicity are the presence of an antigenic determinant on the surface of a body cell of some kind and the concomitant presence of homologous antibody in the circulation. The antigen may be part of the normal cell, as in the foregoing cases, or it may be an antigenic or haptenic substance that has attached to a normal cell, thereby altering its immunologic nature.

Hemolytic anemia is sometimes associated with the continued use of drugs that have an affinity for red blood cells. Phenacetin, chlorpromazine, penicillin, and other drugs may combine with the cell surfaces and incite the formation of antibodies specifically reactive with the drugs. Intravascular hemolysis then occurs, aided by complement. Blood cells or tissue cells that adsorb or otherwise react with antigenic bacterial components may be damaged in vivo when they encounter circulating antibodies against the bacterial constituents.

Thrombocytopenic purpura is a disease in which platelets are destroyed in a similar way. It is characterized by the formation of purple patches on the skin and membranes, hemorrhage from the mucous membranes, and marked decrease in the number of platelets. Platelets react with a drug such as Sedormid (a sedative sometimes used to relieve excitability and mild insomnia) and become antigenic. The antibodies formed react specifically with the drug, and since it is situated on the platelets, the latter are destroyed. This reduces blood clotting activity, so small subcutaneous hemorrhages form.

HYPERSENSITIVITY

In contrast to the foregoing, direct evidence of in vivo humoral antigen-antibody reactions is relatively easy to secure in certain hypersensitivities, including anaphylaxis, various allergies, and local and general complex-mediated reactions, such as the Arthus phenomenon and serum sickness.

Hypersensitivity is a state of increased reactivity to a foreign agent usually acquired by prior exposure to the same or a chemically related substance. The term *allergy* is often used synonymously, although when introduced by von Pirquet in 1906 it had a broader connotation and designated any altered reactivity, decreased as well as increased, to foreign substances. It thus included immunity as well as hypersensitivity. The term allergy is still employed in Europe in this sense, but in the United States it frequently indicates a clinical condition in which humans respond in an exaggerated and often unfavorable manner to an agent that has little, if any, effect on the majority of individuals.

Substances that induce hypersensitivity differ widely in chemical nature. Some are frankly antigenic, such as foreign serum and egg albumin. Others, like plant pollens, possess feeble antigenicity. Still others, like the drugs cited above, are completely nonantigenic per se, but may combine with and alter the specificity of proteins. In view of the heterogeneity of the agents that produce hypersensitivity, the term *allergen* is employed as a general designation.

Sensitization, or induction of the hypersensitive state, requires one or more exposures to the allergen, followed by a latent period. After the latent period, a reaction is elicited by another exposure to the allergen. The nature of the hypersensitivity acquired is determined by the chemical composition of the allergen, the sensitizing route (injection, ingestion, inhalation, and so forth), the physiology and anatomy of the host, and other factors. The specific response observed depends upon the type of hypersensitivity and the mode of contact with the eliciting dose.

Hypersensitivity reactions were originally divided into two categories, immediate and delayed, according to the apparent speed with which a sensitive individual displays a detectable response to the inciting agent. It later became evident that the two types of reaction differ in fundamental mechanism: the former are antibody-mediated, whereas the latter are cell-mediated.

Immediate Hypersensitivities

In immediate-type hypersensitivities, the response usually occurs within minutes after application or absorption of the allergen, although gross effects may not be detectable for hours and may persist several days. Immediate reactions are associated with serum antibodies, and passive sensitization of a normal individual can be accomplished by transfer of serum from a sensitive or an immune individual.

The primary reaction is union of the allergen or antigen with antibody associated via its Fc portion with leukocytes, mast cells, or other cells which have been passively sensitized by antibody produced elsewhere within the same individual or introduced from another individual. Cell damage caused by this reaction may produce characteristic symptoms or may lead to release of pharmacologically active substances, which incite some other harmful response, such as dilatation of blood vessels and contraction of smooth muscles. Succeeding events are determined in part by the location of the affected vessels and muscles.

ANAPHYLAXIS

First Observations. Anaphylaxis was apparently first reported in 1839 by Magendie, who noted the sudden death of animals repeatedly injected with egg albumin. Several other investigators observed a similar phenomenon during the nineteenth century, but no systematic study was made until Richet and his collaborators (1898–1902) rediscovered the phenomenon. They attempted to immunize dogs by repeated injections of eel serum or an extract of sea anemone tentacles, both of which are toxic. When the animals were reinjected about 3 weeks later, even with doses sublethal for a normal animal, they became violently ill and often died. Instead of producing a protective immunity, the series of injections induced an unusually sensitive state in dogs, so that amounts too small to affect normal animals caused rapid death. Since this situation appeared to represent the reverse of prophylaxis, Richet designated it *anaphylaxis*. The reaction is known as anaphylactic shock.

Following a communication by Theobald Smith to Ehrlich in 1905, the guinea pig became the animal of choice for anaphylaxis experiments because it was more easily sensitized and shocked than other common experimental animals. Smith observed that guinea pigs prepared by injections of diphtheria toxin-antitoxin mixtures promptly underwent fatal anaphylactic shock when reinjected several weeks later with normal horse serum. Otto, a student of Ehrlich, found that sensitization was independent of the toxin or antitoxin content of the injected material and was induced by horse serum alone. He also noted that sensitized guinea pigs given a number of very small injections of horse serum withstood subsequent doses that usually produced fatal anaphylaxis. Such animals were said to be in an "anti-anaphylactic" or "desensitized" condition.

Rosenau and Anderson sensitized guinea pigs with as little as 0.000001 ml. of horse serum, although larger amounts gave more consistent results. They also found that anaphylaxis possessed the same specificity as precipitation or other serologic reactions and that sensitivity could be transferred passively from mother to offspring.

It thus became apparent that general anaphylaxis as just described is an in vivo antigen-antibody reaction. It may be defined as the acute systemic response of hypersensitive animals to injection of the material to which they are sensitive. It is principally an experimental phenomenon demonstrated in laboratory animals, although anaphylactic reactions occasionally occur in man. Each species exhibits its own characteristic anaphylactic syndrome.

Active Anaphylaxis. Active anaphylaxis takes place in an animal that is first sensitized by injection of antigen and is later shocked by reinjection of the same antigen. It is contrasted with passive anaphylaxis, in which sensitization is accomplished by transfer of serum from another animal.

Production of active anaphylaxis requires three definite steps: (1) injection of the *sensitizing* antigen, followed by (2) the *incubation* or *latent period* leading to the sensitized state, and finally (3) the *eliciting* or *shocking injection.*

Active sensitivity is induced by any antigenic substance, such as a complete protein or protein complex. The route of administration is relatively immaterial: any parenteral injection may be employed. Intraperitoneal or subcutaneous injections are most often used with guinea pigs. Feeding is not usually successful, although it has been said that about 50 per cent of guinea pigs may be sensitized to certain proteins by this method.

The sensitizing dose depends upon the antigen and the animal. A single injection of a soluble foreign protein suffices for the guinea pig, and the amount may be very small. Customary doses of horse serum range from 0.0001 to 0.25 ml. Egg albumin sensitizes in doses of 0.0001 to 1.0 mg. Guinea pigs are rendered sensitive less easily by means of bacterial proteins, pollens, and some other vegetable proteins, of which preparatory injections on consecutive days are often necessary. Dogs usually require more than one injection of any antigenic substance, and rabbits must almost always be injected repeatedly. Sensitization of mice is most effective when an adjuvant, such as mineral oil and killed mycobacteria (complete Freund adjuvant) or pertussis vaccine, is administered with the first injection of antigen, or the antigen is precipitated with alum; adrenalectomy or ionizing radiations also enhance sensitization.

Following the last sensitizing injection, an incubation period of at least 10 to 21 days must elapse before anaphylactic shock can be demonstrated. Once established, the sensitive state may persist for months or sometimes even years. Mild but definite reactions have been elicited 8 months after sensitization of guinea pigs with horse serum.

The specificity of the anaphylactic reaction is of the same order as that of in vitro serologic tests. Hence, the material used for the shocking injection is the same as or is closely related to that employed for sensitization. Certain separated complex haptens, such as bacterial polysaccharides, elicit typical shock as well as the complete antigen of which the hapten was originally a part. Simple haptens, however, have the reverse effect and specifically inhibit shock following subsequent injection of the original complete antigen or complex hapten. Landsteiner employed anaphylactic methods in studying the specificity of azoprotein antigens (see page 133).

Shocking injections are best given by a route that ensures rapid absorption and almost immediate contact with sensitized cells. For this reason intravenous injections are preferred. The reactions after intraperitoneal injections are usually delayed in onset for 15 to 30 minutes.

The shock dose is generally larger than the sensitizing dose, although not necessarily so. For maximum effect it should provide an appreciable concentration in the blood within a period of 30 to 60 seconds. Guinea pigs sensitive to ovalbumin are shocked by 0.1 to 10.0 mg. of the same material.

Symptom Complex in Anaphylaxis. Certain symptoms of anaphylactic shock are common to almost all animals; these include decreased blood pressure, body temperature, and number of circulating leukocytes, and often decreased blood coagulability. These symptoms appear to be associated with attachment of leukocytes and platelets to the endothelium of small blood vessels, and release of pharmacologically active substances, which produce contraction of smooth muscles, capillary dilatation, and edema. In addition to the foregoing general responses, there are special features by which anaphylactic shock in one species differs from that in another but which are constant within the species.

Within a minute after intravenous administration of an adequate shocking dose to a sensitive guinea pig, the animal becomes restless, its hair bristles, it coughs, kicks, and rubs its nose with its forepaws, and its respiration is slow and labored. Convulsions and death follow, often within 2 to 4 minutes after injection. Immediate postmortem examination reveals the heart still beating and active intestinal peristalsis. The lungs are fully inflated, and there may be evidence of visceral congestion.

In the rabbit, systemic anaphylaxis does not always occur. When fatal shock does take place, the preliminary reaction consists of irregular respiration succeeded by panting. The ears become hyperemic and then blanched. The animal collapses and lies outstretched, gives a few convulsive movements associated with passage of feces and urine, and dies suddenly with head thrown back and eyes protruding. At autopsy the right side of the heart is found greatly dilated, and the inferior vena cava, portal vein, and liver are engorged with blood.

Preliminary signs of anaphylaxis in the dog consist of restlessness and excitement, followed by vomiting and passage of urine and feces, the latter often bloody. The animal then collapses in a state of marked muscular weakness, its respiration is slowed, and it becomes comatose and exhibits epileptiform convulsions. Death may occur in one to several hours. Autopsy discloses that the liver is greatly distended and engorged and often contains as much as 60 per cent of the animal's blood. The animal literally bleeds to death, the blood collecting within the vessels of its own liver, a process accompanied by complete collapse of the systemic vascular system. If shock is prolonged, there may be considerable congestion of the gastrointestinal tract.

The symptoms of anaphylactic shock in these three animals share features referable to the distribution of prominent areas of smooth muscle. The bronchial musculature of the guinea pig and the muscles of the rabbit's pulmonary arterioles are unusually well developed. The principal muscles of the intestines are also of the smooth type. In the guinea pig, death is the result of suffocation, even though the lungs are fully inflated. Contraction of the bronchial muscles prevents exhalation. Coughing is associated with attempts to secure oxygen. Engorgement of the right side of the rabbit heart is caused by contraction of the pulmonary arterioles, which prevents passage of blood through the lung to the left side. Death is attributed to heart failure. Defecation, a common reaction in anaphylaxis, is a consequence of the hyperactivity of the smooth muscle of the intestine wall.

Massive edema contributes to certain symptoms of anaphylactic shock: for example, the occlusion of guinea pig bronchioles. Engorgement of the dog liver during shock, attributed to constriction of the hepatic blood vessels, appears to be caused by edema resulting from dilatation of liver capillaries, which retards the flow of blood through this organ. Manwaring et al. observed that symptoms of anaphylaxis were prevented by excluding the liver from the circulation. Furthermore, by joining the liver of a sensitized dog to the circulation of a normal animal, reactions were induced in the latter when the sensitive dog was shocked. These facts indicated that substances released from the liver during anaphylaxis and distributed throughout the body in the bloodstream stimulate contraction of smooth muscles and cause certain other damage. The active material has been shown to contain histamine, long known as a powerful stimulant of smooth muscle activity. It causes contraction of visceral muscles, dilates capillaries, and stimulates salivary, lacrimal, and various other secretions. The dog liver is rich in histamine and releases it during shock. Other substances found or postulated to be active in anaphylaxis will be discussed later (see page 277).

Passive Sensitization.   As early as 1907, Otto showed that it is possible to sensitize a normal guinea pig passively by injection of serum from a sensitized guinea pig. The recipient undergoes a shock reaction typical of its species when homologous antigen is administered. In most cases an incubation period of 6 to 24 hours must elapse before introduction of the shocking dose of antigen. Moreover, passive sensitization of guinea pigs can be accomplished by injection of antiserum from animals, even of certain other species, that have been immunized against soluble antigens. Sensitizing efficacy is directly related to the precipitin titer of the serum; a small amount of high titer anti-egg albumin rabbit serum sensitizes a guinea pig to a shocking dose of egg albumin injected a few hours later. The incubation period in passive sensitization has been explained as the interval required for antibody to become associated with appropriate cells of the animal body.

Desensitization.   A hypersensitive animal that is given several very small (sub-shocking) subcutaneous injections of antigen at closely spaced intervals (e.g., one-half hour) may then be able to tolerate an ordinarily shocking dose without severe reaction. Such an animal is said to be *desensitized*. The total in vivo antigen-antibody reaction is apparently so prolonged that little tissue damage occurs, and the active substances liberated are detoxified rapidly and do not produce a violent reaction. Desensitization is only temporary, lasting no more than a few days or weeks.

The appearance of hypersensitivity is delayed 2 to 4 weeks in a guinea pig sensitized with a dose of soluble antigen considerably larger than required for normal anaphylactic sensitization, or in an animal given several smaller preparatory injections. The "antianaphylactic" or refractory state produced has been attributed to the presence of "blocking" antibody—IgG antibody—in the circulation, which protects against anaphylaxis by combining with antigen before it can reach sensitive cells.

In Vitro Anaphylaxis.   Schultz and Dale found that when strips of intestinal or uterine muscle were excised from sensitized guinea pigs and suspended in a suitable physiologic saline solution, the muscle contracted strongly upon addition of homologous antigen to the solution. This response displays typical antigen-antibody specificity and can be used to distinguish between different proteins. The Schultz-Dale reaction is also extremely sensitive.

The animal that donates the muscle tissue may have been sensitized either actively or passively. It is also possible to sensitize excised normal guinea pig ileum or uterine tissue by suspending it in antiserum. The tissue is washed after an hour or longer and treated with antigen, whereupon contraction occurs.

In the Schultz-Dale test a latent period of a few seconds usually follows addition of antigen to the bath before contraction of the sensitive muscle. The tissue remains contracted for some time (Figure 9–1) and gradually relaxes. If the saline solution is then removed and replaced by fresh solution, addition of more antigen produces no further contraction. This constitutes in vitro evidence of desensitization. The muscle is still physiologically capable of contracting, however, and responds typically to the addition of histamine, acetylcholine, pilocarpine, or various other reagents. Desensitization therefore involves only the antigen-antibody mechanism and does not affect the contractility of the muscle.

Local Anaphylaxis.   Local dilatation of capillaries can be demonstrated in the skin of a guinea pig by the passive cutaneous anaphylaxis (PCA) test. This procedure,

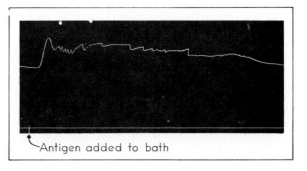

Figure 9–1. Kymograph record of the contraction of an intestinal strip from a guinea pig sensitized with egg albumin. Contraction occurred a few seconds after addition of antigen to the bath, and the muscle did not completely relax for many minutes.

Antigen added to bath

developed by Ovary, consists of administering antigen and a dye such as Evans blue or pontamine blue intravenously to an animal injected intradermally with homologous antiserum 4 to 24 hours earlier. Dilatation and damage to the capillaries in the region of antiserum injection are shown within 15 minutes by escape of the blue dye into the surrounding tissue. Most striking results are seen if the animal is sacrificed and the inner surface of the skin is examined.

Evanescent cutaneous reactions of the "wheal and flare" type may be produced in hypersensitive animals and humans when the appropriate test antigens are injected intracutaneously. An actively sensitized guinea pig reacts to intracutaneous injection of homologous antigen within 5 to 15 minutes. The test area swells and develops erythema and edema of varying intensity, increasing to a maximum within 30 minutes to a few hours, after which the reaction fades and disappears in 2 to 4 hours. Further sensitizing injections cause a higher degree of hypersensitivity in which the reaction is less transient. Under certain conditions evanescent reactivity can be passively transferred by serum from previously immunized or sensitized rabbits or guinea pigs to normal guinea pigs. The latent period following serum injection, the immediate circumscribed reaction to antigen, and the rapid fading indicate an anaphylactic type of reaction occurring within the skin.

Immediate cutaneous reactions in man are more pronounced than in lower animals. They are elicited by intradermal or scratch tests in such allergic conditions as hay fever and food idiosyncrasies. The marked responsiveness of man is associated with a high degree of cutaneous reactivity to histamine, possession of a well developed, superficial lymphatic system, and formation of an antibody called *reagin* that has particular affinity for the skin. Passive transfer of the antibody was first demonstrated by Prausnitz and Küstner in 1921, when they injected serum from Küstner, who was sensitive to fish, into the skin of Prausnitz. Injection of the same site with a protein fish extract a few hours later elicited a prompt and evanescent "wheal and flare" reaction. The *Prausnitz-Küstner* test was formerly employed in the diagnosis of human allergies, in cases in which the patient might react violently to a test allergen; at present the fear of serum hepatitis virus transmission has reduced or eliminated use of the test. The so-called P-K test is performed by injecting a small amount of patient's serum into the skin of a normal person and following it 24 to 48 hours later with the allergen in question introduced into the same area and also into an untreated control area. A positive reaction appears in 10 to 15 minutes, and the control should show no change.

Reagins possess several properties that distinguish them from precipitating antibodies. They are thermolabile, being destroyed at 60° C. in one-half to one hour, and are also inactivated by sulfhydryls (e.g., 0.1 M 2-mercaptoethanol). They do not pass the placental barrier, so cutaneous sensitivity of this type is not congenitally acquired.

Finally, their affinity for cutaneous tissues is marked. Passive skin sensitization may persist as long as 6 weeks.

The "triple response" or "wheal and flare" reaction in man was attributed by Lewis to a histamine-like compound ("H-substance") and perhaps other materials liberated from cells injured directly or by antigen-antibody reaction. Three successive phases follow diffusion of "H-substance" from the site of injury: (1) erythema caused by local dilatation of capillaries, (2) a spreading flare or flush resulting from arteriolar dilatation produced by a local nerve reflex, and (3) formation of a wheal or area of circumscribed edema attributed to increased permeability of the endothelium of small blood vessels.

ALLERGY

Naturally occurring local anaphylaxis in man, which includes many of the disease conditions popularly known as allergies, affects principally the skin, the respiratory tract, and the gastrointestinal tract. Although the sensitive state may seem to arise spontaneously, in most cases it is possible to deduce the manner in which hypersensitivity was incited.

Allergic disorders with demonstrable reagins tend to follow family lines. The role of heredity appeared so striking that Coca subdivided allergies on this basis. Those with marked familial incidence he called "atopic" and others "nonatopic." Heredity does not determine the particular kind of sensitivity displayed, but rather a predisposition toward hypersensitization of some sort. Hereditary factors may influence the nature of the tissue affected and/or the capacity to produce reagin but, in general, the particular sensitivity is determined by the individual's experience.

Allergens, the agents that incite allergic reactions, do not necessarily possess obvious antigenicity. The body areas affected are known as *shock organs* or *shock tissues*. Different allergens normally encounter different organs or tissues, so a variety of clinical forms of allergy occur: hay fever, asthma, urticaria, angioedema, and probably infantile eczema. Serum allergy may occur in individuals "naturally" sensitive to foreign animal proteins such as horse danders, and also frequently develops as a result of active sensitization by injection of foreign serum.

Hay fever is characterized by watery exudation from the mucous membranes of the upper respiratory tract and conjunctivae, the natural consequences of which include violent and often protracted sneezing, nasal discharge, and lacrimation. The allergen is some agent in the surrounding atmosphere that is either inhaled or comes into direct contact with exposed mucous membranes; plant pollens are most commonly incriminated, but house dust, mold spores, and various other substances may also produce the symptoms of hay fever.

Seasonal hay fever is caused principally by pollens. Trees are usually responsible in the spring; in the summer, the grasses such as timothy, rye, and June grass are involved; ragweed and various other weeds are common sources of the offending pollens in the fall. Diagnosis is often based on the seasonal incidence of the disease, and the specific incitant is determined by correlation of symptoms with pollination periods of plants in the locality.

A water-soluble component of plant pollen is the chief cause of hay fever. It is easily extracted in alkaline solution and is used in skin tests for sensitivity. Small superficial scratches made with a sharp instrument are covered with minute amounts of the test liquids. If the reagent is in powdered form, the powder is mixed in a drop of N/10 NaOH over the scratch. Reactions appear in 10 to 30 minutes. Skin tests, although not always reliable, are useful to confirm a diagnosis based on seasonal incidence of the disease.

Specific prophylaxis sometimes attempted consists of desensitization (more correctly called "hyposensitization") before the pollen season starts. The patient receives a series of gradually increasing, very minute doses of an extract of the pollen to which he is sensitive. Injections are timed to culminate just before the beginning of the pollen season, when sufficient "blocking" antibody should be present in the circulation to prevent severe symptoms of the disease.

Local reactions to the injections are common. Systemic or constitutional symptoms occur more frequently in pollen therapy than in any other kind of allergic treatment and usually appear within 1 to 20 minutes. General reactions are controlled by application of a tourniquet above the site of injection to reduce entrance of allergen into the circulation and by administration of adrenaline or ephedrine.

The results of prophylactic treatment are variable. It has been reported that complete or partial relief may be expected in about 85 per cent of patients. Permanent and complete remission may never be obtained, the patient returning year after year for preseasonal injections. In some cases, treatment for two or three seasons leads to remission, and in others treatment for five to ten seasons accomplishes this result.

So-called perennial hay fever occurs throughout the year and bears a clinical resemblance to seasonal hay fever. It is caused by a variety of inhaled or ingested materials, such as animal danders, vegetable powders (orris root, kapok), house dust, foods (milk, eggs, shellfish), and drugs (quinine, aspirin, iodine). In a considerable percentage of cases the cause cannot be ascertained.

Specific treatment includes avoidance of the allergen if possible and attempted desensitization against allergens that cannot be eliminated. Desensitization must be resorted to in cases of allergy to dust.

Asthma is a condition of recurrent or paroxysmal difficulty in breathing, with a wheezing or whistling respiration produced by obstruction of the smaller bronchioles. It is either allergic or nonallergic. The nonallergic type, sometimes called "intrinsic asthma," is produced by unknown factors within the subject. Allergic asthma may be caused by the same inhaled substances as hay fever, together with certain drugs and biologicals inhaled by laboratory workers. Various ingested foods may also incite asthmatic attacks, among them eggs, wheat, and milk.

The specific cause of allergic asthma is determined in the same way as that of hay fever. The history of the patient, including other allergies in himself or his family, may be significant. Skin tests are sometimes performed in an attempt to confirm deductions from the history and physical examination. These tests are positive with 50 to 65 per cent of asthmatic patients. Sensitivities to more than one allergen are common. Negative results are useful because they help to exclude an allergic cause of disease. Another diagnostic procedure, which is applicable to many other hypersensitivities, consists of deliberate elimination followed by diagnostic trial. If, for example, a patient has symptoms while at home but not when taken into the hospital for examination and treatment, it is possible that the causative agent is environmental. He may then be exposed to house dust, animal danders, and other likely allergens to determine whether, under controlled conditions, they induce attacks of asthma. Foods in the customary diet can be tested in the same manner.

Treatment of allergic asthma is similar to that of hay fever. Avoidance of the allergen is always the most desirable method when feasible. Some materials, such as certain foods or drugs, can be avoided without too much difficulty. House dust and pollens, on the other hand, are practically inescapable. In these cases specific desensitization may be attempted as already described, with about the same anticipated effectiveness. For temporary relief of severe symptoms physicians often employ adrenaline, epinephrine, or ephedrine.

Urticaria or hives is a skin disorder characterized by the appearance of crops of intensely itching wheals or welts with raised, often white centers surrounded by an area of erythema. They are usually distributed widely over the body surface and tend to disappear in 1 or 2 days. Allergic urticaria is generally caused by ingestion of the allergen or more rarely by inhalation or contact. Common food allergens include strawberries, citrus fruits, fish and shellfish, eggs, tomatoes, and chocolate.

Angioedema is similar to urticaria, but the lesions are larger and more restricted in distribution. They often occur about the head and neck.

Infantile eczema consists of reddened vesicular or blister-like lesions of the face and neck and the skin inside the elbow and knee joints. The lesions ooze and crust over. The usual allergens are thought to be foods, particularly eggs. There is some question whether infantile eczema is actually an allergy of the immediate type.

Urticaria, angioedema, and infantile eczema are examples of *food sensitivity*. In a very severe case, an extremely small amount of the allergenic food taken into the mouth causes immediate edema and swelling of the lips and tongue so that the patient has difficulty in swallowing. Ordinary urticarial and eczematous reactions are caused by foods that pass through the intestine wall and are carried by the bloodstream to the skin, which is the shock organ. Asthma may be induced by foods that reach the bronchioles, either via the bloodstream following ingestion or by inhalation (e.g., wheat flour in a bakery).

Food allergy in which the alimentary tract constitutes the shock organ is called gastrointestinal allergy. It is characterized by vomiting, cramps, and diarrhea following ingestion of the allergen. The symptoms result from strong contractions of the pylorus and intestinal muscles and from marked edema of the intestinal mucosa. Intestinal reactions may be attributed to unusual sensitivity of this organ or to concentrated exposure to the allergen.

Skin tests are sometimes positive in food allergies but are frequently negative. The Prausnitz-Küstner reaction may be successfully used to determine the allergen responsible for cases of exquisite sensitivity in which direct skin tests might be dangerous. In any event, skin tests provide chiefly contributory evidence regarding the inciting agent, because many patients give positive reactions with foods to which they are not clinically sensitive or fail to react with foods to which they are clinically sensitive. Diagnostic trial is therefore the most accurate procedure. The subject is first allowed a very simple, nonallergenic diet, and then gradually one or more of the suspected foods is added at intervals until typical reactions are obtained.

Avoidance of the responsible food is the most desirable method of treatment. Occasionally, this is almost impossible, as in the case of an infant reactive to milk, eggs, or wheat. In these cases desensitization is sometimes attempted, either parenterally or orally; in the latter method, very small amounts of the food are given repeatedly in pills or capsules until a tolerance is developed.

MECHANISM OF IMMEDIATE HYPERSENSITIVITY REACTIONS

Immediate-type hypersensitivity reactions are a consequence of in vivo antigen-antibody interaction, which apparently damages various cells or tissues or both. The events that follow are determined in part by the fact of damage itself and in part by substances liberated from the damaged tissues.

The evidence for participation of both antigen and antibody in anaphylaxis may be summarized as follows:

1. Only complete antigens or complex haptens can be used to induce anaphylactic shock; injection of simple haptens inhibits shock following subsequent administration of antigen or complex hapten.

2. The incubation period in active anaphylaxis is similar to that in antibody formation.

3. Antibody can be demonstrated in the sera of sensitized animals.

4. Sensitivity can be transferred passively by means of serum or its globulin fractions from a hypersensitive or an immune animal.

5. The specificity of anaphylaxis is the same as that of the in vitro antigen-antibody reactions.

Anaphylaxis was early explained according to a cellular mechanism, which postulated that antigen reacts with "sessile" antibody attached to body cells. Antigen-antibody reaction was assumed to initiate cellular disturbances that induced the characteristic syndrome of anaphylactic shock. Later experimental observations indicated that only certain kinds of antibody can be "fixed" by tissue cells and react with subsequently introduced antigen to incite shock. Use of ^{131}I or a fluorescent dye as a label demonstrated the attachment of antibody to the surfaces of cells and showed that mast cells are important sites of activity. Antibodies of this kind with an affinity for body cells are said to be cytotropic.

IgE. Ishizaka et al. in 1966 identified a unique new class of immunoglobulin in the sera of ragweed-sensitive patients and demonstrated that it possesses reaginic activity. They showed that it was not the same as IgG, IgA, or IgM and named it IgE.

Reaginic antibodies were found to be cytotropic. Following attachment to tissue cells, specific union with homologous antigen leads to release of pharmacologically active substances from these or other cells. IgE antibodies are homocytotropic; that is, they fix to cells of the species in which they were produced. Heterocytotropic antibodies, on the contrary, induce sensitivity only when they fix to cells of species other than their own. For example, injection of rabbit anti-BSA of the IgG class into guinea pigs incites skin sensitivity demonstrable by the PCA test (see page 272). Guinea pigs can also be sensitized passively for PCA by injection of human IgG1, IgG3, or IgG4, but not IgG2.

The cells to which cytotropic antibodies attach differ somewhat according to the species of animal and the class of immunoglobulin. Human IgE has been shown to sensitize various kinds of leukocytes. IgE antibodies of the mouse and rat attach to mast cells. Platelets and macrophages may also be sensitized.

Reaction of antigen and homologous cytotropic antibody in the presence of complement (i.e., in vivo) leads to the formation of C3a and C5a by the usual complement cascade mechanism (see Figure 8–2, page 230). These substances are basic polypeptides with molecular weights of 7,200 and 16,800, respectively. Both have anaphylatoxic activity (Table 8–4, page 231); that is, they release chemical mediators of anaphylaxis from mast and other cells. Anaphylatoxin is also produced via the bypass mechanism, in which various substances such as inulin, endotoxin, and cobra venom initiate a series of steps leading to formation of C3a.

Anaphylatoxin Hypothesis. The anaphylatoxin hypothesis of anaphylaxis developed early but was largely neglected for nearly 50 years. Friedberger (1909) incubated a washed antigen-antibody precipitate with fresh, normal guinea pig serum, removed the precipitate, and injected the supernatant serum into a normal guinea pig, which then displayed the typical clinical and postmortem features of anaphylactic shock. It was postulated that a toxic substance, anaphylatoxin, was formed from the antigen-antibody aggregate by a serum protease with the assistance of complement. It was then proposed that anaphylaxis is the result of a similar reaction between antigen, antibody, protease, and complement in the circulating blood. When it was learned that nonprotein antigens such as bacterial polysaccharides can shock suitably sensitized animals, it appeared that the host's own proteins must constitute the substrate for anaphylatoxin formation.

Later it was found that anaphylatoxin releases histamine from guinea pig tissues. The resemblance between the symptom complex of anaphylaxis and that produced by histamine was noted as early as 1910 by Dale and again by Lewis in 1927. Histamine produces the bronchial muscle contraction and edema characteristic of anaphylaxis. It is now apparent that during anaphylactic shock several substances, including histamine, are released from the cells upon which antigen-antibody reaction takes place and that these substances stimulate the characteristic anaphylactic reaction.

Histamine is a base produced by decarboxylation of the amino acid histidine. It is abundant in the large granules of mast cells, located mainly in connective tissue throughout the body, particularly near small blood vessels. It is also found in various leukocytes and in platelets. Mast cells, leukocytes, and platelets release histamine during anaphylaxis; each mast cell contains about 10,000 times as much as a platelet, so the latter are not ordinarily important sources of histamine during anaphylaxis. As noted previously, histamine dilates capillaries and increases their permeability, incites the contraction of many smooth muscles, and stimulates the glands of exocrine secretion. Its release in anaphylactic shock is very rapid; two-thirds of the total amount set free is released within 1 minute. It is antagonized by antihistaminic drugs.

At least three other pharmacologically active substances appear as a result of antigen-antibody reactions associated with tissue cells. *Slow-reacting substance of anaphylaxis* (SRS-A) is an acidic protein-lipid complex. Minute amounts induce a slow, prolonged contraction of certain smooth muscles, such as the guinea pig ileum and the human bronchiole. Moreover, it is released slowly; for example, Austen and Brocklehurst reported that sensitized guinea pig lung tissue released only 5 per cent of the total SRS-A in the first minute after antigenic stimulation, and complete liberation required 15 minutes. Unlike histamine, SRS-A does not exist preformed in tissue cells but is produced as a result of antigen-antibody reaction. It is resistant to antihistaminic drugs. Its role in anaphylaxis is not clear, but it seems to be an important cause of that part of the bronchial constriction in human asthma that is refractory to antihistamine therapy.

Serotonin (5-hydroxytryptamine) is a base formed by decarboxylation of tryptophan modified by introduction of an —OH group into the indole ring. It contracts certain smooth muscles rapidly and increases capillary permeability. It is present in platelets and in mast cells in various parts of the body. The symptoms of anaphylaxis in the rabbit can be largely attributed to serotonin released from platelets that accumulate in the lung capillary bed.

Bradykinin is a peptide containing nine amino acid residues, first formed by the action of trypsin or snake venom on serum pseudoglobulin and later found to be one of a group of active peptides called plasma kinins (see Figure 9–2). Like SRS-A, it reacts slowly, producing powerful contractions of certain smooth muscles. It has greater

Bradykinin
> Arg-Pro-Pro-Gly-Phe-Ser-Pro-Phe-Arg

Lysyl bradykinin (kallidin)
> Lys-Arg-Pro-Pro-Gly-Phe-Ser-Pro-Phe-Arg

Methionyl kinin (methionyl-lysyl-bradykinin)
> Met-Lys-Arg-Pro-Pro-Gly-Phe-Ser-Pro-Phe-Arg

Kininogen
> (Sialic acid)$_n$-Met-Lys-Arg-Pro-Pro-Gly-Phe-Ser-Pro-Phe-Arg

Figure 9–2.   Amino acid sequences of three kinins and a human kininogen. The number of sialic acid residues in the kininogen is unknown.

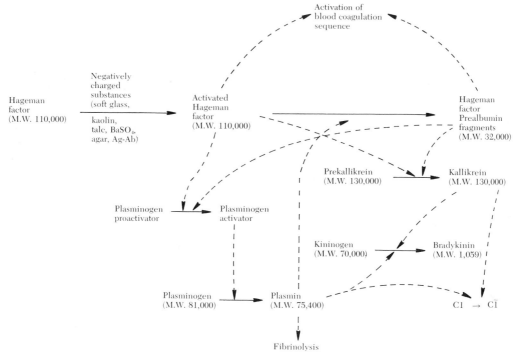

Figure 9–3. Some of the complex series of events that follow activation of Hageman factor. Solid arrows indicate reactions or transformations that are catalyzed by the enzymes or agents, whose participation is indicated by the broken arrows. Approximate molecular weights are given when known.

vasodilator action than any other substance known and markedly increases capillary permeability.

Bradykinin is formed through the enzymatic activity of kallikrein from a precursor, kininogen, which consists of an 11-member peptide, methionyl kinin, plus an unknown number of sialic acid residues (see Figure 9–2). Formation of kallikrein is catalyzed by Hageman factor or Hageman factor fragments (see Figure 9–3). Hageman factor is a γ-globulin present in inactive form in blood plasma. It is activated by certain antigen-antibody aggregates and by exposure to insoluble substances having a negative surface charge, such as soft glass, kaolin, and diatomaceous earth, and possibly by collagen fibers. Activated Hageman factor is a mediator in several very important enzymatic reaction series, including blood clotting, formation and fibrinolytic activity of plasmin, and the liberation of kinins, and it also participates indirectly in the nonimmunologic activation of complement, mediated directly by plasmin or kallikrein.

The four substances just described are active in the body only a few minutes after being released from the cells in which they are normally present or are formed. Histamine, serotonin, and bradykinin are quickly destroyed by enzymes in the body fluids or are metabolized, and SRS-A is apparently adsorbed onto tissues.

The amount of each pharmacologically active substance set free varies according to the animal species and the site of antigen-antibody interaction. Moreover, the sensitivity of different tissues to a given substance also varies, so it is hardly surprising that the manifestations of anaphylaxis vary greatly from one species to another, or even from one individual to another. Acute anaphylactic shock in the guinea pig following intravenous injection of antigen is attributed to histamine and possibly SRS-A released from the lung tissue; contraction of the bronchioles and massive edema resulting from capillary dilatation cause respiratory failure with the accompanying characteristic signs. The protracted shock produced by intraperitoneal injection of antigen may be due to liberation of bradykinin.

In the rabbit, circulatory collapse is accompanied by acute dilatation of the right side of the heart. Histamine and serotonin are released into the pulmonary circulation, probably from damaged platelets, and restrict passage of blood out of the lungs to the left heart. It has been postulated that pulmonary emboli of antigen-antibody precipitates may be more important, their effects being exaggerated by the released pharmacologic mediators. The liver is the principal shock organ in the dog, and release of histamine from its mast cells causes capillary dilatation and edema so that blood accumulates in tremendous quantities; general circulatory collapse ensues. Bradykinin may also participate in the reaction, and heparin liberated from the mast cells markedly reduces clotting of the blood.

In man, death by anaphylactic shock is attributed to laryngeal edema and/or acute pulmonary emphysema. Histamine is responsible for only a limited number of the manifestations of anaphylaxis: itching, urticaria, angioneurotic edema. It seems likely that SRS-A causes bronchospasm, and bradykinin produces intense vasodilatation that leads to vascular collapse.

COMPLEX-MEDIATED HYPERSENSITIVITY

When a soluble antigen and its antibody unite in optimal proportion in vivo, a precipitate forms, and this is promptly disposed of by phagocytosis. However, if there is an excess of either reagent, soluble complexes form. These persist in the tissues and react with complement, liberating chemotactic agents (C3a, C5a, $\overline{C567}$) that attract neutrophils. The latter react with the immune complex and set free lysosomal catheptic enzymes that damage the tissues severely, producing local or general inflammation. Anaphylatoxin is also formed, followed by liberation of histamine from mast cells, leukocytes, and platelets. The net effect of these various enzymatic and toxic activities, compounded by local interference with the blood circulation due to the accumulation of aggregated leukocytes, is intense necrosis and hemorrhage.

There are two common situations in which soluble complexes form. (1) When antibody is present in the blood (i.e., inside the blood vessels) and homologous antigen is injected into a tissue, the antigen diffuses from the site of deposition and produces irritating antigen-antibody complexes in the blood vessel walls. Complement is activated, C3 is bound, neutrophils accumulate, and local vasculitis occurs. Injury to the vessel walls causes edema and hemorrhage. This is the Arthus-type of response. (2) When a large amount of antigen is present in the bloodstream and antibody begins to appear in the course of a normal immune response, at a certain period antigen-antibody complexes form with a moderate excess of antigen. General vascular damage ensues with symptoms of the disease known as *serum sickness*.

Arthus Reaction.   *The Arthus reaction* may be elicited in rabbits by a series of subcutaneous injections of foreign protein at intervals of a few days. There is no untoward response to early injections, but later injections produce local infiltration, which develops into necrosis and abscess formation. A more striking picture is obtained by immunizing strongly with a series of intravenous injections and then challenging by the intracutaneous route rather than subcutaneously.

Macroscopic evidence of reaction may not be apparent for several hours, but microscopic changes begin within 1 hour. Marked but transient leukopenia has been observed within 15 minutes after intradermal injection of antigen; white blood cells and platelets adhered to the endothelium of small blood vessels at the site of injection, where they formed thrombi, possibly aided by a layer of fibrin on the vessel walls. Connective tissue fibrils swelled within an hour, and blood vessels were compressed at the site of subcutaneous injection. Leukocytes were immobilized, and there was massive edema. Twenty-four hours after injection histologic examination showed necrosis of the arterioles and resulting hemorrhage, together with local tissue degeneration, inflammation, and edema.

The intensity of the Arthus reaction in actively sensitized rabbits varies with the concentration of antibody in the serum. The phenomenon is not limited to skin reactions; inflammation and necrosis have been induced in the lung, heart, kidney, peritoneum, testis, brain, and joints.

Reverse Arthus reactions are produced in rabbits by injecting protein intravenously and homologous antiserum by the intracutaneous route either immediately or at any time within the next 3 or 4 days. The intensity of local reaction at the site of antiserum injection diminishes as the interval between injections increases. Reverse Arthus reactions may not be so severe as direct reactions, often producing only severe local edema.

Passive Arthus sensitivity can be induced in normal rabbits by injection of serum from other rabbits sensitized or immunized against foreign proteins. When the antiserum is injected intracutaneously and is followed one-half hour later by antigen intravenously, the reaction occurs at the site of antiserum injection. Antigen administered intracutaneously into the site that originally received antiserum produces a reaction in that location. Antiserum injected intraperitoneally or intravenously sensitizes the entire animal skin so that subsequent intracutaneous injection of antigen elicits a reaction at the site of antigen injection. The significant condition seems to be that antigen and antibody meet in the blood vessel walls, and it makes little difference which reagent is initially within the vessel and which is outside.

It will be noted that no latent or incubation period is needed for passive Arthus sensitization, whereas such an interval is often necessary for passive anaphylactic sensitization. Both types of reaction may be demonstrated in the same animal some hours after antiserum injection. Furthermore, passive Arthus sensitization requires several times as much antibody as fatal anaphylactic sensitization.

Arthus reactions can be elicited in the guinea pig, horse, monkey, and man. Reactions in man occasionally occur during the course of repeated serum inoculations.

Serum Sickness. *Serum sickness* develops 8 to 12 days after injection of a large amount of foreign protein such as antitoxin. It is characterized by general swelling of lymph nodes and is accompanied by an itching, urticarial, or erythematous eruption and often edema of the eyelids, face, and ankles. In severe cases fever and pain in the joints are also noted. The average duration of symptoms is 2 days, but they may persist as long as 2 weeks. During the interval of 8 to 12 days before symptoms appear, antibodies are manufactured, and these react with the persisting foreign protein in the circulation to yield complexes that activate complement, forming C3a and C5a, with the liberation of vasoactive substances. The consequent increase in permeability permits the antigen-antibody complex to deposit locally in the blood vessel walls. Polymorphonuclear leukocytes also accumulate, and severe arteritis follows. When kidney glomeruli are involved, complexes deposit along the basement membrane and bind complement, endothelial cells swell, and glomerulonephritis with proteinuria develops.

As the concentration of antibody increases, the reaction becomes more violent. Continued production of antibody hastens disappearance of the foreign protein, whereupon the reaction subsides. A second injection of the same foreign protein after a considerable interval, when antibody is still present but at a low level, provokes a similar sequence of events 3 to 5 days after the injection. This is the "accelerated" reaction, reminiscent of the "recall" phenomenon in immunized animals reinjected with antigen after a rest period. Reinjection of an individual who is in a *high state of sensitivity* elicits an "immediate" reaction consisting of local response within a few minutes and also generalized reactions within a few minutes to 12 hours. Such reactions, occurring almost exclusively in horse asthmatics, are often severe and sometimes fatal. Death may occur in a few minutes or after as much as 24 hours. This is a typical anaphylactic reaction and is a *serum allergy* rather than *serum sickness*.

Anaphylactic sensitivity to foreign serum proteins can be detected in the human by an intracutaneous skin test with diluted foreign serum. A positive reaction, noted after 10 to 60 minutes, consists of a local wheal and erythema. Cutaneous sensitivity is a danger signal and indicates the strong probability of a serious reaction if the foreign serum is administered to the patient.

SUMMARY OF THE ROLE OF ANTIBODIES IN IMMEDIATE-TYPE HYPERSENSITIVITY

The antibodies that participate in immediate-type hypersensitivities include both classic, thermostable, precipitating antibodies, particularly IgG, and thermolabile, nonprecipitating reagins or IgE antibodies. Both classic and reaginic antibodies may be present simultaneously. The former can be detected by in vitro reactions (e.g., precipitation, agglutination), but the latter are detectable only in vivo. IgG antibodies can cross the placenta and hence appear in the fetus. These antibodies may also be transferred passively in serum from a sensitive individual to the skin of a normal individual, where they persist only a few hours. IgE antibodies, on the contrary, do not cross the placenta and hence do not appear in the fetus or newborn, but when injected into the skin of a normal individual they persist for several days.

Cytotropism is a significant feature of the antibodies in immediate-type hypersensitivity. IgG molecules possess only limited cytotropic properties and are heterotropic; that is, they sensitize tissues of heterologous species. IgE molecules have a strong affinity for cells of individuals of the same species and hence are homocytotropic. It is the combination of cytotropism of the Fc portion of the molecule with the specific antigen-reactivity of the Fab portion that is responsible for the nature of immediate-type hypersensitivity. Union of antigen with its homologous antibody-combining site induces an allosteric or other effect that is transmitted via the Fc region to the cell, which responds in its characteristic manner with liberation of pharmacologically active substances. In some cases, complement is also activated and contributes to the total response.

Additional Sources of Information

Austen, K. F., and E. L. Becker (Eds.): Biochemistry of the Acute Allergic Reactions. 1971. Oxford, Blackwell Scientific Publications.

Becker, E. L.: Nature and classification of immediate-type allergic reactions. *In* Dixon, F. J., and H. G. Kunkel (Eds.): Advances in Immunology, vol. 13, pp. 267–313, 1971. New York, Academic Press, Inc.

Bennich, H., and S. G. O. Johansson: Structure and function of human immunoglobulin E. *In* Dixon, F. J., and H. G. Kunkel (Eds.): Advances in Immunology, vol. 13, pp. 1–55, 1971. New York, Academic Press, Inc.

Cochrane, C. G.: Immunologic tissue injury mediated by neutrophilic leukocytes. *In* Dixon, F. J., and H. G. Kunkel (Eds.): Advances in Immunology, vol. 9, pp. 97–162, 1968. New York, Academic Press, Inc.

Cochrane, C. G., and D. Koffler: Immune complex disease in experimental animals and man. *In* Dixon, F. J., and H. G. Kunkel (Eds.): Advances in Immunology, vol. 16, pp. 186–264, 1973. New York, Academic Press, Inc.

Orange, R. P., and K. F. Austen: Slow reacting substance of anaphylaxis. *In* Dixon, F. J., and H. G. Kunkel (Eds.): Advances in Immunology, vol. 10, pp. 106–144, 1969. New York, Academic Press, Inc.

Ratnoff, O. D.: Some relationships among hemostasis, fibrinolytic phenomena, and the inflammatory response. *In* Dixon, F. J., and H. G. Kunkel (Eds.): Advances in Immunology, vol. 10, pp. 145–227, 1969. New York, Academic Press, Inc.

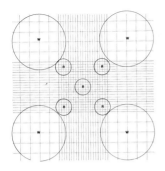

IN VIVO IMMUNOLOGIC REACTIONS: CELL-MEDIATED CYTOTOXICITY

It is generally agreed that T lymphocytes are the major cells responsible for cell-mediated immunologic reactions. In addition to their regulatory role in humoral immunity, T cells stimulated by antigen differentiate into effector cells with various functions.

(1) They mediate delayed hypersensitivity reactions by releasing chemicals such as MIF, cytophilic antibody, interferon, skin-reactive factor, and macrophage chemotactic factor.

(2) They are important in resistance to chronic infections caused by intracellular microorganisms.

(3) They destroy target cells bearing the sensitizing antigen on their cell membrane, whether the antigen is a normal or abnormal constituent of the membrane.

In vitro experiments have demonstrated two different cytotoxicity mechanisms, which are assumed to operate in vivo to some extent. The first is direct interaction of T lymphocytes from immunized donors with membrane antigens via specific receptors. Humoral antibodies either do not participate, or, if they do, they *inhibit* cytotoxic activity by reacting with the membrane antigen and preventing the sensitized T cell from making contact with it. In the second cytotoxic mechanism, IgG antibody is bound specifically, both to a target cell and to a normal lymphoid cell; the Fab regions bind to target cell antigens, and the Fc portion binds to a lymphoid cell possessing a receptor for the Fc region. Cytotoxicity has also been demonstrated with macrophages to which cytophilic antibody is attached via its Fc region.

REGULATION OF CELL-MEDIATED RESPONSES

Phylogenetic studies indicate that cell-mediated immunity developed before humoral immunity as part of the mechanism for maintaining the integrity of the body, and later it became adapted for assistance in the control of chronic, intracellular infections. As high-grade pathogenic organisms evolved, particularly those that are encapsulated or produce toxic by-products, the humoral mechanism developed. Cell-mediated immunity is therefore a function principally of T cells.

Induction of the Cell-Mediated Immunologic Response

Inasmuch as the first important observations of delayed hypersensitivity were those of Koch in tuberculous guinea pigs and humans, it was believed for many years

283

that cell-mediated immunity and the accompanying delayed hypersensitivity developed only in response to microbial antigens. It is now known that the delayed-type reaction can be incited by purified proteins, by simple chemical haptens coupled to protein carriers, or by antigenic, low molecular weight synthetic peptides. Haptenic substances that can couple with proteins include sulfonyl chlorides, catechols, oxazolones, and various halogenated nitrobenzenes. Some of these chemicals couple with proteins so readily that the reaction occurs spontaneously upon contact of the simple chemical with the skin, producing a form of contact dermatitis.

METHODS OF SENSITIZATION

Induction of delayed hypersensitivity is facilitated by use of the intradermal route for injecting antigen and by emulsifying it in Freund's complete adjuvant. (1) Intradermal injection is most effective, and intravenous injection is least effective. The former may produce a state of "partial tolerance," in which subsequent intradermal injections of antigen fail to induce delayed hypersensitivity. (2) Minute quantities of antigen in saline induce delayed skin reactivity, as do antigen-antibody complexes. Skin tests should be performed between 5 and 10 days after sensitization; otherwise the delayed reaction may be prevented by circulating antibody demonstrable by an Arthus reaction. (3) The most satisfactory method of inducing delayed hypersensitivity is to incorporate the antigen in Freund's complete adjuvant. Doses between 1 and 3 μg. suffice. Freund's incomplete antigen, which lacks dead mycobacteria, also induces delayed sensitivity, but the response is not as great, and it is more transient than with complete adjuvant.

As mentioned previously, delayed hypersensitivity can be induced by an antigen containing a simple hapten coupled to a protein carrier. One widely used combination consists of bovine gamma-globulin coupled with dinitrophenol (DNP-BGG). Guinea pigs immunized with DNP-BGG display very strong delayed reactions when tested intradermally 1 week later. However, if they are tested with an antigen containing dinitrophenol coupled with an unrelated protein, such as egg albumin, the delayed skin reaction is usually not obtained. If the original protein, BGG, is coupled with an unrelated hapten, such as O-chlorobenzoyl chloride, a positive skin test is usually secured. This behavior is called "carrier-specificity," in contrast to "hapten-specificity," as obtained in antibody-mediated reactions such as anaphylaxis or the Arthus phenomenon, in which the hapten is the significant determinant.

Passive transfer of delayed hypersensitivity by means of serum is not possible. The sensitive state can, however, be transferred by means of lymphoid cells. Contact sensitivity may be transferred by means of peritoneal exudate cells. Tuberculin sensitivity is transferred by lymph node or spleen cells, as well as by peritoneal exudate cells. Large numbers of cells (several hundred million) must be transferred; sensitivity is demonstrable immediately after intravenous injection, but it persists only a few days unless both donor and recipient are from an inbred strain. Transfer is not successful between species and not always between different strains of inbred animals (e.g., guinea pigs). The transferred cells must be living, and treatment with agents such as actinomycin or mitomycin C, which inhibit RNA synthesis, eliminates the capacity to transfer sensitivity.

The foregoing situation obtains in experimental animals, not in man. A lymphocyte product, discovered by Lawrence and known as "transfer factor," can transfer delayed hypersensitivity from one human to another. Transfer factor is extracted from lymphocytes by lysis or by freezing and thawing and is also released from cells during incubation with antigen in vitro. It is effective in transferring sensitivity to tuberculin, diphtheria toxoid, coccidioidin, and other agents. Transfer factor is a small molecule

(M.W. less than 10,000), comparatively stable at and below room temperature, and is unaffected by trypsin, RNase, or DNase. The mechanism of its activity is not known.

Suppression of Cell-Mediated Responses

Methods used to suppress cell-mediated responses are basically those employed to suppress immunoglobulin synthesis. They are either physical, chemical, or biologic.

PHYSICAL METHODS OF IMMUNOSUPPRESSION

Physical methods include surgical removal of lymphoid tissue and irradiation. Inasmuch as delayed hypersensitivity is a function of thymus-derived cells, thymectomy should prevent the development of delayed-type hypersensitivity. In general this is true, but there are differences between species. Neonatal thymectomy permits mice to retain allografts longer than usual and eliminates the capacity of rats to develop delayed hypersensitivity to tuberculin or BSA. However, guinea pigs and rabbits are little affected by removal of the thymus.

The effects of X-irradiation also differ between species. Doses of 400 to 800 roentgens suppress the development of sensitivity to tuberculin in rabbits, whereas guinea pigs are much more resistant: even doses that will ultimately be lethal have little or no effect on the development of delayed hypersensitivity.

CHEMICAL METHODS OF IMMUNOSUPPRESSION

Since some immunosuppressive chemicals are also powerful anti-inflammatory agents, careful studies are necessary to distinguish the effect of a drug on the *development* of sensitivity from its effect on *expression* of hypersensitivity. In order to do so, administration of the drug must be terminated some days before a skin test of sensitivity. Adrenal corticosteroids are powerfully anti-inflammatory. They are often used to prolong graft survival and to relieve various hypersensitivity conditions. They markedly reduce the transformation of lymphocytes and the number of immunoblasts present in graft rejection and hence prevent both the development and expression of delayed hypersensitivity.

Alkylating Agents. Nucleophilic chemicals such as cyclophosphamide and the mustards are effective because they alkylate nucleic acids and impair their functional activities. Cyclophosphamide is the most effective immunosuppressant of this group; it is widely used in kidney transplant patients, and it markedly inhibits numerous immunologic reactions, including primary and secondary antibody responses, experimental autoimmune disease, allograft rejection, and delayed hypersensitivity. Phenylalanine mustard inhibits tumor allograft rejection in mice but is of minor usefulness in man.

Purine and Pyrimidine Analogues. One of the most widely used immunosuppressive agents in man is azathioprine, which is converted into 6-mercaptopurine (6-MP) in vivo. The latter has long been recognized as an important immunosuppressive agent. It inhibits nucleic acid synthesis by competing indirectly with inosinic acid for the feedback control of phosphoribosylamine synthesis. Azathioprine and/or 6-MP are used in prolonging allograft survival in various animal species and in man, notably in the control of human kidney and heart rejection.

Folic Acid Analogues. The most widely used folic acid analogue is methotrexate, employed in cancer chemotherapy. It inhibits the development of delayed hypersensitivity to simple chemicals as well as proteins, including oxazolone, picryl chloride, egg albumin, and diphtheria toxoid. It also prolongs survival of skin allografts in most animal species. Canine heart and lung transplants have been successfully treated, and tumor allograft rejection is inhibited in mice.

Biologic Suppression of Cell-Mediated Responses. Biologic methods used to suppress delayed hypersensitivity include administration of antiserum against lymphocytes, induction of immunologic tolerance, and specific desensitization.

Antilymphocyte Sera. Inasmuch as the operative cells in delayed hypersensitivity are lymphocytes, antibodies against lymphocytes inhibit or prevent development or expression of delayed hypersensitivity. Antilymphocyte serum (ALS) and its gamma-globulin fraction (ALG) prolong survival of allografts in various animals, including mouse, rat, pig, monkey, and man, and impair the delayed response to allergens such as tuberculin and hapten-protein conjugates. They inhibit the production of immunoglobulin and hence humoral immunity to a greater or lesser extent, since this activity is also a function of lymphocytes.

The effectiveness of ALS or ALG depends upon the cells against which the antiserum is produced and upon the species of animal in which it is raised. Lymphocyte sources that have been used include blood and thoracic duct lymphocytes, cells from patients with chronic lymphocytic leukemia, thymus and spleen cells, and fractions of these various cell populations. Inasmuch as the proportions of T and B cells vary greatly in these preparations, it is not surprising that ALS activities differ widely from one study to another.

Experimental ALS is produced on a laboratory scale in rabbits and other small animals, but for treatment of human graft recipients larger animals, such as the horse, sheep, goat, pig, and calf, are economically more practical. ALG is prepared from ALS by customary purification procedures involving ammonium sulfate or cold ethyl alcohol precipitation and DEAE cellulose chromatography. It contains less extraneous serum protein that might produce toxic reactions in patients.

Standardization of ALG is difficult, because it is species-specific and should therefore be tested in man or closely related primates. Since the principal use of ALG is to control graft rejection, the most desirable test would be assay of graft survival, but this is obviously impossible. The alternative is some sort of in vitro test. A number of tests have been tried, including lymphocyte agglutination, lymphocyte cytotoxicity, MIF production, and inhibition of target cell destruction. One of the most satisfactory tests is based upon inhibition of rosette formation by normal lymphocytes incubated with sheep erythrocytes in vitro. A characteristic of T cells is the formation of rosettes with SRBC, in the absence of complement, and this is inhibited by antiserum against T cells.

As in all prophylactic or therapeutic procedures involving the administration of foreign protein, there is the risk that serum sickness or anaphylactic shock may be produced. The danger is less with ALG than with ALS, because its content of foreign protein is lower. Another hazard associated with use of ALS or ALG arises from their general effect upon the immunologic system. Inasmuch as the principal body defense against various chronic bacterial and viral diseases and against tumors is the T lymphocyte, patients receiving this form of treatment should be guarded carefully against these types of disease. Moreover, unless the antiserum is prepared by immunizing with an extremely pure suspension of T cells, it is likely to contain a sizable proportion of antibodies against B cells, whose function is to assist in the production of humoral immunity against acute bacterial infections.

Induction of Immunologic Tolerance. Induction of tolerance reduces or eliminates development of delayed hypersensitivity in experimental animals. Fetal guinea pigs can readily be made tolerant to bacille Calmette-Guérin (BCG), tuberculin, BSA, and BGG by appropriate injections and thereafter fail to develop delayed hypersensitivity following customary sensitization procedures. They can also be made tolerant to allogeneic tissue such as skin, after which they accept allografts. Precautions should be taken to avoid injecting adult lymphoid cells into fetal or neonatal animals, lest the graft-versus-host reaction be induced. It is also possible to induce tolerance in adult guinea pigs by intravenous injection of doses of BGG totaling 10 μg. in one week.

Combined use of physical or chemical immunosuppressive agents with sensitization also leads to tolerance. Sensitization, accompanied or followed for several days by X-irradiation or administration of purine analogues or alkylating agents, induces a tolerant state. The sensitizing material apparently primes the T cells, which are then more easily inhibited or destroyed by the immunosuppressive agent. An animal so treated remains tolerant for a long time, perhaps until mutation permits development of a new population of cells responsive to the antigen.

DESENSITIZATION

An animal that has been made hypersensitive by injection of antigen in Freund's complete adjuvant can be made comparatively insensitive by intravenous injection of a large amount of the antigen in saline. A single intravenous dose of 1 to 2 mg. of purified protein antigen suffices to desensitize guinea pigs. The desensitized state lasts for several days, the duration increasing with the amount of antigen. Desensitization of man is more difficult.

DELAYED-TYPE HYPERSENSITIVITY AND CELL-MEDIATED IMMUNITY

The cell-mediated immune response, with its accompanying delayed-type hypersensitivity, apparently developed early as a response to localized infectious agents and simple chemicals that could be combatted in hand-to-hand fashion, as in the tubercles of tuberculosis or in skin areas affected by a toxic chemical. The actual sensitizing agent is usually comparatively small, consisting of a low molecular weight substance or the digestion products of microbial cells rather than intact cells. The latter usually stimulate a humoral immune response, as in the case of pneumococci, following which circulating antibodies agglutinate, lyse, or otherwise destroy the dispersed microbial cells.

Infectious agents of concern in cell-mediated immunity produce conditions that are usually not only localized but also chronic and often intracellular. They are exemplified by tuberculosis, brucellosis, certain viral infections (pox, herpes, leukemogenic), and parasitic infestations. Microbial products of low molecular weight released by macrophage activities are accepted by T cells, which undergo blast transformation, replications, and clonal expansion. The resulting population of thymus-derived cells is capable of reacting with and destroying the infectious agent, either directly or by liberating lymphokines that contribute in a variety of ways to defense.

The delayed hypersensitivity response can be demonstrated experimentally in guinea pigs sensitized by the injection of BCG or by application of a simple chemical, such as dinitrochlorobenzene, to the skin. Subsequent challenge a few days later with the purified protein derivative of tuberculin (PPD), in the first case, or with the chemical, in the second case, is followed by a characteristic local cellular response. Mononuclear cells, principally lymphocytes and macrophages, predominate. They accumulate via the vascular system, attach to the inner walls of blood vessels, and migrate through the walls into the surrounding tissues. A large population of proliferating pyroninophilic mononuclear cells resembling blast cells or large lymphocytes develops, and its reaction with the allergen incites the typical delayed hypersensitivity response.

Chronic Infections

BACTERIAL INFECTIONS

Guinea pigs infected with *M. tuberculosis* for several weeks respond to subsequent attempts to superinfect by subcutaneous injection of tuberculosis organisms, with a characteristic local inflammatory reaction appearing in several hours and developing slowly to a maximum at 2 or 3 days. The site gradually heals as the local infection is thwarted. The same type of response is elicited in a tuberculous animal by injecting tuberculoproteins or PPD. Tuberculous humans respond in the same way to cutaneous tests. A tuberculin-positive individual retains sensitivity for many years after onset of the original infection. A positive test therefore indicates either past or present infection, but it does not distinguish between these possibilities except in the case of infants and young children, in whom a positive result is considered diagnostic of active infection. In adults, a negative reaction indicates the absence of tuberculosis (except in overwhelming infections, in which the patient may become "anergic").

Active immunization of man or experimental animals with BCG induces reactivity to tuberculin. There is good evidence that tuberculin conversion (from negative to positive) accompanies actual protection against infection. In one study, 50,000 tuberculin-negative children at approximately age 15 were divided randomly into groups, one of which was immunized with BCG, another being left unvaccinated. In the next 9 years, the incidence of tuberculosis in the vaccinated group was only 20 per cent of that in the control group. It appears, therefore, that the protection is appreciable, although not absolute.

Other infectious diseases in which delayed hypersensitivity is demonstrable by skin reactions include leprosy, brucellosis, deep-seated fungal infections such as histoplasmosis, blastomycosis, and coccidioidomycosis, and various parasitic infestations.

Protective immunization with infectious agents that produce delayed-type hypersensitivity is successful only with living organisms, which are most effective if they can survive intracellularly. It is for this reason that vaccines used to immunize against tuberculosis, brucellosis, and bubonic plague usually consist of living attenuated cultures. Killed vaccines of the same organisms induce strong antibody production, but the host remains essentially unprotected.

The parallel between ability to induce hypersensitivity and protection extends even to the strain of organism. Mackaness reported comparisons of a normal strain of BCG with a streptomycin-resistant mutant and of *Salmonella gallinarum* with *Salmonella pullorum*. In each instance, the first mentioned organism produced both hypersensitivity and protection in mice, whereas the second organism did not incite hypersensitivity or protection against virulent challenge. Both strains of BCG possessed the necessary antigens, but the mutant failed to sensitize and induce protection. In the case of the Salmonella strains, only *S. gallinarum* survived in the mouse, although both organisms possessed sensitizing antigens. It appears, therefore, that survival or multiplication or both within host tissues is required for induction of cell-mediated immunity and hypersensitivity against intracellularly parasitic bacteria. Mackaness concluded that cellular hypersensitivity and acquired cellular resistance are merely different expressions of a common cell-mediated state of reactivity to antigen.

Cellular immunity is also important in brucellosis. This disease is often chronic and prolonged, and it is characterized by the intracellular multiplication of the organisms in monocytes of nonimmune individuals. Serum antibodies are usually present in the circulation as soon as the first symptoms of the disease develop, but their presence does not prevent bacteremia. The antibodies can be detected by agglutination, precipitation, phagocytosis, and bactericidal tests. Only when skin tests with

Brucellergen, a nucleoprotein fraction from Brucella cells, become positive is there evidence of antibacterial defense. Mackaness found that brucellae survived longer in mononuclear cells from nonimmune animals than from actively immunized animals. Cellular immunity was relatively nonspecific, being effective against other varieties of intracellular bacteria.

FUNGAL INFECTIONS

A similar situation obtains in various fungal infections. Circulating antibody in low titer may be produced in infections with *Coccidioides immitis, Cryptococcus neoformans*, or *Histoplasma capsulatum*, but passive transfer of serum from infected to normal animals does not protect the recipients against challenge with the corresponding fungus. Although these antibodies are not protective, their presence in a diseased individual indicates activity of the infectious process. Skin tests with appropriate extracts (e.g., coccidioidin, histoplasmin) demonstrate the development of delayed-type hypersensitivity during these infections, and in some instances its persistence, as indicated by positive skin tests, is correlated with recovery from infection. It appears therefore that cellular immunity affords whatever protection is available. Moreover, hypogammaglobulinemic patients who display a normal cellular response possess satisfactory immunologic defense against pulmonary histoplasmosis, despite their inability to produce antibodies.

VIRAL INFECTIONS

The role of cell-mediated immunity in viral infections is somewhat more complicated than in the infections just discussed. Humoral antibodies are produced in many viral diseases, and they appear to be significant in the immune state, particularly in those instances in which antibodies circulate in the bloodstream and in which viremia is normally part of the disease process. In respiratory infections such as influenza, circulating antibodies are of less significance; secretory IgA antibody on the mucous membranes is much more important than circulating IgG and IgM antibodies.

Delayed hypersensitivity is part of the pathologic response to many viral agents. This is illustrated by the situation in smallpox, knowledge of which has been derived from clinical and pathologic studies of patients and from laboratory study of mousepox (ectromelia) in mice and vaccinia (cowpox) in rabbits. Infection occurs via the upper respiratory tract, where the virus multiplies first in the mucosa and then in regional lymph nodes. Transient viremia distributes the virus to internal organs (e.g., liver and spleen), where it propagates and reinvades the bloodstream. Generalized symptoms then appear, followed by a skin rash due to multiplication of the virus in epidermal cells. The skin rash progresses through a series of changes, beginning with a macular eruption (discolored spots on the skin), which develops to a papular stage (small, circumscribed, elevated areas) and finally to pustules or small, elevated areas containing pus, appearing in the second week of illness. Similar lesions may occur in the mucous membranes of the mouth, pharynx, larynx, trachea, and esophagus, and secondary degenerative lesions also develop in other organs, such as focal necrosis of the liver, kidneys, and adrenals.

There is evidence that the lesions in this eruptive phase of smallpox are not due solely to multiplication of the virus and death of the invaded cells, but that hypersensitivity to the viral antigens is a contributing factor. This has been demonstrated experimentally in infected rabbits, whose antibody response and development of hypersensitivity are inhibited by X-irradiation or appropriate drugs; in these animals virus multiplication is not restricted, but the characteristic pustules do not form.

Active immunization against smallpox is accomplished by intradermal administration of vaccinia virus. Three types of response to the vaccine are elicited, according to the immune status of the individual. (1) The primary response is obtained in an individual with no previous effective immunity. A small papule appearing on the fourth day after vaccination progresses rapidly through the vesicular stage to a pustule. Maximum reaction is reached on the eighth to tenth day. The pustule becomes crusted and may remain 3 or 4 weeks before it sloughs off, leaving a scar.

(2) The accelerated response is given by an individual with some but not complete immunity. It progresses much the same as a primary reaction but more rapidly and less intensely. Maximum reaction is obtained 3 to 7 days after inoculation. Viral multiplication during the response contributes to the development of increased immunity.

(3) The early or immediate response first appears as a papule within 8 to 24 hours; it attains maximum dimensions by 2 to 3 days and usually does not progress beyond the vesicle stage, which suggests a high degree of immunity. This response is essentially a delayed type of allergic reaction. It is due to the host response to viral protein and can be elicited by heat-inactivated (56° C. for 30 minutes) as well as by living virus, in contrast to primary and accelerated reactions, which are elicited only by active virus. The immediate response therefore does not necessarily indicate immunity but, like the tuberculin reaction, implies previous infection. Hypersensitivity may persist longer than effective immunity.

Delayed hypersensitivity occurs in a number of other viral infections, such as measles and mumps. It is detected by a skin reaction to intradermal injection of antigen. It is important in recovery from viral infections like smallpox, but its function in resistance to reinfection is not clearly defined, as indicated by the behavior of patients with immunologic deficiency diseases. Individuals with Bruton's agammaglobulinemia possess a normal cellular immune system, but their humoral system is defective, and they produce little if any antibody. These patients recover without incident from herpes simplex and chickenpox and may be successfully vaccinated against smallpox. These immunologic responses are evidently cellular rather than humoral. In Swiss-type hypogammaglobulinemia, both cellular and humoral mechanisms are impaired. Patients with measles and herpes simplex are seriously threatened, and smallpox vaccination of these individuals may lead to serious consequences, apparently owing to lack of the cellular arm of the immune system.

Contact Dermatitis

Contact dermatitis, including certain forms of *drug allergy*, results solely from contact of the skin with the incitant. Symptoms appear after some delay and consist of inflammatory rashes or eczematous eruptions, often vesicular.

The causative agents are many and varied. They include metals like nickel and mercury; relatively simple compounds such as formaldehyde, picric acid, 2,4-dinitrochlorobenzene, and para-phenylene-diamine (often used in partially oxidized form in dyeing furs); orris root, cosmetics, and insect powders; salvarsan; Novocain; various dyes; and fat-soluble plant extractives such as urushiol, the active principle of poison ivy, and substances from poison sumac, poison oak, and other plants.

Many if not all of these materials are nonantigenic in themselves. For many years, therefore, it was believed that contact dermatitis was separate and distinct from those hypersensitivities in which the allergens are complex, protein-containing substances. An explanation of the sensitizing powers of these simple allergens was provided by the work of Landsteiner (page 131), and others showing that the specificity of proteins may be altered by coupling them with low molecular weight substances such as arsanilic acid. Simple compounds, including degradation products or metabolic derivatives of more complex drugs, combine with constituents of the epidermis, which thus become antigenic and incite an immunologic response.

Although unsensitized individuals may be exposed without ill effects to large quantities of the specific materials, after sensitization has been established even very minute amounts induce the characteristic response. Heredity, frequency and mode of contact, and the chemical properties of the sensitizing agent determine the probability of sensitization.

In both the human and the guinea pig, dermal sensitivity of the delayed type (contact dermatitis) is established in 5 to 20 days by repeated cutaneous or intracutaneous applications of the allergenic chemical. The visible dermatitis reaction is elicited by cutaneous application of the allergen. This type of sensitivity cannot be transferred passively by serum but may be transferred by means of washed living white blood cells, of which the lymphocytes are most important.

The same active sensitizing procedure may produce two different parallel sensitivities: the anaphylactic type and the contact dermatitis type. Certain substances produce chiefly anaphylactic sensitivity, others cause both types, and still others principally delayed sensitivity. Anaphylactic sensitivity can be shown in guinea pigs by intravenous injection of a protein conjugate of the allergen, by passive anaphylactic sensitization with serum from a sensitive animal, and by elicitation of the Prausnitz-Küstner effect using serum from a sensitive animal to produce a local area of sensitization in which an immediate reaction can be produced by a protein conjugate of the allergen.

Diagnosis of contact dermatitis is aided by the usual occurrence of eruptions on exposed surfaces of the body (i.e., not protected by clothing), because direct contact is the only way in which reaction is induced. The presence of vesicles and the absence of a personal or family history of allergy strengthen the diagnosis. Contact dermatitis is more common among men than women and children, inasmuch as many of the responsible agents are used in industry or various trades: paints, lacquers, and metallic substances, for example.

The specific cause of a given case may be indicated by the patient's history. The "patch" test is also used in an attempt to identify the incitant. The test is performed by placing upon the skin a small piece (one square centimeter or less) of linen or blotting paper soaked in a solution of the test reagent or coated with an ointment containing it. This is covered with waterproofed cellophane to prevent drying and is held in position with adhesive tape. The patch is removed after 24 hours, and the area is observed daily for as long as 2 weeks because reactions sometimes develop slowly. A positive test consists of an area of erythema in which vesicles of various size may be present. The most significant reaction is one that closely resembles the patient's original lesion. In a negative test there is no change at the site of the patch.

Specific treatment depends upon knowledge of the causative agent. Avoidance is recommended but is sometimes impractical because this form of allergy is so frequently occupational in nature. In such a case, change of occupation may be the only alternative. Desensitization usually has chance of success only if the excitant is oily in character: for example, plant or pollen oils.

AUTOIMMUNE DISEASES

Autoimmune diseases are those in which the individual mounts an immunologic response to some constituent of his own body. The response may contribute directly to the pathogenesis of the disease. Antibodies that are produced against tissue components may mediate cell or tissue destruction, either alone or in conjunction with complement. This is illustrated by the intravascular agglutination of erythrocytes in an incompatible transfusion and by hemolysis of Rh positive fetal erythrocytes when an Rh negative mother possesses anti-Rh antibodies. In some diseases, tissue damage caused by a physical, chemical, or biologic agent releases a normally sequestered body component so that it can stimulate an immunologic response. Sympathetic ophthalmia is an example: injury to one eye that allows uveal or corneal proteins to get into the circulating blood is followed a few days later by inflammation of the other eye and loss of its sight.

Various body tissues that do not normally come into contact with cells of the immune system incite the immunologic response when injected into the donor animal or another animal of the same inbred genetic line, particularly when they are emulsified in Freund's complete adjuvant. These antigenic materials include spermatozoa, thyroglobulin, lens protein, and myelin of the central nervous system. With the exception of spermatozoa, these antigens are organ-specific rather than species-specific: thyroglobulin from one species incites an immune reaction, even in another species, that causes inflammation of the recipient's thyroid gland.

Several diseases of man appear to be caused by a similar allergic mechanism. For example, a number of cases of encephalomyelitis occurred in individuals who received the early rabies prophylaxis, which consisted of virus cultivated in rabbits and harvested in the form of a spinal cord emulsion. The encephalomyelitis was not associated with the virus content of the vaccine, but represented an allergic response to the myelin of the spinal cord in which the virus was contained.

Thyroiditis

Diseases of the thyroid gland are manifested by enlargement (goiter) and/or by increased or decreased function. Thyroiditis is an acute or chronic inflammation of the thyroid caused by infectious agents or by other unknown but apparently genetic factors.

Hashimoto's disease is the most common of the latter. It is a chronic disease, characterized by moderate, rubbery enlargement of the gland, with mild decrease in activity, extensive infiltration by lymphoid cells, and accumulation of plasma cells, and by the appearance of antibodies against three thyroid-specific antigens. The disease occurs about 30 times as frequently in females as in males, typically at the time of menopause. It was one of the first to be recognized as an autoimmune disease. The operation of genetic factors is indicated by the strong familial incidence of clinically demonstrable cases. It is also suggested by the fact that other diseases presumed to be autoimmune in nature, but unrelated to thyroid disease, occur with greater than normal frequency in patients with Hashimoto's disease; these include rheumatoid arthritis, Addison's disease, Sjögren's disease, and pernicious anemia.

The three thyroid antigens for which antibodies appear in the course of Hashimoto's disease are a microsomal antigen, thyroglobulin of the colloid, and another colloid antigen designated CA_2. The microsomal antigen is localized within the cytoplasm of epithelial cells and is intimately associated with the lipoprotein membrane of microsomes. Its location can be ascertained by immunofluorescence with Hashimoto serum and fluorescent rabbit antihuman serum, using the sandwich technique. It is also detected by complement fixation. The antibody is rapidly cytotoxic for cultured thyroid cells in vitro, but its toxicity in vivo is considered doubtful.

Thyroglobulin is the most abundant antigen. It is a large (M.W. 650,000), iodine-containing molecule and is the principal storage form of thyroid hormones. It comprises more than 75 per cent of the protein in thyroid colloid. Anti-thyroglobulin antibodies are detected by precipitation, by agglutination of antigen-coated latex particles or tanned red blood cells, by immunofluorescence, and by passive cutaneous anaphylaxis.

The other colloid antigen, CA_2, constitutes less than one per cent of the proteins of thyroid colloid and contains no iodine. It is detected by immunofluorescence.

Microscopic examination of thyroid tissue from a case of Hashimoto's disease or from experimental thyroiditis in animals reveals a mononuclear-lymphocytic infiltrate that appears early and is often aggregated into well-developed lymphoid follicles resembling those constituting normal lymph nodes. Large numbers of plasma cells later intermingle with the infiltrate. These cellular changes take place at the expense of normal thyroid structure and interfere with glandular function, so that a moderate hypothyroid condition results.

The symptoms of thyroiditis do not correlate with the titer of antibodies to the three antigens, and passive transfer of serum containing a high concentration of antibodies does not produce thyroiditis in experimental animals. It therefore appears that antibodies are formed as a consequence of tissue damage and do not necessarily cause cellular injury. The predominance of lymphocytes in early lesions suggests delayed-type hypersensitivity, which is confirmed by the fact that thyroiditis can be transmitted via lymphoid cells from a diseased animal to a normal animal. Moreover, the severity of the thyroid lesions correlates well with the intensity of a delayed skin test with thyroglobulin.

The possible pathologic role of delayed hypersensitivity in human chronic thyroiditis is suggested by observations of experimental allergic thyroiditis in guinea pigs and other animals. After injecting thyroglobulin or thyroid extract in Freund's complete adjuvant, delayed hypersensitivity can be demonstrated as soon as the earliest lesions are apparent and prior to the appearance of anti-thyroglobulin antibodies. Moreover, both the intensity of the delayed hypersensitivity reaction and the severity of the thyroid inflammation are reduced by administration of 6-mercaptopurine or by neonatal thymectomy; in neither case is there a significant effect on the anti-thyroglobulin titer. It is also possible to produce a high level of antibody by injecting alum-precipitated thyroglobulin without inducing appreciable thyroid inflammation.

The primary phase of experimental allergic thyroiditis begins within 2 weeks after the sensitizing injection and consists of delayed-type hypersensitivity lesions in which lymphocytes and monocytes accumulate focally around venules. The lesions enlarge and assume an "invasive-destructive" character, gradually impairing the thyroid function. The second phase of the disease process consists of local differentiation and proliferation of plasma cells, which then produce antibodies. The function of the antibodies is not understood; they may act synergistically with delayed hypersensitivity to damage the thyroid further, or they may serve a protective role and help to limit the extent of the lesions in the manner of blocking antibodies. Whatever their function in vivo, the antibodies serve a useful diagnostic role, and the symptoms of disease appear more clearly referable to the delayed-type hypersensitivity reaction.

Experimental Allergic Encephalomyelitis

Injection of brain extract emulsified in Freund's complete adjuvant into an animal induces a disease known as experimental allergic encephalomyelitis (EAE). There is almost no species barrier—brain tissue of most common domestic animals is effective in the usual laboratory animals. Symptoms that appear in the rat 10 to 14 days after sensitization include ascending flaccid paralysis, persisting about 2 weeks and followed by complete recovery. The principal common histologic feature of the brain lesion in all animals consists of focal perivascular areas of inflammation containing lymphocytes, mononuclear cells, and plasma cells. Antibodies are produced that fix complement with brain tissue as antigen, but they do not transfer the disease to normal animals. Passive transfer by lymphocytes has been accomplished. EAE therefore resembles experimental and natural chronic thyroiditis in its histologic and immunologic aspects and, like the latter, appears to be a delayed hypersensitivity.

Brain extracts have been fractionated in an attempt to determine the nature of the antigen responsible for the pathologic response. Lipoproteins, collagen, and myelin antigens have been isolated, and the latter appears to be the most significant. Myelin is a basic protein containing 180 amino acid residues. Tryptic digestion yields an active peptide of 45 residues and M.W. 4,700; it is called *encephalitogen.*

Postvaccinal encephalitis following rabies prophylaxis with rabbit spinal cord emulsions of the virus has been mentioned (see page 292). Its cause is the same as that of EAE. There are other examples of human allergic encephalitis in which the cause appears to be the individual's own brain or spinal cord material altered slightly by infection with neurotropic viruses: vaccinia (smallpox), varicella (chickenpox), herpes zoster, herpes simplex, measles, rubella (German measles), and mumps. It was recently (1969) reported that nearly one-fourth of all cases of encephalitis are associated with childhood viral diseases such as those listed.

TISSUE TRANSPLANTATION

The repair or replacement of damaged tissues by transfer from a healthy donor has been the dream of physicians for centuries. When the mechanical problems were solved, microbiologic problems appeared, to be replaced in turn by immunologic problems. These are currently being studied but are not yet solved.

After the discovery of the blood circulation by William Harvey early in the seventeenth century and the demonstration in 1657 by Sir Christopher Wren, the famous architect, that fluids can be injected into veins, it was only a matter of a few years until blood transfusions were done experimentally in dogs. The first successful human transfusion was performed in 1829 in Guy's Hospital by Dr. James Wardell on a postpartum patient who was hemorrhaging badly. Occasional transfusions were attempted thereafter, but the procedure was plagued by problems associated with coagulation and incompatibility, until Landsteiner's discovery of the ABO blood groups in 1900. The use of blood transfusion increased rapidly thereafter and came into its own during World War II.

Blood transfusion is one of the simplest examples of the transfer of tissue from one host to another. Transfusion reactions are mediated by natural antibodies or by immune antibodies produced as a result of repeated transfusions. Antibodies, in contrast to T lymphocytes, are particularly effective in the destruction of dispersed cells such as blood cells, and cellular immunity plays little if any role. Solid tissues are subject to attack by both circulating antibodies and T cells, and the latter are especially significant.

One of the most common solid tissue transplants is the transfer of skin from one site to another of the same individual in the course of plastic surgery or the repair of burned areas. Other tissues that are frequently transferred include bone and pieces of arteries, cornea, and cartilage; transplants of bone marrow, endocrine tissue, and whole organs such as the kidney, liver, lung, and heart are increasingly common.

Graft Rejection

When skin or other tissue is transferred to an unrelated recipient, the nature of the response varies according to the previous experience of the recipient. (1) If the recipient contains circulating antibodies against antigenic components of the grafted tissue, acute or hyperacute rejection may occur. This is the case when the ABO blood groups of the donor and the recipient are incompatible. As noted earlier (page 212), the A and B antigens are present on *all* body cells. Therefore, if cells bearing the B antigen are transferred to an individual of group O or group A, the anti-B antibody of the recipient can combine with the grafted tissue cells to initiate a cytotoxic reaction. A recipient who has previously received a graft or transfusion of the same ABO group can be expected to possess specifically cytotoxic antibody, possibly in fairly high titer. The circulating antibodies, in conjunction with complement and/or phagocytic cells, destroy the tissue cells so rapidly that the graft never "takes." Grafted skin does not vascularize and appears as a "white graft."

(2) When skin or other tissue is transferred from one individual to another of the same species, it appears to be accepted for a few hours or days; revascularization occurs, and the tissue maintains a healthy color. Solid tissues or organs resume their normal functions, such as urine excretion or hormone production. However, if the donor and recipient are not genetically identical, 5 or 6 days after transplantation the tissue becomes darker and purplish, necrosis occurs, and by 11 to 17 days the graft has been completely sloughed off and rejected. In the case of solid organs, early signs of rejection include loss of function. The tissue becomes increasingly infiltrated by mononuclear cells of various kinds during the rejection process: lymphocytes, monocytes, tissue macrophages, and plasma cells. This response is known as the *first set reaction*.

(3) A host that has undergone a first set reaction is hypersensitive to another graft from the same or a genetically identical donor. If another graft is made from that donor, a *second set reaction* occurs. It is similar to the first set reaction except that rejection is much more rapid. For example, only 6 or 7 days may be required rather than 11 to 17. In some instances the graft does not revascularize, and it resembles the white graft of humoral rejection.

The terminology used to refer to grafts has changed within the past few years. Both systems are given in Table 10–1. *Autograft* is included in both the earlier and the present systems; it refers to a graft from one site of an individual to another site of the same individual. *Syngeneic grafts* are those between two genetically identical indi-

Table 10–1 Transplantation Terminology

Present Term	Previous Term	Relationship of Graft Donor to Graft Recipient
Autograft (Greek, *autos*, self) Autogeneic graft	Autograft	Same individual
Syngraft (Greek, *syn*, with, together) Syngeneic graft Isogeneic graft (Greek, *isos*, equal)	Isograft	Same species, genetically identical (e.g., identical twins, inbred strains)
Allograft (Greek, *allos*, other) Allogeneic graft	Homograft	Same species, genetically dissimilar
Xenograft (Greek, *xenos*, foreign) Xenogeneic graft	Heterograft	Different species

viduals of the same species. Generally, experimental animals that have been inbred by 20 successive brother-sister matings are closely enough related to be considered identical for the purpose of graft transplantation. *Allografts*, formerly homografts, which consist of transplants between nonidentical members of the same species, are sufficiently dissimilar to be rejected by first and/or second set reactions as just described. This response is often called the *allograft (homograft)* reaction. *Xenografts* —transplants of foreign tissue—are usually rejected promptly.

Development of tissue transplantation opened an entirely new area—immunogenetics. The important factor in acceptance or rejection of a graft is its chemical relationship to the tissues of the host, and this is controlled genetically. Therefore, the following rules apply: (1) Autogeneic or syngeneic grafts are accepted without problem. (2) Rejection of allografts can be retarded by appropriate immunosuppressive treatment. This will be discussed later (page 298). (3) The accelerated, second set rejection occurs with any tissues from the same donor but not with tissues from another donor antigenically different from the first. (4) The histologic changes accompanying rejection are typical cell-mediated immune responses: infiltration by lymphocytes, macrophages, and plasma cells. (5) Rejection of grafts is associated with the presence of antibodies and specifically reactive lymphoid cells with an affinity for the donor tissues.

Rejection of dispersed cellular grafts such as whole blood appears to depend upon humoral immunity. Acute rejection of solid transplants often involves both humoral immunity and cellular immunity. The allograft reaction is principally attributed to T lymphocytes and the processes of cellular immunity in which there is either direct attack by activated lymphocytes or production of lymphokines, which mediate destruction of the grafted tissue.

Histocompatibility Antigens

The antigens that participate in transplantation reactions are cell surface components that incite an immunologic response in graft recipients. Since knowledge about them is principally related to their role as determinants of the acceptance or rejection of tissue transplants, they are called *histocompatibility antigens* or *transplantation antigens*.

A tissue or tissue extract may be tested for the presence of histocompatibility antigens by injecting it into a recipient and challenging the recipient a few weeks later with a skin allograft from the same or another appropriate donor. Accelerated rejection of the graft (second set reaction) justifies the conclusion that the injected tissue preparation contained histocompatibility antigens that were also present in the challenge allograft but were absent from the recipient. By this type of procedure, tissues, cells, subcellular components, and chemical fractions of cells can be tested for histocompatibility antigens.

Histocompatibility antigens are composed of protein with a molecular weight between 30,000 and 35,000, containing lipid and 1 to 10 per cent carbohydrate, but the latter components do not seem to contribute to their antigenicity. Some of the principal histocompatibility antigens of man precipitate when mixed with rabbit antiserum against the Fc portion of human IgG and therefore appear to be antigenically identical to human IgG Fc. The histocompatibility antigens are chemically different from the blood group antigens, which owe much of their specificity to their carbohydrate components, so two systems of antigens are involved in the destruction of incompatible cells or tissues—the histocompatibility system and the blood group system. The histocompatibility antigens are present on all nucleated cells, which include the leukocytes of the circulating blood.

The important determinant sites of histocompatibility antigens are presumably distinctive amino acid sequences within the polypeptide chain that determine the folding and stereochemical structure of the molecule. Inasmuch as the amino acid sequence is dictated by the cellular DNA nucleotide code, the immunologic specificity of these antigens is under genetic control.

There have been many genetic studies of histocompatibility antigens in laboratory animals and in man. These indicate the existence of numerous independently segregating gene loci, with multiple alleles at each locus. Fifteen loci have been detected in mice (H-1, H-2, H-3 . . ., and X- and Y-linked loci). In man there appear to be at least 23 loci, in guinea pigs there are seven or eight, and in the hamster only three.

In each animal a single locus controls the antigens that dominate the transplantation reactions of that animal. These are called the major histocompatibility genes. In the mouse, the H-2 locus controls the major histocompatibility antigens, whereas in man the HL-A (human leukocyte antigen) locus controls the major antigens. The difference between a major and a minor locus is that a single strong antigen will usually elicit a maximal allograft reaction; that is, a skin graft is destroyed in about 11 days. A difference at a minor locus may cause rejection of a skin allograft in as much as 100 days.

Most human histocompatibility antigens have been studied in leukocytes. These leukocyte antigens are probably identical to the histocompatibility antigens found on all cells. More than 20 leukocyte antigens have been detected in man, and most of them are in the HL-A system. Three subloci or different mutational sites affecting this system are known, and more than 30 different HL-A alleles have been identified. Many of these are designated by a numerical system (HL-A1, HL-A2, HL-A3 . . .), and antisera for some can be procured and used for detecting the presence of the antigens on leukocytes.

Control of Graft Rejection

HISTOCOMPATIBILITY TESTING

Inasmuch as the success of tissue transplantation depends upon the antigenic similarity between donor and recipient cells, one means of prolonging acceptance of a graft is preliminary testing and selection of the best available donor. If one has access to a suitable set of test antisera, it is possible to ascertain the histocompatibility antigens of the recipient and then search for a donor with as near the same antigens as possible.

Antisera are secured from multiparous mothers. At the time of delivery they usually become inoculated with a small amount of fetal blood, which is almost certainly of a different histocompatibility type than their own. They therefore produce antibodies for at least some of the major fetal antigens that are lacking on their own cells. Tests of leukocyte antigens can be performed by agglutination, cytotoxicity, or complement fixation.

Another test for compatibility is provided by mixing donor and recipient cells in vitro and observing the presence or absence of cytotoxic reactions between the cells. This is the *mixed lymphocyte reaction (MLR)*.

Leukoagglutination. There are several methods for conducting agglutination tests with leukocytes. Defibrinated blood from the patient and prospective donor are collected, and the red blood cells are sedimented and discarded, the supernatant plasma containing leukocytes being collected. The leukocytes are washed, suspended in the desired concentration, and added to the antiserum. In the semimicro test, one or two drops of cell suspension and serum are incubated together in small tubes. Acetic acid may be added to lyse red cells that otherwise interfere with microscopic reading.

Leukocytotoxicity.   The cytotoxicity test depends upon increased permeability induced by the action of complement on lymphocytes that have been treated with antibody. The lymphocytes are purified from defibrinated or heparinized blood; red cells are removed by sedimentation, and granulocytes are allowed to adhere to glass, nylon, or cotton. The remaining cells, principally lymphocytes, are mixed with antibody, and complement is added. Cytotoxicity is indicated by the uptake of a dye such as Evans blue; dead cells take up the dye, while living cells exclude it. This can be observed microscopically, and the percentage of dead cells is readily determined by use of a counting chamber.

The most quantitative indicator of cytotoxicity is ^{51}Cr. The lymphocyte suspension is treated with a radioactive chromium salt, washed, and mixed with antibody and complement. The ^{51}Cr released into the supernate is measured by a gamma counter, and the percentage cytotoxicity is calculated as indicated on page 46.

Mixed Lymphocyte Reaction (MLR).   The mixed lymphocyte reaction depends upon the fact that, when genetically dissimilar lymphocytes are cultivated together, blast transformation and mitosis occur, and each population of lymphocytes reacts with the foreign histocompatibility antigens (principally HL-A in human subjects) of the other population. The test becomes very sensitive when the uptake of tritiated thymidine by actively replicating blast cells is used as the indicator of blast transformation. Leukocytes are prepared from the donor and the recipient in the usual manner and mixed for cultivation. Tritiated thymidine is added, and after appropriate incubation (often 5 days) the amount of tritium fixed by the cultures is determined with a scintillation counter and provides an index of histocompatibility difference between the two individuals. This reaction detects primarily incompatibility of the major transplantation antigens. It does not identify the antigens but indicates their degree of incompatibility.

The test as described is two-directional; that is, lymphocytes from the donor react against those of the recipient and vice versa. It can be made unidirectional by mixing lymphocytes from one individual, often the donor, with mitomycin C to inhibit their mitotic activity before adding the recipient's cells.

Mention may be made again of the graft-versus-host reaction previously described (see page 18). It will be recalled that, when tissue is transplanted from one individual to another nonidentical individual, two rejection processes may occur. The one of major concern is the host rejection of grafted tissue, but the opposite reaction may also occur if lymphoid cells are included in the graft. The transplanted lymphocytes have the potential ability to respond immunologically against the host and reject it. In situations in which the host is immunologically incompetent by reason of age (neonatal) or immunosuppression (irradiation, chemical treatment) so that it cannot reject the graft, the tissue recipient may be seriously damaged. In the newborn the response is called runt disease: the animal fails to grow, its spleen is enlarged, it has diarrhea and anemia and may die. In adult animals, the condition is called homologous or secondary disease.

IMMUNOSUPPRESSION

In transplantation between identical twins or members of an inbred population of experimental animals, there is no problem of rejection because the donor and the recipient possess exactly the same transplantation antigens. In all other transplants, histocompatibility testing permits selection of donors as closely related as possible to the recipient, but the differences between individuals are so great that a perfect match can rarely if ever be achieved. Sibling transplants afford the best chance of success, but even these are ultimately rejected unless immunosuppressive or other measures are taken. Even immunosuppression must be maintained indefinitely, lest the recovering immunologic system develop a population of lymphoid cells capable of reacting specifically with the grafted histocompatibility antigens.

The aim of immunosuppression is to prevent one or more of the steps leading to rejection of a graft, which can be summarized as follows: (1) contact of antigen with lymphoid cells; (2) blast transformation and proliferation of the lymphoid cells; (3) effector activity: sensitized lymphocyte–target cell "combat" or release and action of lymphokines or other pharmacologic mediators.

Interference with contact between the lymphoid cells and the antigen is not yet practical, although some immunosuppressive treatments applied to the donor before transfer of tissue (e.g., a kidney) delay rejection of the graft.

The most important method of suppressing an immune response is to reduce the number of lymphocytes, which can be accomplished by surgical, radiologic, pharmacologic, or immunologic means. Removal of the thymus is effective with experimental animals but is not practical for humans. Drainage from the thoracic duct also decreases the number of circulating lymphocytes. Near lethal total-body X-irradiation is used widely with animals, or lethal doses of X-rays followed by "rescue" with bone marrow or other lymphoid cells of syngeneic or other animals, according to the experimental situation. Local irradiation of particular organs or regions is practiced in man.

Pharmacologic and immunologic methods are most widely applied to the reduction of blastogenesis and/or lymphoid cell proliferation. Several groups of drugs inhibit either antibody production or cell-mediated immunity or both. In general, the antiproliferative compounds bind to macromolecules in target cells and inhibit enzyme or template activity or incorporate into macromolecules and yield inactive products.

Alkylating agents react with nucleic acids and/or nucleoproteins and impair their function. One of the most effective is cyclophosphamide, which inhibits primary and secondary antibody responses, allograft rejection, delayed hypersensitivity, and experimental autoimmune diseases. It is widely used in kidney transplant patients. Various mustards are used in animals, especially to suppress antibody production.

Purine analogues, such as azathioprine, 6-mercaptopurine, and 6-thioguanine, interfere with cell proliferation by inhibiting purine biosynthesis. They inhibit the primary antibody response strongly, and the secondary response to a lesser extent. Azathioprine is one of the most widely used immunosuppressants in man, in whom it inhibits the primary allograft response, as in kidney and heart transplants.

Pyrimidine analogues have not been as extensively studied. In mice, 5-fluorouracil inhibits the primary antibody response to BCG and bacterial vaccines. Arabinosylcytosine inhibits antibody responses, delayed hypersensitivity, and experimental allergic encephalitis.

The *folic acid antagonist*, methotrexate, is widely used in cancer chemotherapy and is also immunosuppressive. It inhibits nucleic acid synthesis by binding to the enzyme that converts dihydrofolate to tetrahydrofolate in the synthesis of purines and pyrimidines. It reduces antibody formation and prolongs allograft survival in animals and in man, although its toxicity somewhat restricts its use in man.

The *actinomycins* interfere with DNA-dependent RNA polymerase activity and hence inhibit protein synthesis. They decrease antibody production in animals but do not affect delayed hypersensitivity reactions, and actinomycin C has been used in man to treat acute kidney rejection.

Alkaloids from the periwinkle, vincristine and vinblastine, arrest cell division in metaphase. They inhibit some antibody responses, delayed hypersensitivity, skin allograft rejection, and inflammatory reactions in animals, often at toxic concentrations. Their use in man is limited.

Adrenal steroids are widely used as immunosuppressants and as anti-inflammatory agents. They apparently inhibit RNA synthesis. In animals they depress antibody production, inhibit various experimental autoimmune diseases, and prolong allograft survival.

Anti-lymphocyte sera (ALS) and *anti-lymphocyte globulin* (ALG) are potent inhibitors of transplantation immune reactions. The use of antihuman ALS in the treatment of kidney allografts in man was first reported in 1967. ALS is obtained primarily by immunization of horses with human lymphocytes from the thoracic duct or from the thymus or spleen. The antibodies react in vitro with lymphocytes, causing agglutination, cytotoxicity in the presence of complement, and in some cases blast cell transformation. In vivo, ALS causes histologic changes in lymphoid tissues and a reduction in the number of lymphoid cells. Its effect upon cell-mediated immunity is much greater than upon humoral immunity, and it appears to be particularly directed toward recirculating "memory" cells derived from the thymus.

ALS is especially effective in prolonging graft acceptance. In animals it is one of the most powerful suppressors of cellular reactivity to bone marrow, kidney, heart, and corneal allografts. Secondary responses are inhibited, and tolerance may even be established. In man, the combined use of ALS with azathioprine and prednisone lowers toxicity and permits reduction of dosage. This treatment is used with renal transplants but is less effective with heart grafts.

Numerous hazards and harmful effects attend the use of ALS and ALG. Although they do not depress antibody production as greatly as they inhibit cellular immunity and delayed hypersensitivity, they markedly reduce the general level of immune response and pave the way for fatal infections, control of which requires massive antibiotic therapy. Another problem arises from the fact that ALS is made in a foreign animal species, usually the horse, so patients often develop severe immediate-type hypersensitivity. Within two weeks after intramuscular injection, patients may have local edema and erythema with induration and pain, and those injected intravenously often develop fever and mild anaphylactic shock. Moreover, the antibodies apparently abrogate the normal surveillance mechanism, and about 2 per cent of patients develop tumors.

IMMUNOLOGIC TOLERANCE AND ENHANCEMENT

In an earlier discussion (page 23), it was pointed out that fetal or neonatal mice injected with nucleated cells from mice of another strain become immunologically tolerant and can later accept skin grafts from mice of the original donor strain. Tolerance can be induced across a major histocompatibility barrier (i.e., H-2). Medawar (1954) concluded that immunologic tolerance is caused by central failure of the immune mechanism as a result of embryonic or neonatal encounter with a specific antigen. Later, it was found that adult animals can be made tolerant, but that much larger doses of allogeneic cells are required, and induction of tolerance is aided by immunosuppression with 6-MP, cyclophosphamide, or ALS.

While it may be theoretically possible to prepare humans for transplantation by a similar procedure, the amount of allogeneic tissue required for induction of tolerance is well nigh prohibitive, and the drastic immunosuppression required severely damages the recipient's entire immunologic system.

Immunologic enhancement is specific immunosuppression attributable to humoral antibodies. In transplantation, it is demonstrated by prolongation of graft survival by antibodies against the graft transplantation antigens. Tissue or organ transplants in experimental animals survive many times longer in recipients immunized either actively by tissue or lymphoid cells of the same donor or passively by antibodies against the donor tissue or lymphoid cells. For example, bilaterally nephrectomized rats survived more than 200 days with transplanted allogeneic kidneys when they were also immunized both actively and passively against spleen and lymph node cells of the same donor.

The mechanism of immunologic enhancement is not clear. It has been attributed to reaction of humoral antibody with determinant sites of the antigen, either preventing them from sensitizing the host or blocking them from contact with sensitized lymphoid cells. There is some evidence that enhancing antibodies are unusually avid and that they prevent the formation of cytolytic antibodies by feedback inhibition. They may also attach to transplant cells and, because of their high avidity, block the transplant from cytolytic antibodies and from lymphoid cells.

PRIVILEGED SITES AND TISSUES

Tissue transplants can be made to certain body sites without the usual likelihood that the graft will be rejected. These areas include the anterior chamber of the eye, the brain, the cornea, and the cheek pouch of the hamster, a saclike cavity just inside the mouth used for storage and transport of food. The principal significant feature of these sites is their lack of lymphatic drainage. As long as grafts into the eye are made carefully without causing undue local damage and inflammation, the tissue is accepted for long periods. The same applies to the brain. In both situations, prolonged tissue survival is related to the absence of lymphatic channels.

The cornea can be transplanted freely from one individual to another with good chance of survival and restoration of vision lost due to corneal injury or defect. A cornea transferred to vascularized tissue is rejected in the usual manner, which indicates that it is the site rather than the tissue that is significant.

There are, however, a number of tissues that appear to be privileged—that is, they can be transplanted to various locations without being rejected. These include bone, cartilage, tendon, heart valves, pieces of aorta, and other large blood vessels. A considerable variety of tissues that have been maintained in culture may also be accepted. The developing fetus is also considered privileged. Some of these tissues—bone, cartilage, and so forth—can even be preserved by freezing or by chemical disinfectants (e.g., 4 per cent formalin) and still be used successfully. Inasmuch as these agents kill the tissue, it is apparent that the transplant provides a matrix about which the host deposits new tissue; steel or plastic pins, tubes, or valves are often used in the same situation with better results and more safely.

The developing fetus has been cited as one of the best examples of immunologically privileged tissue. Except in syngeneic animals, the fetus always contains antigens peculiar to the male and lacking from the mother. The mother does not become sensitized to these antigens and reject them. Other tissues transplanted to the uterine wall are rejected in the customary fashion, so the pregnant uterus evidently possesses some property that protects the fetus. This is presumed to reside in the trophoblast, a layer of tissue that physically separates the uterine wall from the fetus. Each trophoblast cell is covered with mucoprotein, and this layer of material protects the fetus from rejection.

TUMOR IMMUNOLOGY

The immunologic surveillance hypothesis postulates that the immune mechanism evolved as part of the homeostatic system of the body. Its primary function is to assist in maintaining the cellular status quo by destroying or removing aberrant cells—mutated or otherwise altered cells that multiply without being subject to the normal controls that restrict tissues and organs to their most efficient size, shape, and function. The immune mechanism is "turned off" as long as only "self" components or determinants, are present. However, if a single lymphoid cell of the proper kind encounters a foreign component or determinant, the process of *recognition* that it is "not self" triggers the initial steps in the immunologic response. The lymphoid cell is stimulated to replicate, and all of its progeny possess the same recognition characteristic. Differentiation also occurs, leading to the formation of cells with the same recognition ability and, in addition, with some effector function. These cells then mediate the destruction or removal of the "not self" substance, either directly or indirectly (i.e., through the production of pharmacologically active or other chemicals).

Tumor-Specific Antigens

There are many mechanisms by which tissue cells arise or appear that are not subject to the normal homeostatic controls. Somatic mutation may change any one of many characteristics, physical or chemical carcinogens may cause nonlethal alterations, virus invasion may transform a host cell by changing its nucleic acids. There are also tumors that can be transferred from one animal to another by artificial inoculation; if this can be accomplished deliberately without difficulty, it is likely to occur naturally under appropriate conditions.

Tumor cells usually possess antigenic determinant sites that differ from any found on normal cells, and these can be recognized as "foreign" by cells of the immune system. Whether or not this response leads to destruction of the tumor depends on various factors. Most of the distinctive tumor antigens are located on a cell surface, where they are readily recognized. Some resemble major histocompatibility antigens and are strong, whereas others behave like minor histocompatibility antigens and tend to be of little significance.

The antigens of tumors induced by chemical carcinogens resemble the specific transplantation antigens and are very diverse. That is, each tumor has a unique antigen, different from those in tumors induced by the same chemical in other animals. They are called tumor-specific transplantation antigens (TSTA). Each tumor is antigenic, but it induces resistance against only itself; cross-resistance is not engendered.

The antigenic status of virus-induced tumors is just the opposite. All tumors induced by a given oncogenic virus possess the same tumor-specific antigens, so that cross-protection occurs; that is, any animal immunized with a given tumor is protected against any other tumor induced by the same virus. Antigens produced in response to different viruses differ from each other. The antigen in the tumor cells is not viral protein; instead, it is a new protein, presumably synthesized by the host cell after transformation by the virus and incorporation of viral nucleic acid into that of the host. Several kinds of antigens may be produced. Surface or transplantation-type antigens are largely responsible for rejection of transplanted virus-induced tumors. In addition, the T or "neoantigens" are situated intracellularly, sometimes in the nucleus of tumor cells. They are demonstrable by immunofluorescence.

Spontaneous tumors in mice are sometimes nonantigenic or only weakly antigenic. Some are induced by viruses that are transmitted from mother to progeny. Their incidence is great in certain strains of mice. Neonatal contact with the virus induces tolerance to the tumor-specific antigen, so the animals cannot be immunized. Sporadically occurring tumors are sometimes mildly antigenic.

In addition to tumor-specific antigens, a tumor possesses the normal histocompatibility antigens of the animal in which the tumor first arises. Therefore, if the tumor is transplanted to an allogeneic individual, it is rejected in the same manner as a normal tissue allograft. When transplanted into a syngeneic individual, it is accepted, flourishes, and may kill the recipient. The number of tumor cells required for a lethal syngeneic graft is greater if the recipient has been previously immunized against that tumor.

An interesting antigen that occurs in patients with adenocarcinoma of the colon or rectum is called the carcinoembryonic antigen (CEA), because it is also present in embryonic gastrointestinal mucosa and in the liver and pancreas, which are endodermal derivatives of the gut. The carcinoembryonic antigen is a glycoprotein of M.W. 100,000 to 200,000, containing about 50 per cent carbohydrate. It can be detected by the use of rabbit antiserum against an extract of normal intestinal mucosa. The CEA appears to be coded by a normal gene that is expressed temporarily in the fetal endodermal cells and again in the adult if these cells become malignant. Highly sensitive radioimmunoassays for CEA assist greatly in the diagnosis of this form of cancer.

Host Resistance and the Immune Response

A host in which a tumor has arisen or been introduced may develop some degree of immunity, depending upon the rate of growth of the tumor or the size of the transplant. A small or slowly growing tumor can incite a sufficient immune response to retard growth of the tumor and eventually reject it. However, if the tumor is too large or grows too fast, it may overwhelm any developing immunity and be fatal.

Effector Mechanisms in Tumor Immunity

Inasmuch as tumors possess specific antigenic determinants that differ from any others possessed by the host, it is to be expected that both humoral antibodies and specifically sensitized lymphoid cells will be produced. However, as in the case of tissue transplantation, the antibodies are generally not harmful to the tumor and in fact may enhance its growth. Anti-tumor protective immunity appears to be a function of specifically reactive lymphoid cells, particularly thymus-derived cells. This conclusion is supported by the observation that slowly growing tumors are often infiltrated with large numbers of lymphoid cells. Moreover, the success or failure of immunity depends in part on the cellular immunocompetence of the animal. Adult mice whose thymus glands have been removed surgically or who have been treated with ALS produce tumors when treated with oncogenic polyoma virus. Similarly, humans with a defective immune system have an unusually high incidence of various cancers; recipients of kidney allografts who have received prolonged immunosuppressive treatment are about 4,000 times as likely to develop lymphomas as the normal population.

Immunologic Escape of Tumors

If the normal surveillance mechanism breaks down or unusual circumstances supervene, tumor cells escape from control. Occasional clones therefore develop into clinically significant tumors when (1) the tumor-specific antigens are poorly immunogenic; (2) the host's ability to mount a cell-mediated immune response is depressed, as in very young or aging individuals; (3) "enhancing" or "blocking" antibody protects tumor antigens from attack by specifically reactive lymphocytes; or (4) variant tumor cells emerge that have a high growth rate or unusual resistance to immune cytotoxicity and hence produce new tumor cells faster than the host can eliminate them.

Immunotherapy of Human Tumors

One of the problems in the therapy of tumors arises from the fact that most agents used to kill or even to inhibit the growth and multiplication of tumor cells also kill or inhibit normal cells, including those of the lymphoid system. The treatment regimen must therefore be very carefully regulated so as not to do more harm than good. In conventional therapy, it has been found unnecessary to kill every last cancer cell, provided that the normal immune system is not too seriously damaged.

"Autoimmunization" of patients with antigenic material from their own tumors is an attempt to stimulate the immune system specifically. Viable cells have been used, but they are dangerous because, if the treatment fails, they may develop into another tumor. Therefore, cells killed by irradiation or chemical treatment are used. This form of immunization has been partly successful, but it is attended by the risk that formation of enhancing antibody can lead to the undesired effect.

Another approach to tumor therapy is an attempt to magnify the nonspecific aspects of the patient's immune system. Living BCG injected into an animal tumor incites an intense cell-mediated immune reaction. The lymphocytes that congregate at the site produce lymphokines, some of which destroy the tumor nonspecifically. Activated ("angry") macrophages may also destroy tumor cells. Favorable results with BCG in experimental animals appear to warrant its trial in man.

Additional Sources of Information

Alexander, P., and G. H. Fairley: The allergic response in malignant disease. In Gell, P. G. H., and R. R. A. Coombs (Eds.): Clinical Aspects of Immunology, 2nd ed., pp. 499–539. 1968. Oxford, Blackwell Scientific Publications.

Amos, D. B.: Genetic and antigenetic aspects of human histocompatibility systems. In Dixon, F. J., and H. G. Kunkel (Eds.): Advances in Immunology, vol. 10, pp. 251–297. 1969. New York, Academic Press, Inc.

Billingham, R., and W. Silvers: The Immunobiology of Transplantation. 1971. Englewood Cliffs, N.J., Prentice-Hall, Inc.

Burnet, Sir Macfarlane: Auto-immunity and Auto-immune Disease. 1972. Lancaster, Lancs., Medical and Technical Publishing Co., Ltd.

Gorer, P. A.: The antigenic structure of tumors. In Taliaferro, W. H., and J. H. Humphrey (Eds.): Advances in Immunology, vol. 1, pp. 345–393. 1961. New York, Academic Press, Inc.

Habel, K.: Antigens of virus-induced tumors. In Dixon, F. J., and H. G. Kunkel (Eds.): Advances in Immunology, vol. 10, pp. 229–250. 1969. New York, Academic Press, Inc.

Hauschka, T. S.: Tumor immunity. In Rose, N. R., et al. (Eds.): Principles of Immunology, pp. 417–438. 1973. New York, Macmillan Publishing Co., Inc.

Hellström, K. E., and I. Hellström: Lymphocyte-mediated cytotoxicity and blocking serum antibody to tumor antigens. In Dixon, F. J., and H. G. Kunkel (Eds.): Advances in Immunology, vol. 18, pp. 209–277. 1974. New York, Academic Press, Inc.

Lance, E. M., P. B. Medawar, and R. N. Taub: Antilymphocyte serum. In Dixon, F. J., and H. G. Kunkel (Eds.): Advances in Immunology, vol. 17, pp. 1–92. New York, Academic Press, Inc.

Paterson, P. Y: Experimental allergic encephalomyelitis and autoimmune disease. In Dixon, F. J., and J. H. Humphrey (Eds.): Advances in Immunology, vol. 5, pp. 131–208. 1966. New York, Academic Press, Inc.

Shulman, S.: Thyroid antigens and autoimmunity. In Dixon, F. J., and H. G. Kunkel (Eds.): Advances in Immunology, vol. 14, pp. 85–185. 1971. New York, Academic Press, Inc.

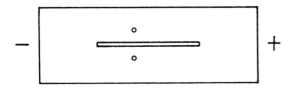

CHAPTER ELEVEN

APPENDIX: EXPERIMENTS IN SEROLOGY

I. INTRODUCTION

The first requirement for success in serologic work is the ability to follow instructions and exercise good technique. The student should become familiar with each experiment before he begins work and should then concentrate on the required manipulations. With adequate practice and constant attention to details nearly everyone can acquire sufficient facility to work rapidly and accurately and obtain proper results.

The aims of laboratory experiments in serology are twofold: first, to provide familiarity with various technical procedures, and secondly, to illustrate fundamental principles. The student must develop skill in injecting and bleeding laboratory animals and handling pipettes and other serologic equipment. He should learn how to set up and read the various tests and should understand the basic principles of the reactions and factors that affect their outcome. He should also learn the importance and significance of proper controls.

Serologic work requires clean equipment, although strictly aseptic technique is not always necessary. However, the materials are often dangerous because of their infectious nature and must be handled carefully and disposed of properly to avoid serious accident.

The procedures outlined in the following sections are intended as experiments or demonstrations for teaching purposes and are not to be considered "standard methods." In many particulars they are subject to considerable variation, according to the preference of the instructor and his experience with the materials available. He will usually find that preparation for each experiment requires one or more "trial runs" to establish a suitable choice of reagents or range of concentrations that can be expected to yield the desired result. No attempt is made to indicate all the possible experimental variations.

The methods suggested in the first few sections are described in considerable detail; later, when the student should have mastered most of the fundamental techniques, directions are given in briefer form.

II. BLOOD COUNTS

1. Total Red Blood Cell Count

a. Clean the (middle left) finger with 70 per cent alcohol. Prick with a lancet and squeeze gently to secure a drop of blood. Wipe off the first drop with dry cotton and secure another fairly large drop.

b. Draw blood to the mark 0.5 of a red cell pipette, using a suction tube.

c. Immediately draw diluting fluid to the mark 101, rotating the pipette while filling it. (Toisson's solution is commonly used: 0.5 per cent NaCl, 4.0 per cent Na_2SO_4, 15 per cent glycerin.)

d. Holding the pipette horizontally, shake it up and down for 1 to 2 minutes, finally giving it a few horizontal shakes.

e. Discard 3 or 4 drops and fill a hemacytometer chamber. Allow the cells to settle a few minutes.

f. Count the cells in 80 *small* squares of the ruled area (see Figure 11–1), using the high dry (43 to 45×) objective of the microscope. The ruled area is divided into nine large squares, each 1 mm. on a side. The central large square is subdivided into 25 medium-sized squares, each of which is further subdivided into 16 small squares. Count the corpuscles in five groups of 16 small squares, preferably the four corner groups and the center group. Count only cells within the squares or touching the lines above and to the left.

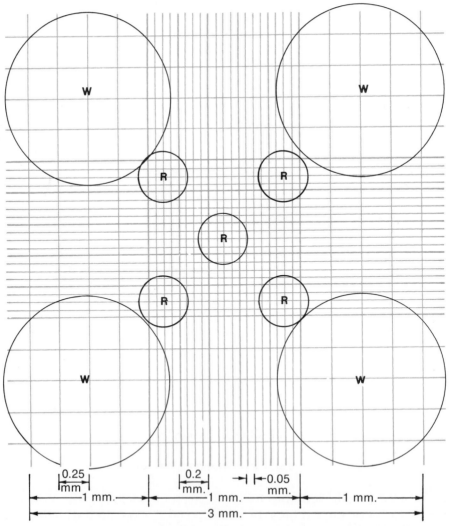

Figure 11–1. Hemacytometer rulings showing areas in which red cells (R) and white cells (W) are counted.

g. Multiply the total count obtained by 10,000 (i.e., add four zeros). This gives the number of red blood cells per cubic millimeter of blood.

Explanation: The small squares are 1/20 mm. on a side, and the chamber is 1/10 mm. deep. The volume of blood dilution in one small square is therefore 1/4,000 cu. mm. Since 80 small squares are counted, the red cells in 80/4,000 or 1/50 cu. mm. are found. The blood was diluted 0.5/101 or approximately 1/200, so the count as obtained represents the cells in 1/10,000 cu. mm. of whole blood. Hence the count is multiplied by 10,000 to give the red cells per cu. mm. of blood.

2. Total White Blood Cell Count

a. Use the same procedure as for red cells except that a white cell pipette is employed, filled to the mark 0.5 with blood and to the mark 11 with white cell diluting fluid (0.5 per cent acetic acid containing a little crystal violet; the acid dissolves the red cells and makes the white cells stand out as highly refractile bodies).

b. Count with the low power (10×) objective the white cells in the four corner *large* squares of the ruled area. The total number, multiplied by 50, gives the white blood cells per cubic millimeter of blood.

Explanation: The large squares are 1 mm. on a side, and the chamber is 1/10 mm. deep, so the volume of diluted blood in one such square is 1/10 cu. mm., and in four squares it is 4/10 cu. mm. The blood was diluted 0.5/11, or approximately 1/20. The count obtained represents the white cells in 4/200 or 1/50 cu. mm. of blood. Hence the count is multiplied by 50 to give the white cells per cu. mm. of blood.

3. Differential White Blood Cell Count

a. Have available three *clean* microscope slides.

b. Prepare and puncture the finger as usual and place a small drop of blood near one end of each of two slides.

c. Use the other slide to spread the blood into thin films. Hold it at an angle of about 30° and draw it along the slide from position 1 to position 2, as shown in Figure 11–2. When the drop is reached, capillarity will cause the drop to flow along the edge of the spreader slide. Immediately push the spreader away from the drop to position 3 and remove. Blood follows the spreader and makes a thin, even film. It should dry almost immediately in air. Do not heat. Thicker smears are produced when the spreader is held more nearly vertical.

d. Stain with Wright's stain:

(1) Cover the film with 10 to 15 drops of stain. Let stand 1 minute.

(2) Add an equal amount of Wright buffer (KH_2PO_4, 1.63 g., Na_2HPO_4, 3.2 g.,

Figure 11–2. Preparation of blood smear. Start with spreader slide at 1, draw it to position 2 and let drop of blood spread, then push spreader quickly to 3 and remove.

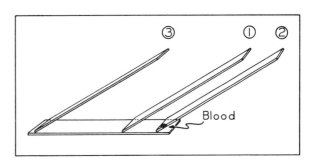

distilled water, 1 liter), dropwise, and let stand until a greenish metallic sheen or scum appears on the surface (usually in 2 to 3 minutes). Wash with running water until the smear appears pink. Dry in air.

3. Observe under oil with the 95× objective. Pink cells are erythrocytes; those with purple nuclei are white blood cells. Examine 100 WBC in order as found and classify, recording the number of each kind. These numbers represent the percentages of the various types in the circulating blood. Use a standard hematology or diagnostic laboratory manual, such as Bray (1946) or Kolmer et al. (1951) as an aid in classification of the following:

(1) polymorphonuclear neutrophils
(2) eosinophils
(3) basophils
(4) lymphocytes
(5) monocytes

III. PREPARATION OF IMMUNIZING MATERIALS

1. Bacterins

Bacterins are suspensions of bacteria used for stimulating the production of antibodies in humans and animals for prophylactic or therapeutic purposes, or for the production of antisera. A suitably prepared bacterin contains a definite number of bacterial cells (e.g., 500,000,000 or 1,000,000,000 per ml.) and is usually sterile. Preparation of a bacterin includes the following steps: (a) mass cultivation of the bacteria, (b) suspension in saline and dilution to the requisite concentration, and (c) sterilization and preservation.

a. Inoculate two to five slants of a suitable agar medium heavily (i.e., over the entire surface) with the organism to be employed and incubate under proper conditions to secure heavy growth. *Salmonella typhosa*, for example, grows well on nutrient or trypticase soy agar in 12 to 18 hours at 32 to 37° C.

b. Add approximately 2 ml. of saline (0.85 per cent NaCl) to each slant and gently loosen the bacterial growth with a sterile loop. Gram stain the suspensions, pool those that appear pure in a sterile test tube containing glass beads, and shake well to break up clumps.

c. Several methods are available for counting the bacteria in a suspension.

(1) Wright method:

(a) Prepare a Pasteur pipette by drawing an 8-inch piece of 7-mm. glass tubing and breaking so that the constricted capillary portion is about 3 inches long. Mark the pipette approximately 1 inch from its tip.

(b) Using a rubber bulb, draw 4 per cent sodium citrate solution to the mark and let in a bubble of air.

(c) Take up blood from a finger prick to the mark and let in another bubble of air.

(d) Draw up the bacterial suspension to the mark.

(e) Expel the contents of the pipette onto a clean microscope slide and mix by alternately aspirating into the pipette and expelling five or six times.

(f) Deposit a drop on one end of each of two or three microscope slides. Spread as directed above (II,3,c) and stain by Wright's method.

(g) Count the bacteria and red blood corpuscles separately in several oil immersion fields until about 200 corpuscles have been counted. Assuming that normal blood contains 5,000,000,000 RBC per ml., calculate by simple proportion the number of bacteria per ml. of the stock suspension.

(2) Hemacytometer method:

(a) Dilute the bacterial stock suspension 1:200 with filtered weak crystal violet in a red cell pipette.

(b) Fill a hemacytometer counting chamber and allow the cells to settle.

(c) Count the bacteria in 80 small squares (five groups of 16, as in the total red cell count) and multiply the total by 10,000,000 to obtain the number of bacteria per ml.

(3) Opacity method:

(a) Dilute the bacterial stock suspension as necessary (e.g., 1:5, 1:10, etc.) to get an optical density (OD) reading near the center of the spectrophotometer scale, using light at a wavelength of 530 mμ.

(b) Read the OD and refer to a graph such as that in Figure 11–3 to determine the number of bacteria per ml. in the dilution. Multiply by the reciprocal of the dilution to calculate bacteria per ml. of stock suspension.

d. Calculate the amount of stock suspension required to prepare 30 ml. of bacterin containing one billion cells per ml. as follows:

$$\text{ml. stock to use} = \frac{30 \times 1,000,000,000}{\text{bacteria/ml. in stock suspension}}$$

e. Pipette the required amount of stock suspension into a sterile vaccine bottle (e.g., Army Medical School type), add sufficient preservative to yield the desired final concentration, and make up to 30 ml. with saline. Cap the container with a sterile vaccine bottle stopper. Merthiolate (1:10,000) is a good general sterilizing and preserving agent, although formalin (0.5 per cent) may be preferred. The preservative may be added to the saline used to prepare the original bacterial suspension and to dilute it, if desired. Some bacterins are sterilized by heating in a waterbath for 30 minutes at a temperature between 55 and 65° C.

f. Test the bacterin for sterility. Heated preparations may be tested immediately, chemically disinfected bacterins after 1 or more days. Using a sterile syringe and needle withdraw a sample of the bacterin and inoculate suitable broth and agar media (e.g., thioglycollate broth and trypticase soy agar slant). If no growth appears in 4 days the preparation is considered ready to use.

g. Label the bottle showing the name of the organism, the name of the person who prepared the bacterin, and the date. Store in the refrigerator when not in use.

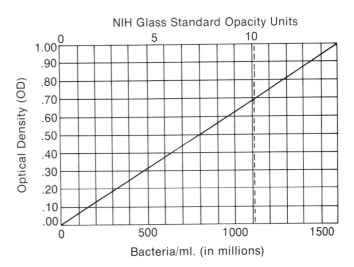

Figure 11–3. Standard optical density curve calibrated against an NIH powdered glass standard. Similar curves can be calibrated against BaSO$_4$ standards or against bacterial suspensions standardized by direct microscopic count.

2. Erythrocytes

A 50 per cent suspension of washed red blood cells is satisfactory for production of antiserum in experimental animals.

a. Draw blood of the desired species aseptically. Defibrinate it by shaking with glass beads or use one of the following to prevent clotting: heparin (0.1 mg. per ml. of blood), sodium citrate (3 mg. per ml.), or potassium oxalate (2 mg. per ml.). A satisfactory mixture contains 2.4 per cent ammonium oxalate and 1.6 per cent potassium oxalate; it is used in the proportion of 0.05 ml. per ml. of blood, either as the solution or dried in the bottom of a vial or test tube. Blood that must be stored may be preserved in the refrigerator for as long as 10 weeks with an equal volume of Alsever's solution:

Glucose	2.05%
Sodium citrate	0.80%
Sodium chloride	0.42%
Citric acid	0.055%

b. To prepare cells for injection, centrifuge the desired quantity of blood at moderate speed, remove the supernatant liquid by aspiration with a Pasteur pipette attached to a water pump, and wash the cells three times by suspending in 0.9 per cent NaCl, centrifuging, and discarding the supernatant liquid. After the final centrifugation suspend the cells in an equal volume of 0.9 per cent NaCl. (Saline containing 0.9 per cent NaCl, rather than 0.85 per cent NaCl, is often used with red blood cells because it is more nearly isotonic with the cell contents.)

3. Protein Solutions

Solutions containing about 1 per cent protein are satisfactory for inoculation into laboratory animals. Serum diluted 1:7 with saline contains about this concentration of protein. Dissolve egg albumin and other dried proteins by adding a little saline and mixing with a glass rod to make a thick paste; dilute the paste gradually. Stirring is preferable to shaking, which creates a troublesome foam. Add a preservative if desired.

4. Use of Adjuvants

Aluminum hydroxide and paraffin oil are frequently incorporated into materials for animal inoculation. They reduce the number of injections required and often increase the antibody response.

A. ALUM PRECIPITATION

Prepare 50 ml. of the bacterin or other immunizing agent and its preservative (if any) in double strength. Add 2.33 ml. of 10 per cent $AlCl_3$ and sufficient 20 per cent NaOH to bring the reaction to pH 7. Dilute to 100 ml. with saline.

B. OIL-IN-WATER EMULSION (FREUND ADJUVANT)

Freund's incomplete adjuvant contains 8.5 volumes of light paraffin oil and 1.5 volumes of an emulsifier (Arlacel A). The complete adjuvant also contains 10 mg. per ml. of dried *Mycobacterium tuberculosis* or *M. butyricum*. Both adjuvants can be obtained commercially.

Protein solutions or other antigens are emulsified with Freund adjuvant as an oil-in-water emulsion by mixing equal volumes of the reagents, using a syringe with an 18 gauge needle to aspirate and expel the mixture repeatedly as vigorously as possible. Test the emulsion by allowing a drop to fall onto the surface of water. If the drop remains perfectly formed and does not spread over the surface, the emulsion is ready for use.

IV. INOCULATION AND BLEEDING OF ANIMALS

Laboratory animals are usually as cooperative as humans if treated properly. There should be no confusion or unnecessary noise in the operating room. Animals should be handled firmly but gently, and the student should know beforehand what he is going to do so that he will not fumble around unnecessarily and irritate the animal.

Observe animals closely during the period of experimentation for signs of an unfavorable reaction to the inoculated material. Such signs include loss of weight resulting from loss of appetite, listlessness and apathy, and fever. If an animal under immunization shows such signs, suspend injections until its condition improves or decrease the doses.

Syringes of 1 ml. (tuberculin), 2 ml., 5 ml., 10 ml., 20 ml., and 50 ml. capacity are required. In addition, adapters for connecting hypodermic needles to rubber tubing are useful. The size of needle varies with the intended use (see Table 11–1).

Sterilize syringes and needles by autoclaving or boil for 20 minutes. It is advisable to keep on hand a reserve supply of sterile needles. They may be slipped into pieces of 6- or 7-mm. glass tubing slightly longer than the needles, placed point down in plugged test tubes, and sterilized in the autoclave. Check needles for sharpness before sterilization. Examine them with a hand lens and test by drawing them between the fingers. Animals respond very poorly to barbed and dull needles. Needles can be sharpened, if not in too bad condition, with a very fine sharpening stone, or they may be "touched up" by rubbing on a flat glass surface.

Before filling a syringe from a vaccine bottle, disinfect the stopper (e.g., with 70 per cent alcohol). Retract the plunger of the syringe to the same volume as the vaccine to be withdrawn, insert the needle through the thin central portion of the stopper, and force air from the syringe into the bottle. Invert bottle and syringe, and with the bottle uppermost take slightly more than the desired quantity of vaccine into the syringe. Return entrapped air bubbles to the bottle and bring the plunger to the required volume.

After each use a syringe and needle must be thoroughly cleaned. If it is undesirable (because of the virulence of the inoculum) to separate the barrel and plunger immediately, withdraw the plunger almost completely from the barrel to prevent sticking. Boil syringes and needles contaminated with infectious material before cleaning. All equipment used with blood must be thoroughly rinsed with water

Table 11–1 *Sizes of Hypodermic Needles for Various Purposes*

Purpose	Gauge	Length
Intravenous injection of rabbits	25–27	⅜–½ in.
Subcutaneous injections	23–26	¾–1 in.
Intraperitoneal injections	20–24	1 in.
Bleeding rabbits from the heart	18	1½–2 in.
Bleeding guinea pigs from the heart	22	1–1½ in.

immediately—otherwise it will have to be soaked for some time in a detergent to loosen and remove clotted blood.

1. Rabbits

Young adult rabbits (2 to 4 kg.) are usually preferred for production of antisera. Inoculations may be intravenous, intraperitoneal, or subcutaneous; the intravenous route is commonly employed.

A variety of schedules is used for routine production of antibacterial sera in rabbits. One that gives satisfactory results with killed suspensions of gram-negative rod bacteria consists of the following intravenous injections:

> 1st day: 0.1 ml.
> 4th day: 0.3 ml.
> 8th day: 0.5 ml.
> 11th day: 1.0 ml.
> 15th day: 2.0 ml.

Serum of high titer is usually secured 3 to 5 days after the last injection.

Closely spaced intravenous injections of living bacteria are satisfactory with many kinds of organisms. Stock saline suspensions having the turbidity of an agglutination test antigen (see page 315) are employed. Fresh stock suspensions are prepared as indicated below and refrigerated when not in use. The injection schedule is as follows:

> 1st day: 0.1 ml. fresh stock suspension diluted 1:100
> 2nd day: 0.2 ml. suspension diluted 1:100
> 3rd day: 0.3 ml. suspension diluted 1:100
> 4th day: 0.1 ml. fresh stock suspension undiluted
> 5th day: 0.2 ml. suspension undiluted
> 6th day: 0.3 ml. suspension undiluted
> 11th day: 0.5 ml. fresh stock suspension undiluted
> 16th day: trial titration; if titer is satisfactory, bleed from the heart; otherwise inject 0.5 ml. fresh undiluted stock suspension and titrate after an additional 5 days.

Prepare anti-erythrocyte sera in rabbits by a series of twice weekly intravenous injections of 1 ml. of 50 per cent suspension of washed red blood cells. Three or 4 days after the fourth injection titrate the animal's serum, and if the titer is not satisfactory give additional inoculations. Another injection routine consists of four daily intravenous injections of 1 ml. of 10 per cent red blood cells per kg. body weight, followed by six injections every second day. Peak titer is usually found about 2 weeks after the first injection and is often maintained for several days.

Inject 1 per cent protein solutions intravenously once or twice a week; the number of injections is determined by the results of trial titrations of the animal's serum. After the first 2 weeks, make injections following a rest period of a week or more by the intraperitoneal route to reduce the likelihood of anaphylactic shock. Intravenous injections usually consist of 1 ml. amounts; intraperitoneal doses may be 2 to 3 ml.

One or two 0.5 ml. subcutaneous injections of antigens emulsified in paraffin oil usually suffice to produce antisera of high titer. Three or 4 weeks after the first injection perform a trial titration, and if the antibody titer is not as high as desired give a second injection.

Anti-BSA may be prepared by using 1 ml. of emulsion containing 50 mg. of the protein in Freund's complete adjuvant. Five doses of 0.2 ml. each are injected subcutaneously into separate sites. Eight weeks later a trial bleeding is made. Further injections are not usually required.

A. INTRAVENOUS INJECTION

The marginal vein of the rabbit ear is readily accessible. It is located at the outer edge of the dorsal side of the ear. Reserve one ear for injections, the other for bleeding. The first injection of a series is always made as near the tip of the ear as possible, succeeding injections being made closer toward the animal's head, so that scar tissue will not prevent injected material from entering the circulation.

Hold the animal on the lap facing the operator. Shave the skin over the vein with a sharp razor blade and rub vigorously with 70 per cent alcohol. A right-handed person usually finds it more convenient to inject the animal's left ear. Hold the ear with the left hand so that the middle finger supports the area to be injected, the little finger holding the tip of the ear down out of the way. Insert the inoculating needle, bevel up, in the direction of blood flow (toward the heart) through the skin and into the vein at a very acute angle (almost parallel) to the vein so that it does not pass completely through. Inject the inoculum slowly. When the vein is entered correctly the inoculum can be seen passing toward the heart as it partially replaces the blood. If the needle is not within the vein, the antigen will produce a blanched, raised area in the neighboring tissue. Gentle massage should be used to force the material out of the needle puncture, and injection should be attempted at another site. After the inoculation is completed, firmly apply cotton moistened with alcohol and withdraw the needle. After a few moments remove the cotton. If bleeding occurs, replace the cotton and hold for several minutes.

B. SUBCUTANEOUS INJECTION

The back is a convenient site for subcutaneous inoculation. Clip and shave the hair on one side of the back and disinfect the area with alcohol. Pinch up a fold of skin between the thumb and forefinger, insert the inoculating needle into the ridge between the finger and thumb for about one-half inch, and release the skin. Inject the inoculum slowly; a raised bleb shows that the injection was properly made. Wash the area again with alcohol.

C. INTRAPERITONEAL INJECTION

Have an assistant hold the animal firmly, head down. Clip the hair in the median abdominal line and disinfect with alcohol. Pinch up a fold of skin and peritoneum between the thumb and forefinger, insert the needle into the ridge of skin and through the fold of peritoneum, release the peritoneum and skin, and make the injection. There should be no bleb of injected fluid. Wash the area with alcohol.

D. BLEEDING FROM THE EAR VEIN

Small amounts of blood are easily secured from the marginal vein of the ear, and with patience even as much as 50 ml. may be taken. Usually the vein is punctured and the blood allowed to flow, although a syringe and needle are sometimes employed. The first bleeding of a series is made from a site near the base of the ear, succeeding punctures being made more and more distal from the head.

Hold the animal on the lap facing away from the operator. Rub the ear vigorously to promote strong circulation of blood, and if necessary place a drop of xylol on the tip of the ear to produce mild inflammation. If xylol is used, it must be removed before the animal is returned to its cage, lest prolonged inflammation cause permanent damage and destroy the future usefulness of the ear. Xylol is removed by washing at least three times with liberal amounts of alcohol, wiping each time with cotton.

Shave the area to be punctured and wash with alcohol. Rub petrolatum over both sides of the ear to prevent blood from sticking to the fur. Place an artery clamp (Dieffenbach) over the vein proximal to the site to be punctured. Hold the ear so that the middle finger of the left hand supports the site of puncture and make a short quick jab with a sharp instrument; this may be a piece of broken microscope slide or capillary pipette, or a metal lancet. Some operators make a small snip with scissors or a scalpel or razor blade. Collect the desired amount of blood in a centrifuge tube, then move the artery clamp distal to the puncture and hold dry absorbent cotton firmly over the puncture until bleeding stops.

Allow the tube of blood to stand at room temperature until clotting occurs. Then loosen the clot from the wall of the tube with a fine glass rod. The tube may be centrifuged immediately to throw down the clot or refrigerated overnight to allow the clot to retract and express the clear, straw colored serum. Remove the serum carefully with a pipette. A rubber tube with mouthpiece or a rubber bulb on the pipette permits close observation while the serum is withdrawn.

E. BLEEDING FROM THE HEART

Large quantities of blood are secured from the heart or from the jugular vein. Cardiac bleeding is usually simpler and can be repeatedly performed on the same animal if proper technique is used. Blood is drawn into a large syringe, or the needle may be attached by rubber tubing to a bottle fitted with a suction tube. If an assistant is available, anesthesia is not necessary, although it is usually helpful. Ether is often used, but great care must be exercised because rabbits are easily killed by an overdose. Nembutal or another barbiturate is frequently preferred. The dose by intravenous injection is about 1 ml. of a 4 per cent solution of Nembutal per kg. of body weight, or the solution may be injected until the animal no longer gives an eye reflex. An animal anesthetized with Nembutal remains asleep for about 2 hours.

Clip the area over the sternum and disinfect with alcohol and tincture of iodine. Locate the area of maximum pulsation, usually about midway of the sternum and slightly to the left, and insert the needle between two ribs, advancing it in a straight line toward the right shoulder. When the heart is entered, blood will appear in the syringe or tubing connected to the needle, and may be slowly aspirated. Fifty milliliters may safely be removed from an average rabbit; 80 to 120 ml. can usually be secured when it is not intended to save the animal. If difficulty is experienced in finding the heart, withdraw the needle almost completely and reinsert in another direction. Twisting the needle within the pericardial cavity is likely to tear the heart and cause immediate death.

After the blood has clotted, loosen the clot from the wall of the container with a glass rod and refrigerate for 24 to 48 hours. The clot usually retracts sufficiently to permit removal of clear serum by pipette. The last serum withdrawn may contain red blood cells and require centrifugation.

Serum is stored frozen in glass or plastic bottles or it is refrigerated. If not frozen, it must be preserved. Merthiolate (1:10,000) or phenol (0.5 per cent) are satisfactory. A stock 1 per cent solution of Merthiolate is prepared by adding 1 g. of the dry powder to 100 ml. of 1.4 per cent borax. Add this solution at the rate of 1 ml. per 100 ml. of serum.

Phenol dissolved in ether (equal parts by weight) is used in the proportion of 0.9 ml. per 100 ml. serum.

2. Guinea Pigs

Subcutaneous and intraperitoneal inoculations of guinea pigs are most commonly used. The procedures are very similar to those employed with rabbits.

A single operator can bleed guinea pigs from the heart if they are anesthetized. Ether is satisfactory. Hold an ether cone over the animal's nose until it stops kicking. Lay the animal on its back with the cone partially over its head, disinfect the area over the heart, insert the needle between two ribs at the point of maximum pulsation and advance it slowly, exerting slight negative pressure with the plunger of the syringe. As soon as the heart is entered, blood will appear in the syringe. Average guinea pigs yield about 5 ml. of blood without ill effects. If subjected to ether for only a few minutes they recover quickly.

3. Mice

Intraperitoneal injections are usually employed with mice and can be done without assistance. Hold the mouse by its tail with the right hand and let it try to run away. Grasp it firmly between the ears with the thumb and forefinger of the left hand and turn it over. Use the little finger of the left hand to hold the tail down and keep the body taut. Disinfect the abdomen with 70 per cent alcohol. Hold the animal's head down so that the intestines fall forward, and make the injection in the posterior region of the abdomen. A quick jab of the needle is usually followed by sudden contraction and relaxation of the abdominal wall, which indicates that the peritoneum has been entered.

Intravenous injections are easily made with a small needle into the tail veins. A light beneath the tail permits the operator to find the vein readily.

V. AGGLUTINATION

Agglutination tests are performed with particulate antigens such as bacterial cells or erythrocytes. Methods for preparing test antigens and setting up tests will be described.

1. Tube Agglutination

Tube agglutination tests are performed by mixing a constant amount of antigen suspension with increasing dilutions of antiserum, incubating, and reading the degree of clumping in each tube.

A. PREPARATION OF BACTERIAL TEST ANTIGENS

For most purposes a bacterial culture is grown on a slant of suitable agar medium inoculated heavily in a zig-zag manner with a loop or slightly bent needle. After incubation the organisms are washed off with saline and diluted to a turbidity that can best be determined by trial. The suspension should be sufficiently dense so that when added to serum in the actual test a faint but definite turbidity is evident. At a distance of 6 or 8 feet from a north window the strips of wood separating the panes are just visible through the suspension contained in an ordinary culture tube.

Test antigens for flagellar agglutination are either living or killed with formalin (0.5 per cent). Prepare somatic antigens of motile bacteria by heating heavy suspensions at 100° C. for 30 minutes before diluting with saline to the proper turbidity. Suspend nonmotile bacteria in saline containing 0.5 per cent formalin. Living or formalized (0.5 per cent) organisms are used for Vi agglutination.

B. SETTING UP THE TEST

Arrange in a serologic rack enough agglutination tubes (10 × 75 or 11 × 100 mm.) to exceed the expected titer of the serum and add one tube for a control. Pipette saline into each tube, 0.9 ml. into the first tube and 0.5 ml. into each of the others. Carefully measure 0.1 ml. of antiserum into the first tube with a 1 ml. serologic pipette (graduated to the tip). Mix the contents by aspirating most of it into the pipette and blowing out three to five times. This tube contains a 1:10 dilution of the serum. With the same pipette, transfer 0.5 ml. to the second tube, mix as before, and continue transfers in like manner to and including the next to the last tube. Discard 0.5 ml. from this tube. Each tube contains one-half the concentration of antiserum in the tube preceding (i.e., the dilution series is as follows: 1:10, 1:20, 1:40 . . .). Reserve the last tube as a control. Carefully measure 0.1 ml. of test antigen with a graduated pipette into each tube including the control. Shake the rack thoroughly and incubate.

It is frequently necessary to prepare more than one identical series of dilutions of the same antiserum. This is most conveniently done, and with greatest accuracy, by preparing all series of dilutions simultaneously. If only four or five such series are required, "master dilutions" can be prepared in the front row of agglutination tubes and pipetted into the other rows ("internal master dilutions"). When more rows of dilutions are needed, "external master dilutions" are prepared in larger test tubes. The use of master dilutions can best be illustrated by a diagram (Figure 11–4). Dispense saline into tubes in the front row and into the last tube of each row as indicated by the figures within the various tubes. Add antiserum to the first tube in the front row and mix. Pipette 0.5 ml. quantities into the two tubes behind it, and 1.5 ml. into the second tube of the front row. Continue mixing and transfers through the next to last tubes, and discard 1.5 ml. as indicated. Then add appropriate antigens to all tubes in each row.

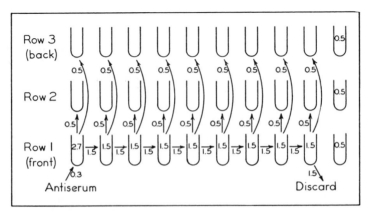

Figure 11–4. Preparation of triplicate simultaneous serial dilutions of antiserum using "internal" master dilutions. Figures within tubes indicate the amount of saline (ml.) initially added. Figures accompanying arrows represent the volumes (ml.) transferred. (Dilution series: 1:10, 1:20, 1:40 . . . 1:2,560, Control.)

C. INCUBATION

There is not complete uniformity with regard to incubation time and temperature for various kinds of agglutination. However, it is suggested that flagellar agglutination tests be incubated 2 hours at 37° C., read, reincubated for 12 to 18 hours at 55° C., and read again. Take the highest reading as the flagellar agglutinin titer of the serum. Incubate somatic agglutination tests 12 to 18 hours at 55° C. Tests for Vi agglutinin are incubated 2 hours at 37° C., read, and kept at room or refrigerator temperature overnight before final reading. In this case also the highest value obtained is considered the titer of the serum.

D. READING AGGLUTINATION TESTS

A good light source (for example, a gooseneck lamp) and a dark background are desirable for reading agglutination tests. Examine each tube first without shaking; then shake or flip to suspend the sediment. A 4+ (++++) reaction is one in which all cells are clumped at the bottom of the tube and usually resuspend as distinct granules, flakes, or flocculent masses in an otherwise clear fluid. In a negative (0 or −) reaction there is no clumping except normal sedimentation of individual cells, so shaking the tube causes little if any change in turbidity. Intermediate degrees of agglutination are graded 3+, 2+, and 1+. Somatic agglutination usually produces fine granules, whereas flagellar agglutination usually appears in the form of flocculent masses, but all gradations between these extremes may be observed. Considerable practice is necessary to develop facility and confidence in reading tests.

2. Microscopic Slide Agglutination

The formation of clumps of agglutinated bacteria can be observed directly with the microscope when antiserum diluted sufficiently is mixed with homologous bacteria. Employ a broth culture or saline suspension of a motile organism such as S. typhosa. Dilute the corresponding antiserum to about 1/10 or 1/20 of its titer as determined by tube agglutination (for example, a serum having a tube titer of 10,240 or 20,480 can be used in a dilution of 1:1,000). Mix on a cover glass one small (2 mm.) loopful each of the bacteria and the antiserum dilution and prepare a hanging drop, sealing it with petrolatum. Observe with the high dry objective of the microscope for 1 hour or longer and note the gradual cessation of motility and formation of loose clumps. It is desirable also to prepare a control slide consisting of bacteria and saline and compare the two preparations.

3. Macroscopic Slide Agglutination

The identification of unknown bacteria, particularly members of the Enterobacteriaceae, is often hastened by macroscopic slide agglutination. Antisera diluted only slightly (e.g., 1:5 or 1:10, according to their titers) are employed and are mixed with very heavy suspensions of the bacteria. Suspend the growth from a heavily inoculated agar slant evenly in about 2 ml. of saline. Mix one small drop (e.g., from a Pasteur pipette) of diluted antiserum with an equal amount of bacterial suspension within a paraffin or wax pencil ring on a microscope slide or other glass surface, and rock and tilt the slide for 1 to 5 minutes. Agglutination is shown as fine or coarse granulation. Always include a control consisting of saline and bacterial suspension for each organism tested.

This procedure is adaptable to large scale operation. Several bacteria can be tested against one or more antisera simultaneously. Plates of window glass can be employed, and a simple device for making rings with melted paraffin can be fashioned from a piece of wire bent into a ring about three-quarters of an inch in diameter, with a handle several inches long. The wire ring should be wrapped with string. In use, it is dipped into the melted paraffin and then touched momentarily to the glass plate, where the paraffin cools and hardens almost immediately. After the required number of horizontal and vertical rows of rings have been prepared, each bacterial antigen (for example) is placed in the rings of a horizontal row and each antiserum in the rings of a vertical row. A piece of glass 4½ inches by 6 inches is large enough to test six organisms in each of eight antisera.

VI. HEMAGGLUTINATION: BLOOD GROUPING

It is customary to determine the blood group and Rh type of persons who are to receive blood transfusions and of prospective donors. Test sera should be secured from a reliable laboratory.

1. Determination of ABO Group

Slide agglutination is considered less delicate than test tube methods and is more likely to show rouleaux formation, but it is commonly used because it is more rapid and convenient and less equipment is required.

Collect a large drop of blood from the finger in 1 ml. of 0.9 per cent NaCl in a small test tube. Divide a microscope slide in half with a marking pencil. Place a drop of anti-A serum in the left half of the slide, and a drop of anti-B serum in the right half. Add a drop of the blood cell suspension to each half of the slide but separate from the serum. Mix serum and cells with a wooden applicator or toothpick, using a fresh stick for each serum. Rock and tilt the slide to hasten agglutination; reaction will usually be apparent within 30 seconds to 2 minutes. Occasionally the reaction in anti-A will be slow because cells of subgroup A_2 react less strongly, so the slide should be kept 20 minutes before being discarded. Microscopic examination helps to decide some doubtful cases and to distinguish agglutination from rouleaux formation. The blood group of the cells is determined from reactions in the two sera as follows:

AGGLUTINATION OF RBC IN		
ANTI-A	ANTI-B	CELLS OF GROUP
−	−	O
+	−	A
−	+	B
+	+	AB

If anti-A_1 (adsorbed anti-A) serum is available, the subgroup of A or AB cells can be determined by a second test. Mix a drop of the cell suspension and a drop of the anti-A_1 serum on a slide and observe agglutination in the same manner. Interpret the results as follows:

Agglutination of A or AB RBC in anti-A_1	Cells of Group
+	A_1 or A_1B
−	A_2 or A_2B

2. Determination of Rh Type

Most Rh typing sera in use today require fresh whole blood or oxalated blood rather than saline suspensions of erythrocytes because they contain albumin agglutinins, which will not react properly in the absence of protein or certain other substances. The directions supplied with the testing serum must be followed carefully. One procedure used to determine the $Rh_o(D)$ type of red blood cells will be described.

Warm a microscope slide on a substage lamp and collect on it a large drop of blood directly from the finger. Add a drop of anti-Rh_o(anti-D) serum and mix with an applicator stick, spreading the mixture over an area about ¾ × 1½ inches. Keep the slide warm (37 to 45° C.) and tilt it back and forth. Look for clumping detectable with the naked eye. Positive reactions begin to appear in 30 seconds and should be complete in 2 minutes. Do not examine slides with the microscope or after drying.

Additional sera are required to determine the other Rh types.

3. Cross-match (Direct Compatibility) Tests

Cross-match tests are used directly before transfusion to determine that the blood of the donor is compatible with that of the recipient; otherwise transfusion reactions might occur, even though the two bloods are of the same group, because of other intragroup factors. The test with recipient's serum and donor's cells is most important, but many laboratories also include a test with patient's cells and donor's serum.

Slide tests are commonly performed. Secure specimens of venous blood from the recipient and from the prospective donor, allow them to clot, and remove the sera. Also prepare RBC suspensions by collecting a drop of blood from each individual in 1 ml. of saline. Mix one drop of recipient's serum and one drop of donor's cell suspension on the left half of a slide, as in blood group determination, and mix donor's serum and recipient's cells on the right half of the slide. Cover the slide with half a Petri dish to retard drying and read after 15 and 30 minutes. If the cells at the left agglutinate, the prospective donor is unsuitable for the patient in question, because his erythrocytes would be promptly agglutinated by antibodies in the circulation of the recipient. The cells at the right will not agglutinate if the two blood specimens are perfectly compatible.

Tube tests of compatibility may be more reliable than slide tests. A complete test includes mixtures containing 2 drops each of (a) recipient's serum and donor's cells and (b) donor's serum and recipient's cells, together with control tubes containing each serum and its own cells. The cells are often suspended in 20 to 30 per cent bovine albumin to detect albumin agglutinins. Centrifuge at moderate speed for 3 minutes, shake to resuspend the cells, and read. There should be no agglutination in any tube if the donor's blood is compatible with that of the recipient. (See also Table 7–17, page 222.)

VII. ADSORPTION OF AGGLUTININS

Adsorption of agglutinins is used to compare the antigenic structures of two or more bacteria. A laboratory demonstration of the principles of adsorption can be performed with a mixture of antisera against unrelated bacteria (e.g., S. typhosa and Escherichia coli), which is adsorbed with each organism separately, followed by titration of residual antibodies for each organism. A more practical demonstration consists of the reciprocal adsorption of antisera for two related bacteria, such as S.

typhosa (antigenic formula: 9,12:d:---) and *S. pullorum* (antigenic formula: 9,12:---:---). A suggested procedure for this experiment will be described.

1. Preparation of Adsorbing Antigens

Inoculate four thick (30 to 40 ml.) trypticase soy agar plates heavily all over the surface with *S. typhosa*, and four plates with *S. pullorum*. Employ cotton swabs for this purpose, and secure the inoculum by removing the entire growth from one slant culture for each plate. Incubate the plates at 37° C. for 48 hours. Add about 2 ml. of saline to each plate and gently loosen the growth with a bent glass rod. Use a Pasteur pipette with rubber bulb to pool the thick suspensions in centrifuge tubes so that there is one tube of each organism. Centrifuge at high speed to pack the cells. Remove the supernatant fluid, discarding it into a tube or flask to be sterilized.

2. Adsorption

Prepare 4 ml. each of 1:20 dilutions of antityphoid and antipullorum sera. Add 2 ml. of diluted antipullorum serum to the tube of *S. typhosa* cells, and 2 ml. of diluted antityphoid serum to the tube of *S. pullorum* cells. Suspend the cells in the sera by means of a wire loop, and incubate the tubes in a waterbath at 37° C. for 30 minutes to 1 hour. Centrifuge the two tubes at high speed. Remove the sera to appropriately marked test tubes. These are known as "adsorbed sera."

3. Titration of Unadsorbed and Adsorbed Sera

Prepare simultaneous duplicate serial dilutions of the original unadsorbed 1:20 antityphoid and antipullorum sera, using internal master dilutions. Start with a 1:40 dilution (tube 1 in the front row receives 1 ml. of saline and 1 ml. of 1:20 antiserum), and continue through as many dilutions as needed to indicate the titers of the sera. Prepare similar dilutions in duplicate of the adsorbed sera. Eight rows of tubes in all will be required.

Prepare test antigens of the usual turbidity for agglutination from 24-hour trypticase soy agar slants of the two organisms. Add typhoid antigen to all tubes in one row of each unadsorbed and each adsorbed serum, and pullorum antigen to the remaining rows of tubes. Incubate overnight at 50° C. and read. Tabulate the results in a form like that of Table 11–2.

VIII. PRECIPITATION

Additional procedures, including quantitative determination of precipitin, are found in the books by Campbell et al. (1970), Kabat (1961), and Williams and Chase (1967–1971).

1. Ring (Interfacial) Test

This sensitive precipitin test is used to detect and identify proteins and other antigenic materials. The reagents are carefully added to small test tubes so that they do not mix but form a sharp interface. Undiluted antiserum constitutes the bottom layer in

Table 11–2 *Form for a Reciprocal Adsorption Experiment*

Antiserum	Adsorbing Antigen	Test Antigen	Serum Dilutions					Control (Saline)
			1:40	1:80	1:160	1:320	etc.	
Anti-typhoid	None	Salmonella typhosa						
		Salmonella pullorum						
Anti-pullorum	None	Salmonella typhosa						
		Salmonella pullorum						
Anti-typhoid	Salmonella pullorum	Salmonella typhosa						
		Salmonella pullorum						
Anti-pullorum	Salmonella typhosa	Salmonella typhosa						
		Salmonella pullorum						

each tube, with serial dilutions of antigen forming the upper layer. Reaction is rapid with antisera of high potency. For this experiment any antigenic protein such as egg albumin or animal serum may be employed, together with homologous antiserum.

Use a pipette with capillary tip to place undiluted antiserum in each of a series of 6 × 50 mm. tubes to a depth of 6 to 10 mm. The exact amount is not critical, but the quantities should be reasonably uniform. In a separate series of larger test tubes prepare decimal dilutions (1:10, 1:100, 1:1000 . . .) of the antigen solution (e.g., 0.9 ml. saline + 0.1 ml. antigen, etc.). With a Pasteur pipette and rubber bulb, transfer antigen dilutions (and saline for a control tube) to the precipitin tubes containing antiserum. Insert the tip of the pipette into the precipitin tube and touch it to the inside wall a few millimeters above the antiserum. Carefully expel antigen so that it runs slowly down and forms a layer over the serum, withdrawing the pipette at the same rate. The layer of antigen should be one to two times as deep as that of antiserum. The same pipette may be used throughout if the control tube (saline over antiserum) is prepared first, the *most dilute* antigen tube next, and so on.

Examine the tubes after 10 and 30 minutes and 1 and 2 hours at room temperature. They may also be refrigerated overnight and observed again. The first sign of reaction is a thin line of white precipitate between the layers, which gradually broadens and increases in intensity. The precipitate later falls to the bottom of the tube and may be dislodged by flipping, as in reading agglutination tests. Grading the reactions (+, + + . . .) is difficult, but after some experience a fairly uniform system may be evolved. The titer is indicated by the reciprocal of the highest antigen dilution that gives a detectable reaction.

2. Optimal Ratio Titration

When antiserum and antigen are mixed, each lot of antiserum reacts most rapidly with its antigen when the two reagents are in a certain definite proportion. This may be demonstrated with a purified protein such as bovine serum albumin (BSA) and rabbit anti-BSA serum. Antigen dilutions to be employed must be determined by preliminary rough titration with each antiserum. A 1:100 dilution (i.e., 1 per cent solution) in saline is a convenient working stock solution.

Prepare triplicate simultaneous serial dilutions of BSA in 0.5 or 1.0 ml. amounts in agglutination tubes. Start with 1:500, for example, and continue through 7 or 8 tubes (see Table 11–3). Prepare external master dilutions of rabbit anti-BSA: 1:2, 1:4, 1:8. To each BSA dilution in the front row, add an equal amount of 1:2 anti-BSA; to each tube in the middle row, add 1:4 antiserum; and to each tube in the back row, add 1:8 antiserum. Note the time antiserum was added to each row. Shake the rack and allow to stand at room temperature, observing each tube every few minutes. Note the tube in each row in which opalescence or other evidence of reaction first appears. The most significant reaction is the appearance of discrete floccules. At the end of 1 or 2 hours grade the amount of precipitate in each tube. Compare the dilutions of antigen that reacted most rapidly and most strongly with each dilution of antiserum.

3. Passive Hemagglutination

It was noted previously (Table 4–1, page 83) that tannic acid–treated erythrocytes coated with a protein constitute a sensitive indicator for the presence of antibody corresponding to the protein. A solution containing as little as 0.005 μg. of antibody-N per ml. will agglutinate suitably prepared red cells. Two procedures are described in detail by Campbell et al. (1970, p. 279 ff.) and by Nowotny (1969, p. 143 ff.). Another procedure, employing Bacto-Formocells Rabbit (Difco Laboratories, Detroit, Michigan), is the following:

A. PREPARATION OF TANNED RED BLOOD CELLS

Wash Formocells four times with 4 volumes of normal saline. Determine their volume and dilute with 39 volumes of normal saline (2.5 per cent RBC). Add an equal volume of 1:2,000 tannic acid (Merck or Mallinckrodt) in saline and incubate in a waterbath at 37° C. for 10 minutes. Centrifuge and wash once with buffered saline at pH 5.6 (PBS 5.6) (100 ml. saline + 6 ml. M/15 Na_2HPO_4 + 94 ml. M/15 KH_2PO_4, adjusted if necessary). Resuspend in PBS 5.6 at 5 per cent concentration of RBC.

B. PREPARATION OF COATED RED BLOOD CELLS

Mix 1 volume of 5 per cent tanned RBC and 1 volume of protein solution (0.01 per cent bovine serum albumin, 0.005 per cent human serum albumin, or 0.1 per cent egg albumin, in normal saline) and stand at room temperature for 30 minutes with occasional gentle mixing. Centrifuge and wash the cells once in 4 volumes of 1:200 normal rabbit serum (NRS) (normal rabbit serum diluted 1:200 with normal saline). Centri-

Table 11–3   *Plan of a Precipitin Optimal Ratio Experiment*

Anti-BSA	Dilution of BSA							
	1:500	1:1,000	1:2,000	1:4,000	1:8,000	1:16,000	1:32,000	etc.
1:2								
1:4								
1:8								

fuge and resuspend the cells in 1 volume of 1:200 NRS (to make 5 per cent coated tanned RBC). This may be preserved by addition of Merthiolate to a concentration of 1:10,000 and stored at 2 to 8° C.

C. ANTISERUM TITRATION

Prepare a series of doubling dilutions of the antiserum in 10 × 75 mm. tubes, using 1:200 NRS as diluent and final volumes of 0.5 ml. Include a control tube with diluent only. To each tube add 0.05 ml. of the coated RBC suspension and shake the rack to mix well. Allow to sediment at room temperature and read after 2 hours and again overnight (see Figure 7–2, page 187).

+ Compact, granular mat of agglutinated cells covering bottom of tube or smooth mat with folded or ragged edges.

± Diffuse film of agglutinated cells surrounded by a narrow ring of cells.

− Heavy ring of cells or a uniform smooth dark button of cells in center of tube.

4. Ouchterlony Gel Diffusion Test

Gel diffusion precipitation methods permit resolution of the soluble antigenic components of a mixture and are useful in studying the purity and identity of the antigens in a natural material. Single or double diffusion procedures can be used. The Ouchterlony double diffusion method will be described.

Heat to dissolve 0.85 g. of a refined grade of agar such as Ionagar No. 2 (Consolidated Laboratories, Inc., Chicago Heights, Ill.) in 99 ml. of borate saline prepared by adding 5 ml. of borate saline buffer, pH 8.4–8.5 (boric acid, 6.184 g.; sodium tetraborate, $Na_2B_4O_7 \cdot 10 H_2O$, 9.536 g.; NaCl, 4.384 g.; distilled water to 1.0 liter) to 94 ml. of 0.85 per cent NaCl. Add 1.0 ml. of 1 per cent Merthiolate and pour into Petri dishes to a depth of about 2 mm. (approx. 15 ml. agar).

When the agar is hard, cut holes in a convenient pattern using a cork borer 7 mm. in diameter. A useful pattern consists of a central hole with six circumferential holes spaced so that the distance from the edge of the center hole to that of the peripheral holes is 1 cm. The agar can be removed from the holes by sucking with a pipette attached to a vacuum line. It is often considered desirable to coat the plates with a thin layer of agar, which is allowed to dry, before pouring the 15 ml. portion.

Fill the central well with antiserum, using a Pasteur pipette, and fill the peripheral wells with antigens (e.g., homologous, related, and unrelated, in alternating sequence). Store the plates at room temperature and observe daily for lines of precipitate between the antiserum and antigen wells. Troublesome condensation may be avoided by placing a tightly fitting piece of filter paper in the lid of the Petri dish. Positive reactions may appear in less than 24 hours, but observations may be continued for a week or longer.

Precipitation occurs more rapidly—within a few hours—in the micro method performed on ordinary 1-inch by 3-inch microscope slides covered with 2.5 ml. of 0.85 per cent Ionagar. Holes spaced about 4 mm. apart are cut with a Pasteur pipette 2 mm. in diameter using a rubber bulb or vacuum line to remove the agar. The wells are easily filled with melting point capillaries or hematocrit tubes (ca. 1 mm. ID); when the capillary is touched to the antiserum or antigen, it fills partially by capillarity, and when it is then touched to the agar hole, the reagent automatically fills the hole. A fresh capillary (or end) must be used for each reagent. After the wells are filled, the slides are supported over moist filter paper in Petri dishes while lines of precipitate form.

A glass slide with agar containing lines of precipitate may be dried, stained, and preserved as follows: Remove untreated protein by immersing the slide in saline for several hours, changing the saline several times during this period. Saturate a piece of filter paper the size of the slide with distilled water and place it over the slide so that no air bubbles are trapped beneath the paper. Allow the paper and agar to dry and then remove the paper. Stain by immersing the slide 10 minutes in 0.2 per cent acid fuchsin in a mixture of 10 per cent acetic acid and 50 per cent methyl alcohol, and wash with two or three changes of acetic acid–methyl alcohol solution during a period of 15 to 20 minutes. Dry the slide in air. A solution containing 0.1 per cent amidoschwarz in a mixture of 10 per cent acetic acid and 90 per cent methyl alcohol also stains satisfactorily in 1 minute. The slide is then washed with several changes of 2 per cent acetic acid.

5. Immunoelectrophoresis

Immunoelectrophoresis combines electrophoretic separation of substances of different electric charges with separation by double diffusion in agar gel and thus produces a high degree of resolution of the antigenic constituents of a mixture such as serum. Both macro and micro procedures are available; the latter are rapid and require only minute amounts of reagents.

An electrophoresis apparatus like that pictured in Figure 3–3 may be used. The buffer reservoirs at each end are filled with barbital buffer, pH 8.2 (500 ml. N/10 sodium barbital, 150 ml. N/10 HCl, 350 ml. distilled water).

Prepare a microscope slide by covering it with 2.5 ml. of 0.85 per cent Ionagar in barbital buffer, pH 8.2. When the agar is hard, cut holes and a trough as shown in Figure 11–5. The holes are made with a Pasteur pipette, using suction to remove the agar. The trough may be cut by use of two single-edged (e.g., Gem) razor blades taped together so that their cutting edges are about 1 mm. apart; the agar is removed by use of a fine Pasteur pipette attached to a vacuum pump.

Fill the wells with antigen, using a 1-mm. capillary, as described in the micro-Ouchterlony method (p. 323). Place the slide between the buffer reservoirs with the polarity indicated in Figure 11–5. Connect the ends to the buffer solutions by 1-inch strips of filter paper moistened with buffer. One end of each paper strip should cover about 0.5 cm. of the agar on the slide; the other should hang down into the buffer.

Connect a direct current power supply and adjust it to apply 4 to 6 volts per cm. (i.e., about 45 volts across the slide) at about 5 ma. per slide. After about 45 minutes disconnect the current and remove the slide.

Fill the trough with antiserum. Place the slide in a level position above moistened filter paper in a Petri dish and allow the pattern of precipitation to develop for 24 hours. Dry the agar and stain and preserve the precipitate lines as described previously (see above).

IX. HEMOLYSIS

The necessity for both complement and amboceptor in hemolytic reactions and the order in which they combine with erythrocytes can be demonstrated by a simple

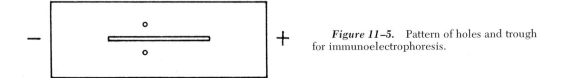

Figure 11–5. Pattern of holes and trough for immunoelectrophoresis.

experiment. Preparation of the red blood cell suspension and preliminary titrations will first be described.

It is important that all reagents used in complement reactions, including barbital buffered saline, red cells, amboceptor, and complement, be kept in the refrigerator or ice bath except when actually being used.

1. Barbital Buffered Saline

Buffered saline containing calcium and magnesium ions gives higher titers in hemolysis experiments than plain saline. Its composition and preparation are as follows:

Barbital (5,5-diethylbarbituric acid)	2.875 g.
Barbital sodium (sodium 5,5-diethylbarbiturate)	1.083 g.
$CaCl_2$	0.083 g.
$MgCl_2$	0.238 g.
NaCl	42.500 g.

Dissolve barbital in 250 ml. of hot distilled water and add the other reagents in order. Cool and dilute to 1,000 ml. Refrigerate this stock solution. Dilute as needed, or at least once a week, by adding four parts of distilled water to one part of stock buffer. Final pH should be 7.3 to 7.4 Store diluted solution in the refrigerator.

2. Red Blood Cell Suspension

Sheep red blood cells are usually employed in hemolytic and complement fixation experiments. Either defibrinated or citrated blood secured from the jugular vein of a sheep (or purchased from a reliable laboratory) is satisfactory. Dilute sufficient blood for the day's work with 5 to 10 volumes of saline (0.9 per cent NaCl) and centrifuge at moderate speed just long enough to deposit the cells. Discard the supernatant liquid, resuspend the cells in saline, and centrifuge again. Repeat this process twice more. Measure the final deposit of packed cells and dilute with 50 volumes of saline. This provides a 2 per cent suspension of red blood cells. (Some laboratories prefer a 5 per cent suspension.) The suspension must always be shaken immediately before it is used, because erythrocytes settle rapidly in saline.

The erythrocyte suspension may also be standardized by use of a spectrophotometer or colorimeter. The cells in an accurately prepared suspension of known concentration are lysed by distilled water, and the optical density (OD) of the resulting solution is determined against a distilled water blank at a wavelength of 530 mμ in the spectrophotometer. The OD reading thus ascertained is used for standardization of future suspensions.

It has been found that 1 ml. of a 1 per cent suspension of sheep red cells lysed with 4 ml. of distilled water has an OD of 0.300 (cells of other species may give different readings). To prepare 2 per cent sheep cells, make a slightly more concentrated suspension (e.g., 2.5 per cent) and lyse three 0.5 ml. aliquots with 4.5 ml. of distilled water. Determine the average of their optical densities and calculate the further dilution required according to the equation:

$$\text{Final volume} = \text{Initial volume} \times \left(\frac{\text{Average OD}}{0.300} \right)$$

Determine the OD of the adjusted suspension and readjust if necessary. A suspension that is too dilute may be concentrated by centrifugation and removal of part of the supernate.

3. Amboceptor Titration

Sheep amboceptor is prepared by immunizing rabbits with sheep erythrocytes; it may be purchased from various laboratories. It is very stable, so it needs to be titrated only occasionally. Amboceptor is usually preserved with an equal volume of neutral glycerin, a fact to be taken into account when preparing dilutions (e.g., 1:500 amboceptor is prepared by adding 0.2 ml. of preserved amboceptor to 49.8 ml. saline).

Complement is also required. Guinea pig serum is ordinarily used. Fresh serum is secured by bleeding at least three males or nonpregnant females from the heart under light ether anesthesia (or without anesthetic if an assistant is available), and removing and pooling the sera after clotting has occurred. Serum from each animal should be tested individually for hemolytic activity, although in practice this is not always done. Complement can be preserved for some time in a freezer. Lyophilized complement is available from many suppliers; it is reconstituted according to directions supplied.

Table 11–4 illustrates the titration of amboceptor. Pipette diminishing amounts of amboceptor to the bottoms of agglutination tubes, using a 1-ml. serologic pipette graduated in hundredths. Add increasing amounts of saline, followed by complement diluted 1:20 and the red cell suspension. Shake the rack of tubes just sufficiently to disperse the cells uniformly and place in a 37° C. waterbath for 30 minutes. Read the degree of hemolysis in each tube. Complete hemolysis (+ + + +) consists of apparent dissolution of all cells, the hemoglobin imparting a clear red color to the liquid. The smallest amount of amboceptor yielding complete hemolysis is considered the unit of amboceptor. For many purposes two units are employed, the serum being diluted so that they are contained in a volume of 0.1 ml. For example, if the unit were 0.04 ml. of 1:500 amboceptor, two units would be 0.08 ml. of 1:500 or 0.1 ml. of 1:625 amboceptor.

4. Complement Titration

Complement is very unstable and must be titrated each day. The procedure is illustrated in Table 11–5. Decreasing amounts of complement diluted 1:40 are pipetted into agglutination tubes, together with increasing amounts of saline. One-tenth millili-

Table 11–4   *Amboceptor Titration*

Tube	Amboceptor (1:500)	Saline	Complement (1:20)	RBC (2%)	
1	0.10 ml.	0.20 ml.	0.1 ml.	0.1 ml.	
2	0.09 ml.	0.21 ml.	0.1 ml.	0.1 ml.	
3	0.08 ml.	0.22 ml.	0.1 ml.	0.1 ml.	
4	0.07 ml.	0.23 ml.	0.1 ml.	0.1 ml.	
5	0.06 ml.	0.24 ml.	0.1 ml.	0.1 ml.	Waterbath at 37° C. for 30 min.
6	0.05 ml.	0.25 ml.	0.1 ml.	0.1 ml.	
7	0.04 ml.	0.26 ml.	0.1 ml.	0.1 ml.	
8	0.03 ml.	0.27 ml.	0.1 ml.	0.1 ml.	
9	0.02 ml.	0.28 ml.	0.1 ml.	0.1 ml.	
10	0.01 ml.	0.29 ml.	0.1 ml.	0.1 ml.	
11	0.00 ml.	0.30 ml.	0.1 ml.	0.1 ml.	

Table 11–5 Complement Titration

Tube	Complement (1:40)	Saline	Amboceptor (2 units)	RBC (2%)	
1	0.13 ml.	0.17 ml.	0.1 ml.	0.1 ml.	Waterbath at 37° C. for 30 min.
2	0.12 ml.	0.18 ml.	0.1 ml.	0.1 ml.	
3	0.11 ml.	0.19 ml.	0.1 ml.	0.1 ml.	
4	0.10 ml.	0.20 ml.	0.1 ml.	0.1 ml.	
5	0.09 ml.	0.21 ml.	0.1 ml.	0.1 ml.	
6	0.08 ml.	0.22 ml.	0.1 ml.	0.1 ml.	
7	0.07 ml.	0.23 ml.	0.1 ml.	0.1 ml.	
8	0.06 ml.	0.24 ml.	0.1 ml.	0.1 ml.	
9	0.05 ml.	0.25 ml.	0.1 ml.	0.1 ml.	
10	0.04 ml.	0.26 ml.	0.1 ml.	0.1 ml.	
11	0.03 ml.	0.27 ml.	0.1 ml.	0.1 ml.	
12	0.02 ml.	0.28 ml.	0.1 ml.	0.1 ml.	

ter of amboceptor containing two units is added to each tube, followed by red cells. Hemolysis is read after 30 minutes in the 37° C. waterbath. It is sometimes desirable, as in preparation for complement fixation tests, to allow a period of primary incubation of the complement-saline mixtures before addition of amboceptor and red cells, because this more nearly duplicates the conditions of the final test. The smallest amount of complement yielding complete hemolysis constitutes one unit. Two units are often employed, and the guinea pig serum is diluted to contain this quantity in 0.1 ml.

5. Role of Amboceptor and Complement in Hemolysis

The role of the two principal reagents in hemolysis can be shown by the following simple experiment:

a. Set up four 10 × 75 mm. tubes as shown in Table 11–6, adding the reagents column by column. Shake and incubate in the waterbath at 37° C. for 30 minutes. Read hemolysis. This part of the experiment demonstrates that both complement and amboceptor are necessary for hemolysis.

b. Centrifuge tubes A and B at moderate speed. Carefully transfer the supernatant liquids to clean agglutination tubes and label these A_s and B_s, respectively. Treat tubes A, A_s, B, and B_s as indicated in Table 11–7. Shake and incubate at 37° C. as before. Read hemolysis. From the results it is possible to decide in what order complement and amboceptor combine with red cells.

6. Quantitative Effect of Amboceptor (or Complement) Dosage on Hemolysis

A spectrophotometer may be used to determine the percentage hemolysis in each of a series of mixtures of sheep erythrocytes, homologous amboceptor, and comple-

Table 11–6 Participation of Complement and Amboceptor in Hemolysis

Tube	Complement (2 units)	Saline	Amboceptor (2 units)	RBC (2%)
A	—	0.3 ml.	0.1 ml.	0.1 ml.
B	0.1 ml.	0.3 ml.	—	0.1 ml.
C	0.1 ml.	0.2 ml.	0.1 ml.	0.1 ml.
D	—	0.4 ml.	—	0.1 ml.

Table 11–7   *The Order with Which Complement and Amboceptor
Unite with Red Blood Cells*

Tube	Complement (2 units)	Saline	Amboceptor (2 units)	RBC (2%)
A (RBC)	0.1 ml.	0.6 ml.	—	—
A$_S$ (supernate)	0.1 ml.	—	—	0.1 ml.
B (RBC)	—	0.6 ml.	0.1 ml.	—
B$_S$ (supernate)	—	—	0.1 ml.	0.1 ml.

ment. Either amboceptor or complement may be varied, the other reagent being constant (or both may be varied in a "checkerboard" experiment). A procedure employing various amounts of amboceptor and constant complement will be described.

Unless the strength of the reagents is already known, preliminary titration is necessary. This may be accomplished by the procedure in sections 3 and 4 above. Since the experiment is to be conducted in a volume of 5.0 ml., consisting of 1.0 ml. 2 per cent sheep cells, 2.0 ml. diluted complement, and various amounts of amboceptor and saline, the dose of complement to employ (i.e., two times the amount needed to lyse 1.0 ml. of 2 per cent cells) is approximately 20 times greater than the unit determined according to Table 11–5. For example, if 1 unit of complement for 0.1 ml. of 2 per cent red cells is 0.08 ml. of a 1:40 dilution, 2 hemolytic units for 1.0 ml. of 2 per cent cells is 1.6 ml. of 1:40 or 2.0 ml. of 1:50 complement. Amboceptor will be supplied as decreasing volumes of a solution containing sufficient antibody in 2.0 ml. to lyse 1.0 ml. of 2 per cent cells. The amount to employ is therefore ten times as great as that calculated from Table 11–4. If lysis of 0.1 ml. of 2 per cent cells requires 0.02 ml. of 1:500 amboceptor, 1 hemolytic unit for 1.0 ml. of cells is 0.2 ml. of 1:500 or 2.0 ml. of 1:5,000 amboceptor.

Set up 12 Wassermann tubes (13 × 100 mm.) as shown in Table 11–8. After adding the saline, amboceptor, and cells to all tubes, mix thoroughly by inverting each tube three times against the thumb or index finger. Following the last inversion, squeeze the finger over the edge of the tube to return fluid to the tube and then wipe the finger on a clean towel. Let the tubes stand 10 minutes at room temperature, add complement, and

Table 11–8   *Quantitative Effect of Amboceptor Dosage on Hemolysis*

Tube	Barbital Buffered Saline	Amboceptor (1 hemolytic unit/2 ml.)	RBC (2%)		Complement (2 hemolytic units)		Optical Density (OD)	Percentage Hemolysis: $\left(\dfrac{OD_x}{OD_b} \times 100\right)$ °
A	2.0 ml.	—	1.0 ml.	Room temperature for 10 min.	2.0 ml.	Waterbath at 37° C. for 30 min.	Set to 0	
B	Distilled water 4 ml.		1.0 ml.		—			100
1	1.9 ml.	0.1 ml.	1.0 ml.		2.0 ml.			
2	1.8 ml.	0.2 ml.	1.0 ml.		2.0 ml.			
3	1.7 ml.	0.3 ml.	1.0 ml.		2.0 ml.			
4	1.6 ml.	0.4 ml.	1.0 ml.		2.0 ml.			
5	1.5 ml.	0.5 ml.	1.0 ml.		2.0 ml.			
6	1.4 ml.	0.6 ml.	1.0 ml.		2.0 ml.			
7	1.3 ml.	0.7 ml.	1.0 ml.		2.0 ml.			
8	1.2 ml.	0.8 ml.	1.0 ml.		2.0 ml.			
9	1.1 ml.	0.9 ml.	1.0 ml.		2.0 ml.			
10	1.0 ml.	1.0 ml.	1.0 ml.		2.0 ml.			
11	0.0 ml.	2.0 ml.	1.0 ml.		2.0 ml.			

*OD_x = optical density of test solution.
OD_b = optical density of lysed 2% RBC (ca. 0.600).

mix as before. Incubate at 37° C. in the waterbath for 30 minutes. Centrifuge all tubes at 700 × g. for 10 minutes (2100 r.p.m. with a 14-cm. radius of rotation). Decant the supernates into spectrophotometer tubes or cuvettes.

Set the OD of the instrument to 0 with tube A, using a wavelength of 530 mμ. Read the OD of tube B and of tubes 1 to 11. Calculate the percentage hemolysis in each tube according to the formula:

$$\text{Hemolysis (\%)} = \left(\frac{OD_x}{OD_b} \right) \times 100$$

in which OD_x is the optical density of the test solution and OD_b is the optical density of lysate from 1.0 ml. of 2 per cent RBC (normally 0.600). Plot the results in a graph with amboceptor volumes on the horizontal axis and percentage hemolysis on the vertical axis.

X. BACTERIOLYSIS

Bacteriolysis can be demonstrated with some strains of S. *typhosa* and *Vibrio cholerae*. With most samples of complement a dilution of 1:20 or 1:25 gives satisfactory results in the procedure outlined, together with a 1:500 dilution of antibacterial serum having an agglutinin titer of about 10,000. Use young (5- to 6-hour) nutrient broth cultures grown at 37° C.

Prepare four Wassermann tubes (13 × 100 mm.) as indicated in Table 11–9. Mix the contents of the tubes by flipping and incubate in the waterbath at 37° C. for 2 hours. At the end of each 30 minutes observe the tubes with the naked eye, prepare a smear from each, and stain 15 seconds with gentian violet. Examine with the oil immersion objective. Agglutination may be noted in one or two tubes and bacteriolysis in one tube. Bacteriolysis is shown by irregular staining and bloated or otherwise abnormal cells, and ultimately by disappearance of formed cells. Occasionally complete dissolution is apparent upon macroscopic inspection of the tube.

XI. COMPLEMENT FIXATION

Complement fixation is conveniently demonstrated with a protein-antiprotein system, such as crystallized egg albumin or foreign serum protein. The procedure with bovine serum albumin will be outlined.

The 1 per cent solution of BSA employed in the precipitin test will be satisfactory. Inactivate anti-egg albumin serum by heating in a waterbath at 56° C. for 30 minutes shortly before using. Employ two periods of incubation in titrating complement (see

Table 11–9   Bacteriolysis

Tube	Complement (1:20)	Antiserum (1:500)	Saline	Young Broth Culture
1	—	—	1.0 ml.	0.5 ml.
2	—	0.5 ml.	0.5 ml.	0.5 ml.
3	0.5 ml.	—	0.5 ml.	0.5 ml.
4	0.5 ml.	0.5 ml.	—	0.5 ml.

page 327 and Table 11–5), incubate the complement-saline mixtures at 37° C. for 1 hour, add amboceptor and sheep cells, and return to the 37° C. waterbath for an additional 30 minutes. Prepare sensitized RBC by mixing equal volumes of 2 per cent RBC and amboceptor diluted to contain two units in 0.1 ml. Keep them cold until needed.

The complement fixation test is set up as illustrated in Table 11–10. Prepare decimal dilutions from the stock 1 per cent BSA solution in any convenient amounts. The actual test is performed in agglutination tubes. Pipette BSA dilutions into these tubes as indicated, using a single pipette and beginning with the greatest dilution, rinsing the pipette in each succeeding dilution before transferring. Note that tube 6 (antigen control) receives 0.1 ml. of the lowest dilution employed in any of the tests. Add antiserum, complement, and saline where needed, mix by shaking the rack, and incubate for 1 hour before adding the sensitized red blood cells. Shake sufficiently to suspend the cells evenly and reincubate. Read the tests 5 to 10 minutes after the cells in tube 8 (hemolytic control) are completely lysed. Tubes 6 through 9 are controls and must always be included in a complement fixation test. There should be complete hemolysis in all except tube 9, which should show no hemolysis. Complete hemolysis in the test indicates no fixation of complement and is recorded by the symbol − or 0. Absence of hemolysis represents complete fixation and is designated + + + + .

Complement fixation is most widely used in various modifications of the Wassermann test for syphilis. Details of the procedure vary from one laboratory to another; for example, in some laboratories the final volume of reagents is 0.5 ml., and in others it is 3.0 ml. Specific methods can be found in such references as Wadsworth (1947); Kolmer, Spaulding, and Robinson (1951); and Davidsohn and Wells (1962).

XII. PHAGOCYTOSIS

Phagocytosis can be shown by use of artificially opsonized staphylococci. Normal or immune opsonins are demonstrated in suitable human or animal sera.

1. Phagocytosis of Artificially Opsonized Staphylococci

The antigen is prepared from well grown, heavily inoculated nutrient or trypticase soy agar slants of *Staphylococcus aureus*. Wash the organisms from each slant with

Table 11–10   Complement Fixation

Tube	Egg Albumin (0.1 ml.)	Inactivated Anti-Egg Albumin Serum (1:5)	Complement (2 units)	Saline	Waterbath at 37° C. for 1 hour	Sensitized RBC (2%)	Waterbath at 37° C. for 15–30 min.
1	1:1,000	0.1 ml.	0.1 ml.	—		0.2 ml.	
2	1:10,000	0.1 ml.	0.1 ml.	—		0.2 ml.	
3	1:100,000	0.1 ml.	0.1 ml.	—		0.2 ml.	
4	1:1,000,000	0.1 ml.	0.1 ml.	—		0.2 ml.	
5	1:10,000,000	0.1 ml.	0.1 ml.	—		0.2 ml.	
6	1:1,000	—	0.1 ml.	0.1 ml.		0.2 ml.	
7	—	0.1 ml.	0.1 ml.	0.1 ml.		0.2 ml.	
8	—	—	0.1 ml.	0.2 ml.		0.2 ml.	
9	—	—	—	0.3 ml.		0.2 ml.	

about 2 ml. of saline. Pool and add an equal volume of 1 per cent chrome alum in saline. Incubate 2 hours at 37° C. Centrifuge at high speed to pack the cells, discard the supernatant liquid, and wash the cells twice by centrifugation with saline. Resuspend the organisms in saline to a concentration of about 500,000,000 cells per ml.

In an agglutination tube mix 0.2 ml. heparinized human blood and 0.2 ml. staphylococcus antigen. Incubate in the waterbath at 37° C. for 30 minutes. With a Pasteur pipette transfer single drops to the ends of several microscope slides, smear with a spreader slide as in preparing blood films, and stain by the Wright method. Examine with the oil immersion objective and count the bacteria ingested by each of the first 25 polymorphonuclear leukocytes encountered. The average number of bacteria ingested is the phagocytic index.

2. Opsonizing Antibodies in Serum

Opsonins for Brucella or *S. aureus* can be detected in suitable human or animal sera. The pooled sera of at least five apparently normal individuals should be used as a control.

Cultivate the organisms on an appropriate agar medium and suspend them in saline. Wash the cells three times by centrifugation with saline, and finally resuspend them to a concentration of about one billion bacteria per ml. in saline, or preferably in Krebs-gelatin solution, the composition of which follows:

Gelatin (6% in 0.9% NaCl)	50 parts
0.9% NaCl	50 parts
1.15% KCl	4 parts
1.22% CaCl$_2$	3 parts
2.11% KH$_2$PO$_4$	1 part
3.82% MgSO$_4$·7H$_2$O	1 part
5% NaHCO$_3$	4.6 parts

Mix in an agglutination tube 0.1 ml. of heparinized human blood, 0.1 ml. of patient's serum, and 0.1 ml. of bacterial suspension. Prepare a similar (control) tube containing 0.1 ml. quantities of heparinized human blood, pooled normal serum, and bacterial suspension. Incubate at 37° C. in the waterbath for 30 minutes. Make smears from each tube by the usual blood smear technique, stain by the Wright method, and examine with the oil immersion objective. Determine the phagocytic index of each preparation. Calculate the opsonic index of the patient's serum by dividing its phagocytic index by that of the normal serum.

XIII. TOXIN-ANTITOXIN REACTIONS

Laboratory demonstrations of the action of toxins and antitoxins depend upon the nature and properties of the materials available. Tetanus toxin, toxoid, and antitoxin can be used to demonstrate determination of the M.L.D. of toxin, neutralization of toxin by antitoxin, and immunization by toxoid. Similar experiments can also be arranged with diphtherial products. Either mice or guinea pigs may be employed with tetanus toxin. Mice are preferable from the standpoint of expense and offer the advantage that statistically better experiments can be arranged without too great cost. Guinea pigs are usually employed with diphtheria toxin. It should be pointed out that in the titration of diphtheria and tetanus toxins and antitoxins for control purposes guinea pigs are always used.

1. M.L.D. of Tetanus Toxin

Unless the potency of the toxin is known, preliminary trial with widely spaced doses will be necessary. Prepare decimal dilutions of toxin from 1:100 to 1:1,000,000 using a diluent consisting of 0.5 per cent NaCl containing 1 per cent peptone to increase the stability of the toxin. Inject pairs of mice (approximately 20 g. in weight) intramuscularly in the right hind leg with 0.5-ml. amounts of the various toxin dilutions. Observe the mice at frequent intervals during 5 days, noting the time when paralysis and/or death of each animal occurs. Determine the approximate M.L.D. of the toxin from the average death time of the pair of mice that received the smallest fatal dose by reference to Table 11–11. For example, if both mice injected with 0.5 ml. of 1:100,000 toxin survived, and the mice injected with 1:10,000 toxin died after 40 and 44 hours, respectively, the 1:10,000 toxin contained about 4.5 M.L.D. One M.L.D. is therefore 0.5 ml. of 1:45,000 toxin.

Prepare three toxin dilutions, one consisting of the estimated M.L.D. dilution and the others differing by about 10 per cent above and below, and repeat the inoculations and observations using 10 mice for each dose. In the above example, dilutions of 1:40,000, 1:45,000, and 1:50,000 might be employed.

2. Neutralization of Toxin by Antitoxin

Antitoxin of known potency can usually be secured because it is very stable. Dilute tetanus antitoxin to contain 0.4 antitoxic unit per ml. Prepare a dilution of the tetanus toxin previously titrated in saline-peptone so that each milliliter contains 10,000 M.L.D. For example, if 1 M.L.D. is represented by 0.5 ml. of 1:45,000 toxin, 10,000 M.L.D. is contained in 1.0 ml. of 1:9 toxin.

Into each of six test tubes or shell vials pipette 1.0 ml. of the antitoxin dilution, add saline-peptone as indicated in Table 11–12, and then toxin, mixing the contents of each tube immediately. Allow the mixtures to stand 1 hour at room temperature, inject 0.5 ml. amounts of each intramuscularly into two or more mice as before, and record reactions during the next 5 days. From the observed death times calculate the indicated free toxin (in M.L.D. units) in as many mixtures as possible, and subtract

Table 11–11　Death Time of Mice and Dosage of Tetanus Toxin*

T†	No. of M.L.D.‡	T	No. of M.L.D.	T	No. of M.L.D.
12	282	60	2.3	108	1.10
18	45	66	2.0	114	1.05
24	18	72	1.74	120	1.00
30	9.8	78	1.55	126	0.96
36	6.3	84	1.41	132	0.93
42	4.5	90	1.30	138	0.90
48	3.4	96	1.21	144	0.87
54	2.8	102	1.15	150	0.85

*Modified from Ipsen, 1941. Arch. Exp. Path. Pharmak., 197:536.
†T = Death time (hours).
‡1 M.L.D. of tetanus toxin is defined for this table as the dose which kills a 20-gram mouse in 120 hours.

Table 11–12   Neutralization of Tetanus Toxin by Antitoxin

Antitoxin (1:) (1 ml. = 0.4 unit)	Saline- Peptone	Toxin (1:) (1 ml. = 10,000 M.L.D.)	Dose per Mouse (0.5 ml.)	
			Antitoxin	Toxin
1.0 ml.	0.92 ml.	0.08 ml.	0.1 unit	200 M.L.D.
1.0 ml.	0.87 ml.	0.13 ml.	0.1 unit	325 M.L.D.
1.0 ml.	0.80 ml.	0.20 ml.	0.1 unit	500 M.L.D.
1.0 ml.	0.68 ml.	0.32 ml.	0.1 unit	800 M.L.D.
1.0 ml.	0.50 ml.	0.50 ml.	0.1 unit	1250 M.L.D.
1.0 ml.	0.00 ml.	1.00 ml.	0.1 unit	2500 M.L.D.

from the corresponding doses of toxin injected to determine the quantity presumably neutralized by 0.1 unit of antitoxin.

3. Immunizing Action of Toxoid

Inject each of four mice subcutaneously in the back with a dose of tetanus toxoid containing 20 flocculating units (Lf). Inject an equal number of mice with 2 Lf of toxoid. After 14 days challenge all mice by intramuscular injection of 10 M.L.D. of tetanus toxin, and at the same time inject a third equal group of (unimmunized) mice with the same dose of toxin, as a control. Observe the animals during 5 days and compare the survival time of mice immunized with the two dosages of toxoid.

4. Flocculation of Toxin or Toxoid by Antitoxin

Flocculation can be demonstrated with diphtherial or tetanal antitoxin and homologous toxin or toxoid. Varying amounts of antitoxin are mixed with a constant amount of toxin or toxoid, incubated, and observed constantly. The first mixture that shows visible flocculation is called the *indicating mixture* and is, in general, neutral when tested by animal inoculation. Toxin mixtures on one side of the indicating mixture are toxic and on the other side are antitoxic. The relationship between toxin and antitoxin in the indicating mixture is expressed by the equation:

$$\text{ml. antitoxin} \times \text{antitoxic units/ml.} = \text{ml. toxin} \times \text{Lf units/ml.}$$

Thus, if the indicating mixture consisted of 1 ml. of toxin and 0.01 ml. of an antitoxin that possessed a potency of 1,000 units per ml., the toxin contained 10 Lf units per ml.

Use an antitoxin of known potency. Unless the approximate Lf value of the toxin or toxoid is known, preliminary titration over a wide range will be necessary to establish the zone in which an end point can be expected. Measure antitoxin into agglutination or Wassermann tubes, the amounts varying from tube to tube by increments of 25 to 30 per cent (e.g., 0.010 ml., 0.013 ml., 0.016 ml., 0.020 ml., 0.025 ml., etc.). Add toxin in constant amounts of 1 to 4 ml. rapidly to each tube. Shake the rack of tubes and incubate in a constant temperature waterbath at about 42° C. Cloudiness and a fine granular precipitate may appear within a very few minutes in certain tubes, and eventually flocculation should occur in one or more tubes. The flocculation time may vary from a few minutes to several hours. Toxoids and some toxins, particularly those with a low Lf value, flocculate slowly and may require a higher incubation temperature. Calculate the approximate Lf value of the toxin or toxoid from the equation above.

If toxin rather than toxoid is employed, conclude the experiment by centrifuging the indicating mixture and one or two mixtures on either side and injecting the supernatant liquids into experimental animals to test for residual toxicity.

XIV. MOUSE PROTECTION TESTS

Protection tests in mice are readily performed using S. *typhosa* and anti-typhoid serum, either from rabbits or from humans who have received typhoid immunization. One group of mice is inoculated with the immune serum and an equal number of mice with normal serum of the same species. One hour later each group of animals is divided into smaller groups containing two or more mice, which are then inoculated with graded doses of living typhoid bacteria suspended in mucin. The animals are observed during the next 6 days and deaths are noted. The LD_{50} values calculated for each type of serum treatment provide an indication of the protective potency of the immune serum under the conditions of the experiment.

Twenty-eight mice are needed for the protection test. Inoculate 14 mice intraperitoneally with 0.5 ml. amounts of immune serum; similarly inoculate the remaining mice with normal serum.

Suspend the growth from a heavily inoculated trypticase soy agar slant of S. *typhosa* that has been incubated 18 to 20 hours at 37° C. in 10 ml. sterile saline. Prepare serial decimal dilutions in sterile saline from 1:10 to 1:100,000,000. Plate 1 ml. quantities of the 1:10,000,000 and 1:100,000,000 dilutions for a count of the viable bacteria in the suspension.

Pipette 4.5 ml. of sterile 5 per cent mucin into each of seven shell vials or other suitable containers of 10- to 15-ml. capacity. [To prepare the mucin solution, suspend 5 g. of mucin (e.g., Granular Mucin, Type 1701-W, The Wilson Laboratories, Chicago) in 100 ml. distilled water, heat in a boiling waterbath to aid solution, filter through several thicknesses of cheesecloth, and sterilize by steaming 30 minutes on each of three successive days.] To each vial add 0.5 ml. of one bacterial dilution from 1:10 to 1:10,000,000, thus giving final dilutions in mucin from 1:100 to 1:100,000,000. Use a separate pipette for preparing each mucin dilution, and mix the bacteria and mucin thoroughly.

One hour after the serum injections inoculate each mouse intraperitoneally with 0.5 ml. of one of the mucin dilutions of typhoid bacteria. A syringe fitted with a 1-inch 22 to 24 gauge needle will be found useful for this purpose, because the inoculum is quite viscous. Pick the mice by pairs at random and inoculate two from each serum treatment with each dosage of bacteria. Keep each pair of mice in a separate cage or jar and observe at frequent intervals during the next 6 days, recording the time of death of each animal. At the end of the period of observation tabulate the results (see Table 11–13); calculate the LD_{50} of typhoid bacteria for animals treated with normal serum and compare with a similar figure for animals treated with immune serum.

It may also be of interest to perform agglutination tests to confirm the absence (or low normal titer) of typhoid agglutinins in the normal serum, in contrast to the immune serum.

XV. ANAPHYLACTIC SHOCK

It is difficult to give detailed directions for anaphylactic experiments because of differences in the materials available and the natural biologic variation of animals. Until familiarity with these variations has been gained, experiments should be planned

Table 11–13   Mouse Protection Test

Bacterial Dilution in Mucin (0.5 ml.)	Number of Bacteria Injected	Normal Serum (0.5 ml.) TIME OF DEATH (HOURS)		Immune Serum (0.5 ml.) TIME OF DEATH (HOURS)	
1:100					
1:1,000					
1:10,000					
1:100,000					
1:1,000,000					
1:10,000,000					
1:100,000,000					

in duplicate or triplicate to increase the chance of providing a satisfactory demonstration.

1. Active Anaphylaxis

Sensitize one or more guinea pigs by intraperitoneal injection of 1 to 5 mg. of foreign protein contained in about 1 ml. of saline. Horse serum or egg albumin is satisfactory for this purpose. Three weeks later administer the shocking injection of the same protein. The dose should be about ten times that of the sensitizing injection and should be introduced directly into the bloodstream, either intravenously or by cardiac puncture. Intracardial injections without anesthetic are not difficult if the animal is properly held on its back with its front legs stretched forward and outward. Insert the needle as in bleeding from the heart, and when gentle aspiration brings blood into the syringe, inject the contents into the heart. In a typical anaphylactic reaction the animal begins to cough and gasp for breath within a few moments, may scratch its face with its forepaws and make convulsive movements. In a fatal reaction the animal collapses and dies, often within 2 to 4 minutes. Immediately perform an autopsy, noting especially the continued heartbeat and intestinal peristalsis and the inflated condition of the lungs.

2. Passive Anaphylaxis

Guinea pigs can be sensitized passively by means of rabbit precipitating antiserum. The dosage depends upon the titer of antibodies in the antiserum and must be determined by trial for each serum. As little as 0.1 ml. of high titer antiserum may suffice. Inject the antiserum intraperitoneally and allow about 1 day to elapse before attempting to elicit anaphylactic shock. The shocking material is the antigen homologous to the antiserum (i.e., egg albumin will produce shock in a guinea pig passively sensitized with rabbit anti-egg albumin serum), and the dose should be the same as used to elicit active anaphylaxis. If the animal dies perform an autopsy and look for the usual signs.

3. Histamine Shock

Inject a guinea pig intracardially with about 0.25 mg. (1 ml. of 1:4,000 solution) of histamine in saline. The response may be indistinguishable from fatal anaphylaxis. Perform an autopsy and observe the customary signs.

4. Action of Antihistamines

Sensitize guinea pigs as usual and wait 3 weeks. Demonstrate the hypersensitive condition of at least one animal by inducing anaphylactic shock. Inject an antihistaminic drug intraperitoneally into one or more of the remaining sensitive animals. The dose required may vary from 1 to 10 mg. per kg. and may be dissolved in a small amount of saline. After 15 to 30 minutes inject a shocking dose of antigen intracardially. The anaphylactic reaction may be prevented entirely, may be mild and nonfatal, or may consist of greatly delayed death (e.g., one-half hour).

5. Passive Cutaneous Anaphylaxis

Anti-BSA serum prepared as suggested in section IV, 1 (page 313) by injecting rabbits with BSA in Freund's complete adjuvant has been found satisfactory for this demonstration.

Remove the hair from the backs of white guinea pigs with an electric clipper and wipe the skin with 70 per cent alcohol. Inject three sites intradermally with 0.1-ml. amounts of the following:

(a) Anti-BSA undiluted
(b) Saline
(c) Anti-BSA diluted 1:10 with saline

Three to 6 hours later inject intravenously or intracardially 1 ml. of BSA-Evans blue solution (equal volumes of 0.25 per cent BSA and 2 per cent Evans blue). Observe the sites previously injected with antiserum or saline continuously for 30 to 45 minutes. A positive reaction consists of blueing of the injection area, usually reaching a maximum in 5 to 10 minutes. It is more vividly shown on the subcutaneous surface of the skin, so the animal may be sacrificed and the skin reflected for inspection.

XVI. IMMUNOPLAQUE DEMONSTRATION

Production of antibodies by individual lymphoid cells can be demonstrated by the following procedure.

1. Inject a mouse intraperitoneally with 1 ml. of 5 per cent washed sheep RBC, and 3 to 7 days later sacrifice it, together with a normal control mouse.

2. Remove the spleens to Petri dishes containing 5 ml. MEM (minimal essential medium containing Hanks's basal salts solution). (Use only siliconized glassware and keep glassware and reagents cold in an ice bath.) Dice the tissue and tease it gently with a rubber policeman to make a lymphocyte suspension. Strain through nylon to remove gross particles.

3. Centrifuge cold at 270 g for 10 minutes. Wash the sediment of cells once with 5 ml. MEM and resuspend the packed cells in 1 ml. MEM.

4. Dilute the cell suspension 1:10 with WBC diluting fluid in a WBC pipette. Count the cells in 80 small squares of a hemacytometer and multiply the total by 5×10^5

to calculate the number of cells per ml. of suspension. Dilute the spleen cell suspension with MEM to 25×10^6 cells per ml.

5. Wash sheep RBC three times with saline and make a 6 per cent suspension in MEM. Dilute 1:100 with saline or MEM in an RBC pipette and count the cells in 80 small squares of a hemacytometer. Multiply the total by 5×10^6 to calculate the number of RBC per ml. Dilute to 12×10^8 per ml. with MEM.

6. Prepare two slides by attaching three cover glasses, 22 mm. square, to 1×3 in. microscope slides with 4×22 mm. strips of double stick Scotch tape, as shown in Figure 11–6.

7. Prepare the following mixture:
   0.2 ml. spleen cell suspension
   0.2 ml. sheep RBC
   0.2 ml. 1:3.3 complement

8. Using a Pasteur pipette, fill the three chambers of a prepared slide with the mixture containing immune spleen cells, and the chambers of the other slide with the normal spleen cell mixture. Seal the edges with Vaspar (equal parts of Vaseline and paraffin oil) and incubate at 37° C. for 30 to 60 minutes.

9. Observe plaques with the naked eye, a hand lens, and the low power and/or high dry objectives of the microscope. Look for the lymphoid cell in the center of each plaque. Assuming that each slide contains 0.1 ml. of mixture, calculate how many PFC (plaque-forming cells) were present in each spleen.

XVII. FLUORESCENT ANTIBODY DEMONSTRATION

Any combination of bacteria and antiserum can be used to demonstrate the indirect fluorescent antibody technique. A procedure employing *E. coli* and homologous rabbit antiserum will be described.

1. Prepare smears of *E. coli* and *P. vulgaris* (as control) at opposite ends of a microscope slide and fix by heat. Add a loopful of anti-*coli* serum to each smear and incubate the slide 30 minutes at room temperature in a moist chamber (Petri dish with moistened filter paper).

2. Rinse with FA buffer at pH 7.2 (commercially available: contains NaCl, 7.65 g.; Na_2HPO_4, 0.724 g.; KH_2PO_4, 0.21 g.; per liter), and wash 10 minutes in a Coplin jar or beaker with two changes of FA buffer.

3. Cover each smear with 1 drop of anti-rabbit FA serum (commercially available) and incubate 30 minutes at room temperature in the moist chamber. Rinse and wash as before with FA buffer. Blot dry, add a drop of FA mounting fluid (borate buffered glycerine at pH 7.4, available commercially) to each smear, and cover with a cover glass.

4. Examine each smear under oil (nonfluorescing) at ca. $1,000 \times$ magnification, using UVL (mercury vapor lamp) and suitable filters. Focus on a fluorescing particle of debris and then look for fluorescent bacteria. The smear of *P. vulgaris* serves as a negative control and should show minimal fluorescence.

Figure 11–6.· Immunoplaque demonstration slide. Double-stick Scotch tape strips, 4×22 mm., are used to attach 22-mm. square cover glasses to the slide, making three chambers where RBC, sensitized lymphocytes, and complement interact.

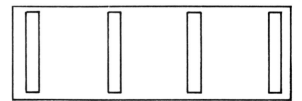

Additional Sources of Information

Bray, W. E.: Synopsis of Clinical Laboratory Methods. 1946. St. Louis, Mo., C. V. Mosby Company.

Campbell, D. H., J. S. Garvey, N. E. Cremer, and D. H. Sussdorf: Methods in Immunology, 2nd ed. 1970. New York, W. A. Benjamin, Inc.

Davidsohn, I., and J. A. Wells (Eds.): Clinical Diagnosis by Laboratory Methods, 13th ed. 1962. Philadelphia, W. B. Saunders Company.

Kabat, E. A.: Kabat and Mayer's Experimental Immunochemistry, 2nd ed. 1961. Springfield, Ill., Charles C Thomas, Publisher.

Kolmer, J. A., E. H. Spaulding, and H. Robinson: Approved Laboratory Technic, 5th ed. 1951. New York, Appleton-Century-Crofts.

Nowotny, A.: Basic Exercises in Immunochemistry. 1969. Heidelberg, Springer-Verlag.

Wadsworth, A.: Standard Methods, 3rd ed. 1947. Baltimore, The Williams and Wilkins Company.

Williams, C. A., and M. W. Chase (Eds.): Methods in Immunology and Immunochemistry, Vols. 1–3. 1967–1971. New York, Academic Press, Inc.

INDEX

Note: Page numbers in *italics* indicate illustrations; page numbers followed by (t) indicate tables.

339